AF687193

Current Diagnosis and Treatment in Rheumatology

Current Diagnosis and Treatment in Rheumatology

Editor: Sullivan Princeton

AMERICAN
MEDICAL PUBLISHERS
www.americanmedicalpublishers.com

AMERICAN
MEDICAL PUBLISHERS
www.americanmedicalpublishers.com

Cataloging-in-Publication Data

Current diagnosis and treatment in rheumatology / edited by Sullivan Princeton.
p. cm.
Includes bibliographical references and index.
ISBN 979-8-88740-030-3
1. Rheumatology. 2. Joints--Diseases--Diagnosis. 3. Joints--Diseases--Treatment.
4. Connective tissues--Diseases--Diagnosis. 5. Connective tissues--Diseases--Treatment.
I. Princeton, Sullivan.
RC927 .C87 2023
616.723--dc23

© American Medical Publishers, 2023

American Medical Publishers,
41 Flatbush Avenue,
1st Floor, New York,
NY 11217, USA

ISBN 979-8-88740-030-3 (Hardback)

This book contains information obtained from authentic and highly regarded sources. Copyright for all individual chapters remain with the respective authors as indicated. All chapters are published with permission under the Creative Commons Attribution License or equivalent. A wide variety of references are listed. Permission and sources are indicated; for detailed attributions, please refer to the permissions page and list of contributors. Reasonable efforts have been made to publish reliable data and information, but the authors, editors and publisher cannot assume any responsibility for the validity of all materials or the consequences of their use.

Trademark Notice: Registered trademark of products or corporate names are used only for explanation and identification without intent to infringe.

Contents

Preface

This book has been a concerted effort by a group of academicians, researchers and scientists, who have contributed their research works for the realization of the book. This book has materialized in the wake of emerging advancements and innovations in this field. Therefore, the need of the hour was to compile all the required researches and disseminate the knowledge to a broad spectrum of people comprising of students, researchers and specialists of the field.

Rheumatology is a discipline of medical science that deals with the study and management of rheumatic diseases. It is involved in the diagnosis and treatment of rheumatic conditions of the musculoskeletal system, autoimmune diseases, soft tissues and inherited connective tissue disorders. Some common rheumatic diseases are arthritis, dermatomyositis, sarcoidosis, scleroderma, vasculitis, lupus erythematosus, Lyme disease and fibromyalgia. It involves the diagnosis of these diseases by performing physical examination tests such as Schober's test, multiple joint inspection, and musculoskeletal examination. X-rays, laboratory tests including erythrocyte sedimentation rate, rheumatoid factor, and anti-citrullinated protein (anti-CCP) antibody tests are also commonly used for diagnosis in rheumatology. The treatment options available for rheumatic diseases include analgesics, non-steroidal anti-inflammatory drugs (NSAIDs), disease-modifying antirheumatic drugs (DMARDs), occupational therapy, and physiotherapy. The severe cases of rheumatic diseases are treated with rheumasurgery or rheumatoid surgery. This book explores the recent trends in the diagnosis and treatment of rheumatic diseases. A number of latest researches have been included to keep the readers up-to-date with the global concepts in this area of medicine. The book aims to serve as a resource guide for students and experts alike and contribute to the growth of the discipline.

At the end of the preface, I would like to thank the authors for their brilliant chapters and the publisher for guiding us all-through the making of the book till its final stage. Also, I would like to thank my family for providing the support and encouragement throughout my academic career and research projects.

Editor

1

Serial whole-body cryotherapy in fibromyalgia is effective and alters cytokine profiles

Philipp Klemm[1*], Johanna Becker[1], Iris Aykara[1], Thomas Asendorf[2], Gabriel Dischereit[1], Elena Neumann[1], Ulf Müller-Ladner[1] and Uwe Lange[1]

Abstract

Introduction: Whole-body cryotherapy (WBC) has shown to be beneficial in the treatment of fibromyalgia (FM). There is cumulative evidence that cytokines play a crucial role in FM. It's unknown whether clinical effects of WBC can be demonstrated at the molecular level and how long the effects last.

Methods: We compared effects of serial WBC (6 sessions (− 130 °C in 6 weeks) in FM patients and healthy controls (HC). Primary outcome was the change in pain level (visual analogue scale 0–100 mm) after 6 sessions. Secondary outcomes were a change in disease activity (revised Fibromyalgia Impact Questionnaire) and pain after 3 sessions and 3 months after discontinued therapy and in cytokine levels (interleukin (IL-)1, IL-6, tumor necrosis factor α (TNF-α) and IL-10). The patients' opinions on the satisfaction, effectiveness and significance of WBC were evaluated.

Results: Twenty-three FM patients and 30 HC were enrolled. WBC resulted in a significant reduction in pain and disease activity after 3 and 6 sessions. No clinical benefit could be measured 3 months after discontinued treatment. Overall, probands were satisfied with WBC and considered WBC to be important and effective. FM patients had significantly different levels of IL-1, IL-6, TNF-α and IL-10 at each reading point compared to HC. Levels of IL-1, IL-6 and IL-10 were significantly altered over time in FM patients. Compared to HC FM patients showed a significantly different response of IL1, − 6 and − 10 to WBC.

Conclusion: Serial WBC is a fast acting and effective treatment for FM. Proven effects of WBC may be explained by changes in cytokines.

Keywords: Whole-body cryotherapy, Fibromyalgia, Cytokines, Physical therapy, Fibromyalgia impact questionnaire

Introduction

Fibromyalgia (FM) is a chronic pain syndrome. It is characterized by widespread pain and somatic symptoms such as fatigue, sleep disorders, cognitive impairment and depressive disorders [1]. Women around the age of 50 are affected more frequently [2, 3]. The global mean prevalence of FM is 2.7% [4]. Not only can FM lead to a high level of individual impairment, but it has been calculated that even a minimal increase in the Fibromyalgia Impact Questionnaire (FIQ) score increases costs in Europe by approximately €865 per year [5]. FM is therefore a problem of high social importance and represents a high economic burden [6].

The pathogenesis of FM is elusive. However, several factors seem to be of importance. These include abnormal pain sensitivity and pain inhibition [7, 8], a disturbed hypothalamic-pituitary-adrenal axis [9, 10] and cytokine dysregulation [11]. In addition, both genetic and environmental factors seem to play a role [7, 8]. Eventually, there is increasing evidence of neurogen- derived inflammatory mechanisms [12]. These affect

* Correspondence: p.klemm@kerckhoff-klinik.de
[1]Department of Rheumatology, Immunology, Osteology and Physical Medicine, Justus-Liebig-University Giessen, Campus Kerckhoff, Bad Nauheim, Germany

peripheral tissues as well as the spinal cord and brain and involve a variety of neuropeptides, chemokines, and cytokines. Both the innate and adaptive immune system appear to be activated in this process [12] and could play an essential role. In neuropathic pain, for example, a balance between pro-inflammatory and anti-inflammatory cytokines is crucial, so that, an imbalance ultimately leads to pain and impaired pain processing [13, 14]. Indeed, in neuropathic pain models, pharmacological blocking of the pro-inflammatory cytokines interleukin (IL-)1, IL-6 and tumor necrosis factor α (TNF-α) has been found to prevent or reverse allodynia and hyperalgesia [15].

Whole-body cryotherapy (WBC) exposes patients to extremely cold dry air in an environmentally controlled chamber or cabin for a short period of time (usually between 1 and 5 min). The exposure to cold air induces vasoconstriction [16] and stimulation of dermal thermoreceptors, which leads to slower nerve conduction [17] ultimately resulting in an analgesic effect. So far, it has been used as a recovery technique after physical exercise [18] and has been successfully tested in inflammatory diseases such as rheumatoid arthritis [19, 20] and ankylosing spondylitis [19, 21]. In addition to its symptomatic and immediate effects, WBC has been shown to affect the immune system. In healthy controls WBC leads to an increase in white blood cell count, especially lymphocytes and monocytes. It also affects the overall oxidative and antioxidative status, which indicates an increased immune capacity [22]. Furthermore, WBC has an influence on cytokine levels: it has been shown to increase IL-6 and IL-10 levels and to decrease IL-1 α levels in healthy individuals [23]. In a pilot study, a significant improvement in IL-1 and TNF-α levels could be observed in patients with inflammatory rheumatic diseases [19]. At the other end of the thermotherapy spectrum, it has been shown that hyperthermia also alters cytokine levels [24]. Nowadays, physical therapy has been shown to change molecular parameters, which explains its profound and beneficial effects in rheumatic diseases [25].

Recently WBC has shown effects in the treatment of FM: it reduces pain [26, 27], fatigue [26] and improves health-reported quality of life [26–28]. Positive effects of serial WBC (10 sessions in 8 days) are still remarkable 1 month after discontinued treatment [28]. An effect on disease activity measured by the revised Fibromyalgia Impact Questionnaire (FIQR) has not yet been reported.

We conducted a controlled, prospective trial to investigate WBC's effects on pain and disease activity and possible changes in molecular parameters (cytokine levels of IL-1, – 6, – 10 and TNF-α) in FM and healthy controls (HC). To evaluate the long-term effects, we also examined relevant parameters 3 months after WBC treatment.

Materials and methods

Participants

Patients with FM and HC were treated at Campus Kerckhoff of Justus-Liebig University Gießen, Dept. of Rheumatology, Immunology, Osteology and Physical Medicine. Eligible participants had to be between 18 and 80 years old. Only patients with primary FM were eligible and the diagnosis of primary FM had to be confirmed on the basis of the 2016 revised 2010/11 diagnostic criteria of FM [29]. HC was not allowed to have a medical history. In the case of women, a commitment not to become pregnant during the trial was obtained. We excluded patients with secondary FM, participants with a disease for which WBC is contraindicated, e.g. unstable coronary disease, heart attack in the last 6 months, active vasculitis or acute infection, participants with a body weight over 120 kg or intolerance to cold. All patients with FM had to be in stable pharmacological and non-pharmacological treatment 4 weeks prior to the start of the study. During the entire study period of 3 months no change in pharmacological treatment or non-pharmacological treatment (such as mind-body-therapy or meditative movement) was allowed. In addition, no physical therapy such as massages or multicomponent therapy was allowed during the entire duration of the study.

Study procedures

In this controlled prospective study, all participants received WBC treatment (6 sessions at – 130° for 3 weeks with 2 sessions/week). Outcomes were measured after 3 and 6 sessions and 3 months after discontinued therapy (follow-up).

WBC treatment was delivered using a cryosauna , SPACE CABIN' (~ 230 V, 50 Hz, serial number: 1050, year of manufacture: 2013) from Cryomed s.r.o., Slowakia. The therapy was delivered to participants in swimsuit/underwear and warm socks. Fingers were placed under the armpits during the treatment to avoid frost-damages. Temperatures between – 110 to – 170 °C can be applied. In this study, a fixed temperature of – 130 °C was selected. The first session was set at 90 s., the second at 120 s and from the third session onwards a time of 180 s (3 min) was set.

Assessments and outcomes

Primary outcome was a change in pain intensity measured by a visual analogue scale (VAS) from baseline after 6 WBC sessions in patients with FM. The measurement of pain intensity with a 10 cm VAS, visually representing the amplitude of pain (0 (best) to 100 (worst) mm) experienced by the subject [30] is well-established for FM [31]. The minimum clinically important difference (MCID) for pain intensity measured with VAS has been reported to be 2.1 points (respectively 21 mm) [32].

The secondary outcome was a change in the baseline pain level (VAS) after 3 sessions of WBC and 3 months of discontinued therapy in patients with FM. In addition, the disease activity measured by the FIQR was assessed after 6 sessions of WBC and after 3 months of discontinued therapy. The FIQR [33] evaluates 21 items in the 3 areas of function (n = 9), overall impact (n = 2), and symptoms (n = 10) of FM. Each item can be rated from 0 (best) to 10 (worst). The domain scores are then divided individually and added in a final step creating a total FIQR score from 0 (best) to 100 (worst). The results of the total FIQR can be adequately compared with the results of older papers reported using the original FIQR [33]. Thus, although no MCID for the FIQR has been reported, the MCID of a 14% change appears important for the FIQR [34].

The study used ELISA to detect changes in cytokine levels (IL-1, IL-6, IL-10 and TNF-α) in FM patients and HC after 3 and 6 WBC sessions and after 3 months of discontinued therapy. To reduce artificially altered cytokine levels, blood samples were immediately cooled and taken to the laboratory. For each sample taken, a time of less than 30 min from collection to centrifugation was recorded. Serum was centrifuged at 3500 rpm at 15 °C for 10 min and plasma was centrifuged at 2850 rpm at 4 °C for 15 min. The samples were stored at – 80 °C until further use. Cytokine levels (IL-10, IL-6, TNF-α and IL-1β/IL-1F2) were measured in sera using Quantikine® ELISAs (R&D Systems) according to the manufacturer' instructions. Optical readings were taken with the SUNRISE (TECAN) system at 450 nm. So far it could be determined that FM patients apparently have different levels of cytokines compared to HC. However, there are neither established ranges of cytokines for FM patients nor a solid correlation between specific concentrations and disease activity [35].

After 6 WBC sessions, the subjective satisfaction, efficacy and significance of WBC were assessed.

Sample size

We calculated that a sample size of 18 will have 89,2% power to detect a difference in pain (VAS 0–10 cm) in means of 1,6, assuming a standard deviation of differences of 2, using a paired t-test with a 5% two-sided significance level. Assuming a dropout rate of 20% we aimed to recruit 20 patients. The considered difference in means and standard deviation are conservative estimates based on previous studies evaluation the reduction of pain (VAS) while treating FM by WBC. Calculations were performed in nQuery 8.

Statistical analysis

Summary statistics (mean, standard deviation, frequencies, and percentages) were used to describe the sample. Differences between groups were tested with t-tests assuming unequal variances. Differences to baseline were tested with t-tests for paired values. All p-values are displayed unadjusted. The global hypothesis was tested by analysis of variance (ANOVA) and p-values less than 0.05 were considered statistically significant. In paired comparisons the p-values are displayed without adjustment, but after Bonferroni-Holm adjustment for multiplicity,they are shown statistically significant. The analyses were performed with R Version 3.6.1.

Results

From July 2014 to July 2015 we screened 89 patients (32 HC and 57 patients with the diagnosis of FM). Of these, 57 participants (26 FM patients, 31 HC) met the inclusion criteria and were enrolled (Fig. 1). The main reason for the exclusion was that FM was in the background of an inflammatory rheumatic disease and was therefore not diagnosed as "primary FM" (Fig. 1). The mean age of the participants was 46±9.8 years, 66% were female.

In FM patients the mean duration of the disease was 13.9±8 years (n=23; disease duration: min. 1 year; max. 35 years). Three FM patients (nausea 1x, unspecific maculae 1x, private reasons 1x) and one HC (1x acute urinary infection) dropped out during treatment. A statistical analysis was therefore carried out with 23 FM patients and 30 controls (Fig. 1).

Primary outcome

The mean (±SD) pain levels measured by VAS in FM patients changed from 5.91±2.3 mm (confidence interval (CI) 4.9 to 6.92) at baseline to 3.43±2.8 mm (CI 2.2 to 4, 7) after 6 WBC sessions (p< 0.0001). The MCID for pain levels of at least 2.1 was achieved.

Secondary outcomes

The mean (±SD) pain levels measured by VAS in FM patients changed from 5.91±2.3 mm (CI 4.9 to 6.92) at baseline to 4±2.7 mm (CI 2.8 to 5,2) after 3 WBC sessions (p=0.0016). The MCID for pain levels of at least 2.1 was not achieved.

3 months after the last WBC session, the pain levels measured by VAS were 71.7±1,89 mm (CI 6.3 to 8), rising to values above the baseline (p=0.0037) (Supplement-Table 1).

Disease activity assessed by FIQ decreased significantly from a mean (±SD) FIQ 60.7±18.4 at the start of the study to mean FIQ 48.5±23 after WBC treatment (p= 0.0006). Three months after discontinued treatment the mean FIQ returned to baseline level of 64.1±15.4 (p=

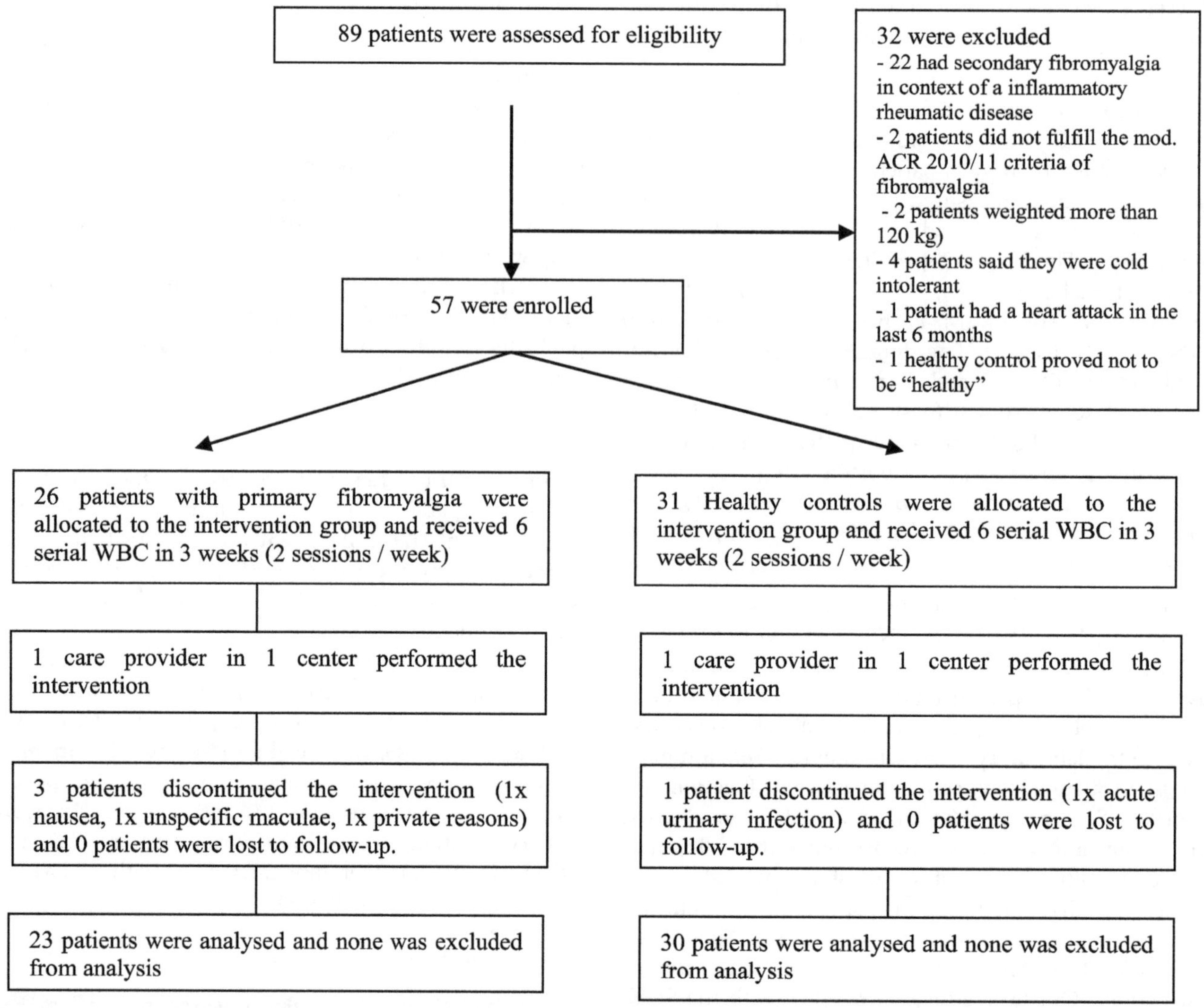

Fig. 1 Trial enrollment and follow-up

0.2142) (Fig. 2 and Supplement-Table 1). The MCID of 14% for a change in FIQ was missed (here 12.2%).

IL-1 levels in FM patients decreased significantly after 3 WBC sessions and after 6 WBC sessions and remained significantly lower compared to baseline 3 months after discontinued WBC treatment. Interestingly, 3 months after the last WBC, IL-1 levels in both groups had decreased compared to baseline, although healthy controls showed no significant change during treatment. In comparison FM patients showed significantly higher IL-1 levels after 3 sessions and 3 months after the last WBC session than healthy controls at the start of treatment (see Fig. 3 and Supplemental Table 2).

IL-6 levels were decreased by WBC in both groups. While IL-6 levels in healthy individuals returned to baseline after 3 months without WBC, FM patients still showed decreased levels. In FM patients, IL-6 levels were significantly reduced by WBC after 3 sessions and after 6 sessions compared to baseline. 3 months after the last treatment IL-6 was also significantly improved. In contrast to healthy controls, FM patients showed significantly decreased IL-6 levels at each reading point compared to baseline (cf. Figure 3 and Supplement-Table 3).

TNF-α levels were not significantly decreased by WBC, neither in FM patients nor in healthy controls (cf. Figure 3 and Supplement-Table 4).

Levels of IL-10 in FM patients were significantly influenced after 3 WBC applications and 3 months after discontinued treatment. Compared to healthy controls, FM patients showed significantly higher IL-10 levels at baseline, after 6 WBC sessions and 3 months after the last WBC application (cf- Fig. 3 and Supplement-Table 5).

Taken together, in an analysis of mixed effects, the concentrations of IL-1, IL-6 and IL-10 as well as pain (VAS) and disease activity (FIQ) were significantly

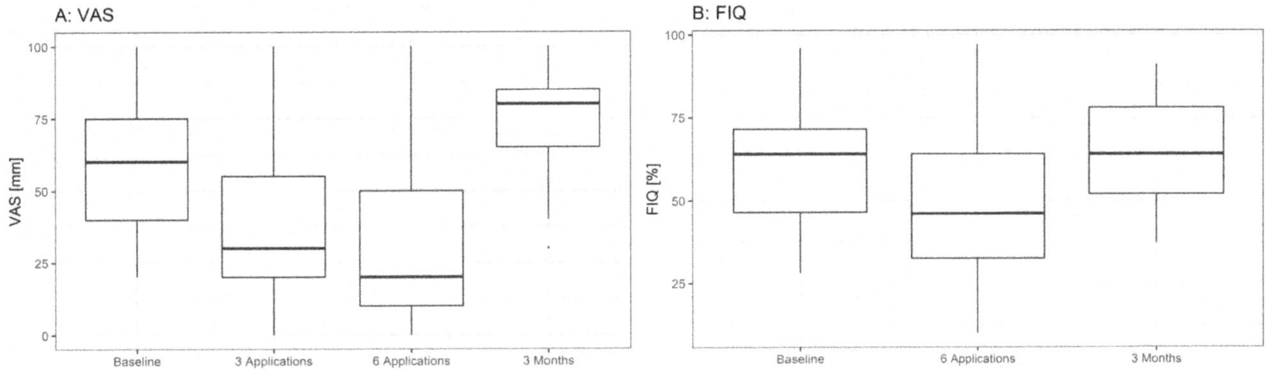

Fig. 2 Course of VAS (**a**) and FIQ (**b**)

altered over time by WBC treatment. FM patients had significantly different levels of IL-1, IL-6, TNF-α and IL-10 at each reading point compared to healthy controls. Most interestingly, FM patients showed a significantly different response to WBC compared to healthy controls in terms of changes in IL1, − 6 and − 10 to WBC over time (cf. Table 1).

Subjective satisfaction, efficacy and significance of WBC

After completing WBC treatment, patients were asked to report on their subjective satisfaction with WBC treatment and on the subjective effectivness and significance of WBC treatment. Most patients were highly satisfied with WBC and perceived WBC as an effective and highly important treatment option (cf. Figure 4).

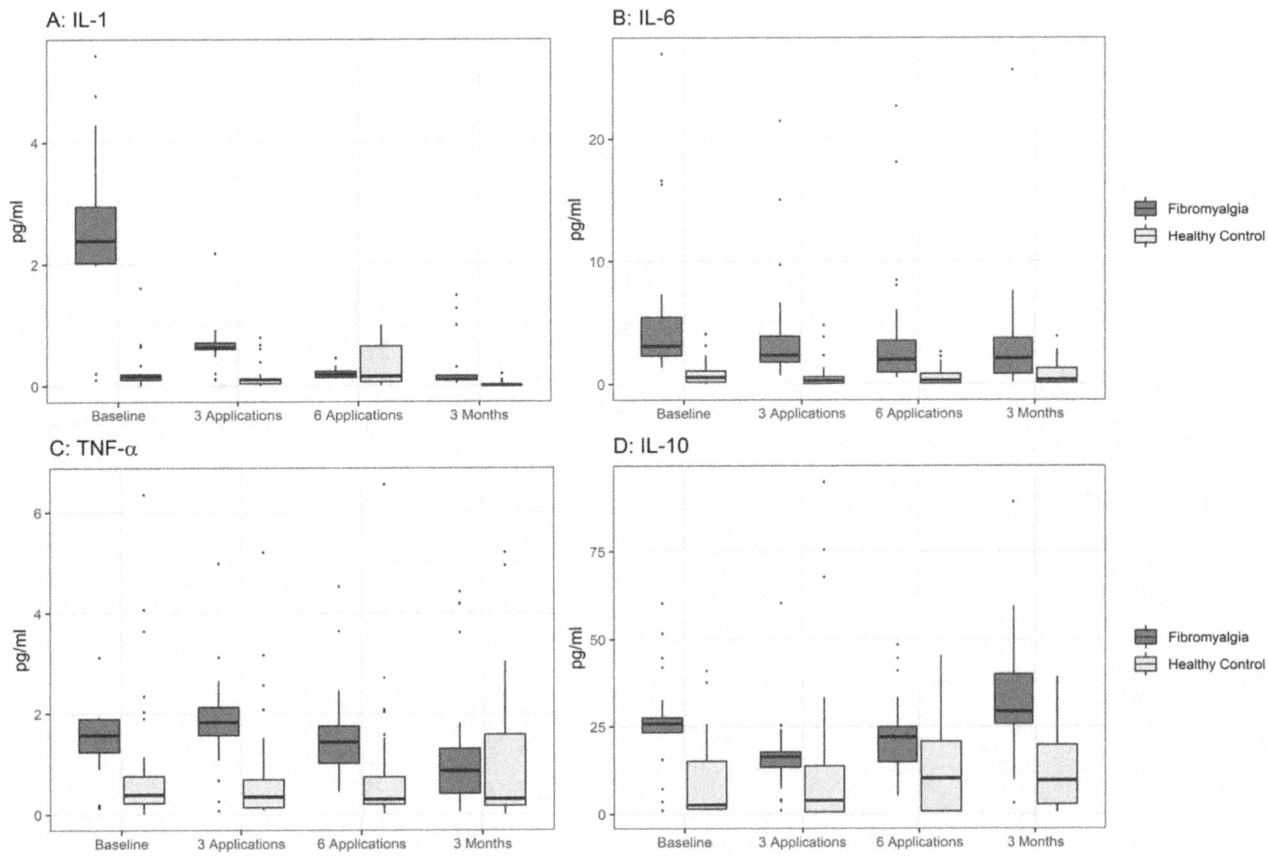

Fig. 3 Course of IL-1 (**a**), IL-6 (**b**), TNF-α (**c**) and IL-10 (**d**)

Table 1 Mixed effects analysis of group effects (Fibromyalgia vs. Healthy Control) and time effects (Baseline, 3 Applications, 6 Applications, 3 Months) as well as interaction. A significant interaction effect indicates differences in value development/performance over time depending on the cohort

	Group Effect	Time Effect	Interaction
IL1	$p < 0.0001$	$p < 0.0001$	$p < 0.0001$
IL6	$p = 0.0005$	$p = 0.0009$	$p = 0.0053$
IL10	$p = 0.0008$	$p = 0.0032$	$p < 0.0001$
TNF-alpha	$p = 0.0096$	$p = 0.8783$	$p = 0.1271$
VAS	–	$p < 0.0001$	–
FIQ	–	$p < 0.0001$	–

Discussion

This trial, which examined the clinical and molecular effects of WBC in FM patients and HC, showed that serial WBC (6 sessions) resulted in a significant and clinically important pain reduction in FM patients. Secondary outcomes showed that disease activity is significantly reduced by WBC and that the effects on pain are significantly manifested after only 3 WBC sessions. The subjects were satisfied with WBC and considered WBC to be important and effective. FM patients had significantly different levels of IL-1, IL-6, TNF-α and IL-10 at each reading point compared to HC. Levels of IL-1, IL-6 and IL-10 were significantly altered over time in FM patients. In comparison to healthy controls, FM patients showed a significantly different response in IL1, – 6 and – 10 levels to WBC.

Three previous studies have already tested the effect of WBC on FM, but with different settings. Bettoni et al. treated recruited patients with mandatory aerobic exercise (cycloergometer or treadmill) for 30 min immediately after WBC treatment [26]. Because aerobic exercise is effective in the treatment of FM [36] and physical activity could have influenced WBC treatment by vasodilatation as opposed to WBC-induced vasoconstriction, the distinct role of WBC in the effects observed in this study was limited. Therefore, we tested without background physical therapy throughout the study and had patients in stable treatment before and during the trial. In the study of Rivera et al. the cross-over design did not work because of too short wash-out periods: patients treated with WBC did not initially return to baseline with regard to VAS and FIQ, so that only results of the first sequence could be reported [27]. Vitenet et al. only treated 11 FM patients with WBC to investigate changes in the Medical Outcome Study Short Form-36 and, which is why the study is limited due to sample size [28]. So far, only Rivera et al. investigated effects of WBC on FIQ [27] and only Vitenet et al. included a follow-up showing

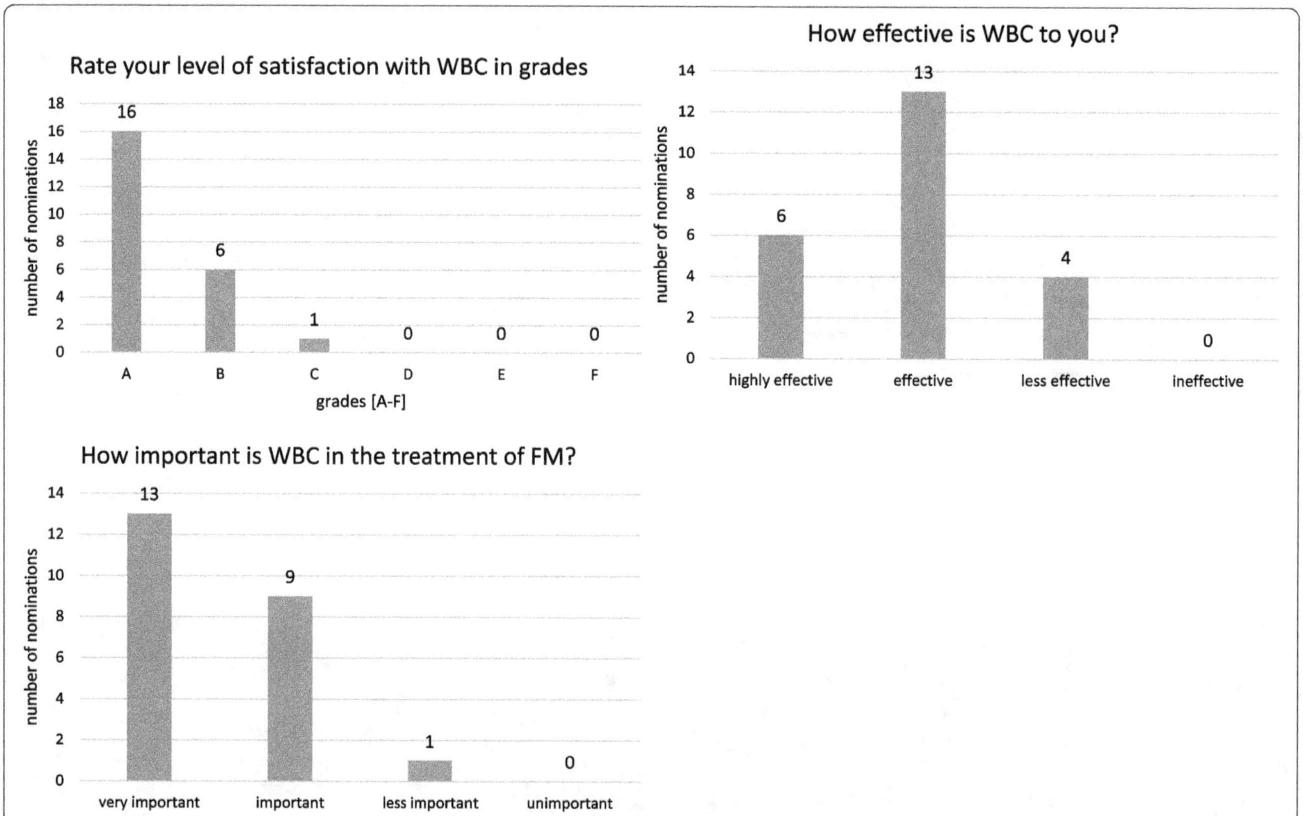

Fig. 4 Patient's report on satisfaction, efficacy, and significance of WBC treatment

effects of WBC 1 month after discontinued treatment [28]. The clinically beneficial effects of WBC in this study appear to be consistent with previous studies.

This study is limited by the absence of an FM control group, that would not receive WBC. As previous studies already tested such settings and thus demonstrated the proposed clinical benefits of WBC, we focused on a slightly different aspect in this study and investigated molecular effects of WBC in addition to the clinical effects. Thus, we first had to confirm the clinical effects of WBC in order to test the molecular effects in comparison to a healthy control group in a second step.

In our study the acceptance of WBC was high, as most patients reported to be highly satisfied with WBC while perceiving WBC as an effective and highly important treatment option. Therefore, WBC seems to be an effective tool to improve disease activity. Interestingly, a reduction of pain and disease activity was reported after only 3 sessions with a prolonged effect with increasing serial applications. Since patients with FM are partially impaired in their ability to work [37] and a minimal increase in the FIQ score increased costs by approximately €865 per year [5], cost-effective WBC can be of great benefit in the treatment of acute exacerbations of FM in an individual, but it can also be important in a social perspective.

Until now, it was not known how long the beneficial effects of WBC on FM would last after treatment. Rivera et al. had problems with their cross-over design as the washout period of 1 week for the first WBC group proved to be too short, confirming an effect of WBC for at least 1 week. Vitenet et al. showed that effects of serial WBC (10 sessions over 8 days) lasted for over 1 month after the last treatment [28]. Our study shows that 3 months after stopping treatment, effects of WBC on pain and disease activity were no longer reduced. Hence, serial WBC (between 6 and 10 sessions in up to 3 weeks) had effects for more than 1 month after termination of WBC treatment, which then decreased over time and were not effective after 3 months.

Overall, WBC seems to be a clinically valid, good and fast-acting treatment for FMS.

In the pathogenesis of FM-related hyperalgesia, central pain amplification, known as central sensitization, plays a major role [8, 38–40]. Additionally, an imbalance of pro- and anti-inflammatory cytokines plays a role in pain induction and maintenance and is known to be altered in FM [11, 35]. Prostaglandin synthesis is increased by IL-1 alone or in combination with TNF-α. It regulates substance P gene expression, thereby lowering the pain threshold in peripheral nerves [41]. In addition, the injected IL-1 causes fever, headache, myalgia and arthralgia [42] – symptoms that FM patients regularly experience. In this context, IL-1RA (IL-1 receptor antagonists) have been found to be higher in FM patients [43]. So far, not all FM patients have been found to have elevated TNF-α [11, 44], but the use of TNF inhibitors has been shown to be less effective in secondary FM [45]. IL-6 can be associated with hyperalgesia, depression stress, fatigue and sympathetic nervous system activation. Several studies have therefore measured IL-6 levels in FM – with varying results. Overall, a meta-analysis by Üceyler et al. favoured the detection of elevated plasma levels of IL-6 in FM [35]. Interleukin-10 (IL-10) inherits many anti-inflammatory properties. The expression of substance P is regulated by IL-10 in a way that the pain threshold is increased. Furthermore, IL-10 decreases the production of IL-1, IL-6 and TNF-α. In addition, WBC has proven to have an influence on cytokines in healthy controls [23].

While previous studies hypothesized the cause of WBC effects in FM [26–28], we found that WBC treatment significantly altered not only disease activity but also levels of IL-1, IL-6 and IL-10 over time. FM patients had significantly different levels of IL-1, IL-6, TNF-α and IL-10 at each reading point compared to healthy controls. These differences in cytokines we found correlate well with a study by Ernberg et al. comparing circulating cytokines between FM and healthy controls with the mentioned findings of Üceyler et al. [35] and Lubkowska et al. [23]. Ernberg et al. investigated the effect of 15 weeks of progressive resistance exercise or relaxation therapy on cytokine levels in FM patients and HC without significant alterations in cytokines and clinical outcomes in FM patients [44]. In accordance with our findings, Ernberg et al. found that FM patients had significantly different levels of cytokines compared to HC, which play a substantial role in inflammation but also pain modulation [44]. As IL-1, IL-6 and IL-10 play an essential role in pain, the observed changes could clearly explain the observed efficacy of WBC.

Conclusion

WBC is effective in FM and reduces the burden of disease. The effects of serial WBC are strongest during application and are diminished 3 months after WBC treatment. Moreover, the significant long-term alteration of IL-1, IL-6 and IL-10 by WBC could explain these beneficial effects.

Acknowledgements

We thank all participants.

Registration

The study was retrospectively registered DRKS00021218 at www.drks.de (German Clinical Trials Register) on the 8th of April 2020.

Authors' contributions

All authors contributed to the study conception and design. Material preparation, data collection and analysis were performed by PK, JB, GD, TA and UL. The first draft of the manuscript was written by PK, UL and IA and all authors commented on previous versions of the manuscript. All authors read and approved the final manuscript.

Author details

[1]Department of Rheumatology, Immunology, Osteology and Physical Medicine, Justus-Liebig-University Giessen, Campus Kerckhoff, Bad Nauheim, Germany. [2]Department of Medical Statistics, University Medical Center Göttingen, Göttingen, Germany.

References

1. Wolfe F, Clauw DJ, Fitzcharles MA, et al. The American College of Rheumatology preliminary diagnostic criteria for fibromyalgia and measurement of symptom severity. Arthritis Care Res. 2010;62:600–10. https://doi.org/10.1002/acr.20140.
2. Wolfe F, Ross K, Anderson J, et al. The prevalence and characteristics of fibromyalgia in the general population. Arthritis Rheum. 1995;38:19–28. https://doi.org/10.1002/art.1780380104.
3. Wolfe F, Smythe HA, Yunus MB, et al. The american college of rheumatology 1990 criteria for the classification of fibromyalgia. Arthritis Rheum. 1990;33:160–72. https://doi.org/10.1002/art.1780330203.
4. Queiroz LP. Worldwide epidemiology of fibromyalgia. Curr Pain Headache Rep. 2013;17:356. https://doi.org/10.1007/s11916-013-0356-5.
5. Spaeth M. Epidemiology, costs, and the economic burden of fibromyalgia. Arthritis Res Ther. 2009;11:117.
6. Knight T, Schaefer C, Chandran A, et al. Health-resource use and costs associated with fibromyalgia in France, Germany, and the United States. Clin Outcomes Res. 2013;5:171–80. https://doi.org/10.2147/CEOR.S41111.
7. Bradley LA. Pathophysiology of fibromyalgia. Am J Med. 2009;122:S22–30. https://doi.org/10.1016/j.amjmed.2009.09.008.
8. Häuser W, Ablin J, Fitzcharles M-A, et al. Fibromyalgia. Nat Rev Dis Primers. 2015;1:15022. https://doi.org/10.1038/nrdp.2015.22.
9. Crofford LJ, Pillemer SR, Kalogeras KT, et al. Hypothalamic–pituitary–adrenal axis perturbations in patients with fibromyalgia. Arthritis Rheum. 1994;37: 1583–92. https://doi.org/10.1002/art.1780371105.
10. Tak LM, Cleare AJ, Ormel J, et al. Meta-analysis and meta-regression of hypothalamic-pituitary-adrenal axis activity in functional somatic disorders. Biol Psychol. 2011;87:183–94.
11. Rodriguez-Pintó I, Agmon-Levin N, Howard A, Shoenfeld Y. Fibromyalgia and cytokines. Immunol Lett. 2014;161:200–3. https://doi.org/10.1016/j.imlet.2014.01.009.
12. Littlejohn G, Guymer E. Neurogenic inflammation in fibromyalgia. Semin Immunopathol. 2018;40:291–300.
13. Ahrens C, Schiltenwolf M, Wang H. Cytokines in psychoneuroendocrine immunological context of nonspecific musculoskeletal pain. Schmerz. 2012; 26:383–8. https://doi.org/10.1007/s00482-012-1153-5.
14. Kiguchi N, Kobayashi Y, Kishioka S. Chemokines and cytokines in neuroinflammation leading to neuropathic pain. Curr Opin Pharmacol. 2012; 12:55–61.
15. Wolf G, Gabay E, Tal M, et al. Genetic impairment of interleukin-1 signaling attenuates neuropathic pain, autotomy, and spontaneous ectopic neuronal activity, following nerve injury in mice. Pain. 2006;120:315–24. https://doi.org/10.1016/j.pain.2005.11.011.
16. Mourot L, Cluzeau C, Regnard J. Hyperbaric gaseous Cryotherapy: effects on skin temperature and systemic vasoconstriction. Arch Phys Med Rehabil. 2007;88:1339–43. https://doi.org/10.1016/j.apmr.2007.06.771.
17. Algafly AA, George KP. The effect of cryotherapy on nerve conduction velocity, pain threshold and pain tolerance. Br J Sports Med. 2007;41:365–9. https://doi.org/10.1136/bjsm.2006.031237
18. Rose C, Edwards KM, Siegler J, et al. Whole-body Cryotherapy as a recovery technique after exercise: a review of the literature. Int J Sports Med. 2017;38: 1049–60. https://doi.org/10.1055/s-0043-114861.
19. Lange U, Uhlemann C, Müller-Ladner U. Serial whole-body cryotherapy in the criostream for inflammatory rheumatic diseases. A pilot study. Med Klin. 2008;103:383–8. https://doi.org/10.1007/s00063-008-1056-5.
20. Bouzigon R, Grappe F, Ravier G, Dugue B. Whole- and partial-body cryostimulation/cryotherapy: current technologies and practical applications. J Therm Biol. 2016;61:67–81.
21. Stanek A, Cholewka A, Gadula J, et al. Can whole-body cryotherapy with subsequent kinesiotherapy procedures in closed type cryogenic chamber improve BASDAI, BASFI, and some spine mobility parameters and decrease pain intensity in patients with ankylosing spondylitis? Biomed Res Int. 2015; 2015:404259. https://doi.org/10.1155/2015/404259.
22. Lubkowska A, Szygula Z, Klimek AJ, Torii M. Do sessions of cryostimulation have influence on white blood cell count, level of IL6 and total oxidative and antioxidative status in healthy men? Eur J Appl Physiol. 2010;109(1):67–72.
23. Lubkowska A, Szyguła Z, Chlubek D, Banfi G. The effect of prolonged whole-body cryostimulation treatment with different amounts of sessions on chosen pro-and anti-inflammatory cytokines levels in healthy men. Scand J Clin Lab Invest. 2011;71:419–25. https://doi.org/10.3109/00365513.2011.580859.
24. Lange U, Dischereit G. Effects of different iterative whole-body hyperthermia on pain and cytokines in rheumatic diseases: a current review. Aktuelle Rheumatol. 2018. https://doi.org/10.1055/s-0044-101543.
25. Lange U, Müller-Ladner U, Dischereit G. Rheumatic diseases and molecular physical medicine – new aspects. Phys Medizin, Rehabil Kurortmedizin. 2017;27:205–10. https://doi.org/10.1055/s-0043-113045.
26. Bettoni L, Bonomi FG, Zani V, et al. Effects of 15 consecutive cryotherapy sessions on the clinical output of fibromyalgic patients. Clin Rheumatol. 2013;32:1337–45. https://doi.org/10.1007/s10067-013-2280-9.
27. Rivera J, Tercero MJ, Salas JS, et al. The effect of cryotherapy on fibromyalgia: a randomised clinical trial carried out in a cryosauna cabin. Rheumatol Int. 2018;38:2243–50. https://doi.org/10.1007/s00296-018-4176-0.
28. Vitenet M, Tubez F, Marreiro A, et al. Effect of whole body cryotherapy interventions on health-related quality of life in fibromyalgia patients: a randomized controlled trial. Complement Ther Med. 2018;36:6–8. https://doi.org/10.1016/j.ctim.2017.10.011.
29. Wolfe F, Clauw DJ, Fitzcharles MA, et al. 2016 revisions to the 2010/2011 fibromyalgia diagnostic criteria. Semin Arthritis Rheum. 2016;46:319–29. https://doi.org/10.1016/j.semarthrit.2016.08.012.
30. Bijur PE, Silver W, Gallagher EJ. Reliability of the visual analog scale for measurement of acute pain. Acad Emerg Med. 2001;8:1153–7. https://doi.org/10.1111/j.1553-2712.2001.tb01132.x.
31. Casale R, Rainoldi A. Fatigue and fibromyalgia syndrome: clinical and neurophysiologic pattern. Best Pract Res Clin Rheumatol. 2011;25:241–7. https://doi.org/10.1016/j.berh.2011.01.016.
32. Mease PJ, Spaeth M, Clauw DJ, et al. Estimation of minimum clinically important difference for pain in fibromyalgia. Arthritis Care Res (Hoboken). 2011;63:821–6. https://doi.org/10.1002/acr.20449.
33. Bennett RM, Friend R, Jones KD, et al. The revised fibromyalgia impact questionnaire (FIQR): validation and psychometric properties. Arthritis Res Ther. 2009;11:R120. https://doi.org/10.1186/ar2783.
34. Bennett RM, Bushmakin AG, Cappelleri JC, et al. Minimal clinically important difference in the fibromyalgia impact questionnaire. J Rheumatol. 2009;36: 1304–11. https://doi.org/10.3899/jrheum.081090.
35. Üçeyler N, Häuser W, Sommer C. Systematic review with meta-analysis: cytokines in fibromyalgia syndrome. BMC Musculoskelet Disord. 2011;12:245.
36. Bidonde J, Busch AJ, Schachter CL, et al. Aerobic exercise training for adults with fibromyalgia. Cochrane Database Syst Rev. 2017. https://doi.org/10.1002/14651858.CD012700.
37. Palstam A, Mannerkorpi K. Work ability in fibromyalgia: an update in the 21st century. Curr Rheumatol Rev. 2017;13:180–7. https://doi.org/10.2174/1573397113666170502152955.
38. Staud R. Abnormal pain modulation in patients with spatially distributed chronic pain: fibromyalgia. Rheum Dis Clin North Am. 2009;35:263–74.
39. Gracely RH, Petzke F, Wolf JM, Clauw DJ. Functional magnetic resonance imaging evidence of augmented pain processing in fibromyalgia. Arthritis Rheum. 2002;46:1333–43. https://doi.org/10.1002/art.10225.
40. Desmeules JA, Cedraschi C, Rapiti E, et al. Neurophysiologic evidence for a central sensitization in patients with fibromyalgia. Arthritis Rheum. 2003;48: 1420–9. https://doi.org/10.1002/art.10893
41. Malcangio M, Bowery NG, Flower RJ, Perretti M. Effect of interleukin-1β on the release of substance P from rat isolated spinal cord. Eur J Pharmacol. 1996;299:113–8. https://doi.org/10.1016/0014-2999(95)00845-4.
42. Janik JE, Miller LL, Longo DL, et al. Phase II trial of interleukin 1α and indomethacin in treatment of metastatic melanoma. J Natl Cancer Inst. 1996;88:44–9. https://doi.org/10.1093/jnci/88.1.44

43. Wallace DJ, Linker-Israeli M, Hallegua D, et al. Cytokines play an aetiopathogenetic role in fibromyalgia: a hypothesis and pilot study. Rheumatology. 2001;40:743–9. https://doi.org/10.1093/rheumatology/40.7.743.
44. Ernberg M, Christidis N, Ghafouri B, et al. Plasma cytokine levels in fibromyalgia and their response to 15 weeks of progressive resistance exercise or relaxation therapy. Mediators Inflamm. 2018;2018:3985154. https://doi.org/10.1155/2018/3985154.
45. Moltó A, Etcheto A, Gossec L, et al. Evaluation of the impact of concomitant fibromyalgia on TNF alpha blockers' effectiveness in axial spondyloarthritis: results of a prospective, multicentre study. Ann Rheum Dis. 2018;77:533–40. https://doi.org/10.1136/annrheumdis-2017-212378.

2

Abdominal symptoms during Sjogren's syndrome

Simon Parreau[1,2*], Jérémie Jacques[3,4], Stéphanie Dumonteil[1], Sylvain. Palat[1], Sophie Geyl[3], Guillaume Gondran[1], Holy Bezanahary[1], Eric Liozon[1], Julie Azaïs[1], Stéphanie Colombie[1], Marie-Odile Jauberteau[2], Véronique Loustaud-Ratti[3], Kim-Heang Ly[1,2] and Anne-Laure Fauchais[1,2]

Abstract

Background: Abdominal symptoms in patients with primary Sjögren syndrome (pSS) are poorly documented. The objective of the study was to describe the abdominal symptoms of patients with pSS and to assess their association with characteristics of the disease.

Methods: One hundred and fifty patients with pSS were evaluated using a composite global symptom score for abdominal symptoms and their severity. Data concerning the clinical and biological characteristics of pSS and abdominal disorders were also collected.

Results: Of the patients with pSS, 95% suffered from abdominal symptoms (median global symptom score 7.5 ± 5.5 points out of 30). More than half of the patients experienced abdominal tension (68%), upper abdominal pain (54%), abdominal discomfort (58%) and/or constipation (54%). Regarding the pSS activity, in relation to European League Against Rheumatism (EULAR) Sjögren syndrome disease activity index score items, general and central nervous system involvement wereassociated with a high global symptom score. The EULAR Sjogren Syndrome Patient Reported Index (ESSPRI) symptom score was positively correlated with the global symptom score ($p < 0.01$). Multivariate analysis showed a significant association between a high global symptom score and SSA seronegativity, gastroparesis, and ESSPRI score ($p < 0.01$ for each).

Conclusions: The majority of patients with pSS suffered abdominal symptoms. There is currently no therapeutic recommendation because of the lack of information on the underlying pathophysiological mechanisms.

Trial registration: NCT03157011. Date of registration: July 17, 2017.

Keywords: Sjögren's syndrome, Abdominal symptoms, Gastroparesis, ESSPRI, ESSDAI, Quality of life

Background

Primary Sjögren syndrome (pSS) is a chronic autoimmune disorder characterized by lymphocytic infiltration of the exocrine glands and loss of secretory function with oral and ocular dryness. It affects predominantly females (female:male ratio 9:1), and the peak frequency of the disease is about age 50 years. The etiology of pSS is unclear [1]. Like other autoimmune diseases, negative impact, pain, and fatigue predominate, reducing the quality of life. Furthermore, abdominal disorders affect approximately 25% of patients with pSS but are poorly documented in the literature [2]. Indeed, epidemiological characteristics vary among studies because of the small number of patients and use of old classification criteria [2]. Also, data concerning the frequency of abdominal symptoms and their associations with clinical and biological manifestations of pSS are contradictory [2]. This heterogeneity led us to conduct a non-interventional prospective study of abdominal symptoms in patients with pSS as defined by

* Correspondence: simon.parreau@hotmail.com
[1]Internal Medicine Department, Limoges University Hospital, 16 rue du Professeur Bernard Descottes, 87042 Limoges, France
[2]EA 3842 - Cellular Homeostasis and Diseases, Faculty of Medicine, University of Limoges, 2 rue du Docteur Marcland, 87025 Limoges, France

the 2016 American College of Rheumatology-European League Against Rheumatism (ACR-EULAR) criteria [3].

Methods

Population

From July 2017 to June 2018, we conducted a single-center study in a French Hospital and University Center. It was a prospective, non-interventional study, and was approved by the Committee for the Protection of Individuals "Sud-Ouest et Outre Mer III" (France). All patients (age > 18 years) followed in our center for pSS were considered for enrollment. All of them fulfilled the 2016 ACR-EULAR classification criteria for pSS [3]. The patients provided written consent after receiving information on the study. The patients' characteristics (age at disease onset, sex, and duration of pSS), clinical manifestations of pSS, associated organ-specific autoimmune disorders, and treatments were recorded. pSS Activity as measured by the EULAR Sjögren syndrome disease activity index (ESSDAI) and pSS symptoms measured by EULAR Sjogren Syndrome Patient Reported Index (ESSPRI) were systematically evaluated concurrently with abdominal symptoms [4]. The data were completely anonymized before being assessed. Blood tests were performed at the time of diagnosis and concurrently with assessment of the abdominal symptoms score.

Evaluation of abdominal symptoms

The patients with pSS were interviewed by a physician using a questionnaire. The questionnaire comprised 10 abdominal symptoms (nausea, vomiting, upper and lower abdominal pain, abdominal discomfort, bloating, diarrhea, constipation, tenesmus, dysuria). Each symptom was scored from 0 (no symptom) to 3 (severe) as evaluated by professional judgement. A global symptom score (GSS), calculated as the sum of all symptom scores, was assigned to each patient (maximum score, 30) [5–13]. This score has been used for another chronic autoimmune disease, systemic sclerosis, as well as for two chronic digestive pathologies (i.e., diverticulitis and functional dyspepsia) [5–13]. Previously diagnosed digestive, pancreatic, and hepatic diseases, as well as treatments for digestive complaints, were systematically recorded in the medical file. Previous diagnosis of gastroparesis was based on international clinical guidelines [14] and irritable bowel syndrome on the Rome IV classification [15]. After completing the questionnaire, only those patients with alarm signs (endoscopy) or signs evocative of gastroparesis (gastric emptying scintigraphy) underwent exploration of the digestive system, in accordance with the French recommendations [16–18].

Statistical analysis

Quantitative variables are presented as means ± standard deviations, and qualitative variables as numbers and percentages. For qualitative variables, a chi-squared or Fisher's exact test was used to compare the groups (SSA +/− SSB patients and seronegative patients). For normally distributed quantitative variables, Student's *t*-test was used to compare groups of two or more classes. For non-normally distributed quantitative variables, the Wilcoxon signed-rank test or the Kruskal–Wallis test was used to compare groups of two or more classes. Univariate analyses between the abdominal symptoms and the other variables were performed. Variables with a value of $p < 0.20$ were included in a multivariate logistic model, simplified by a stepwise elimination method [19], so that the final model included only variables significantly associated with digestive symptoms. Quantitative variables fulfilling the logit linearity assumption were incorporated without modification, or otherwise categorized. The relevance of the model was assessed using Pearson's residual and deviance tests, and its quality by means of a receiver operating characteristic curve. To test the correlation between the GSS score and continuous variables, Spearman's rho was calculated. A supervised discretization will be performed with a decision tree to identify thresholds for the GSS variable. Statistical analysis was conducted using R software (version 3.2.2, rpart package). Values of $p < 0.05$ were considered indicative of significance.

Results

Patients' characteristics and treatments

A total of 150 patients (mean age 63 ± 13 years, male $n = 9$) with pSS were enrolled. Eighty patients (53%) had anti-SSA antibodies and 31 (21%) had anti-SSB antibodies (22%). One hundred and four patients (86%) had a Chisholm score of ≥3 at the time of diagnosis. None of the patients had auto-antibodies, symptoms, or capillaroscopy findings suggestive of an associated systemic sclerosis. The most common systemic involvements, defined in the ESSDAI score, were articular ($n = 107$; 71%) and muscular ($n = 68$; 45%). Twenty-two percent of the patients ($n = 33$) had neurological involvement (central $n = 20$ [13%] and/or peripheral $n = 24$ [16%] with 14 [9%] biopsy-proven small-fiber neuropathies) [20]. Other systemic involvements were hematologic ($n = 30$; 20%), pulmonary ($n = 17$; 11%), cutaneous vasculitis ($n = 11$; 7%) and interstitial nephritis ($n = 8$; 5%) (Table 1). The average ESSDAI score was 3.4 ± 4.8 points out of 123. The average ESSPRI score was 5.9 ± 2.1 out of 10. The latter score is the average of the dryness (6.2 ± 2.4 out of 10), fatigue (6.2 ± 2.4) and pain (5.5 ± 2.7) scores. Hydroxychloroquine was taken by 46% ($n = 70$) of the patients, corticosteroids by 23% ($n = 35$), immunosuppressive drugs by 14% ($n = 22$; including three patients taking mycophenolate mofetil), targeted therapies by 3% ($n = 5$), and intravenous immunoglobulin by 5% ($n = 8$). Symptomatic treatments

Table 1 Characteristics of patients according to serological status

	SSA+ ($n = 80$)	SSA- ($n = 70$)	TOTAL ($n = 150$)	*p-value* [a]
	n (%)			
Male	3 (3.7)	6 (8.7)	9 (6.0)	n.s.
Age at diagnosis, years	51.2 (13.4)	55.0 (11.0)	53.0 (12.5)	n.s.
Mean follow-up, years	10.3 (7.9)	9.6 (6.9)	10.0 (7.4)	n.s.
Salivary gland enlargement	21 (26.3)	19 (27.1)	40 (26.5)	n.s.
Raynaud's phenomenon	29 (36,3)	18 (25.7)	47 (31.1)	n.s.
Articular involvement	56 (70.0)	51 (72.9)	107 (70.9)	n.s.
Muscular involvement	32 (40.0)	35 (50.0)	67 (44.4)	n.s.
Neurologic involvement	15 (18.8)	19 (27.1)	34 (22.5)	n.s.
Cutaneous vasculitis	9 (11.3)	1 (1.4)	10 (6.6)	0.026
Pulmonary involvement	11 (13.8)	5 (7.1)	16 (10.6)	n.s.
Interstitial nephritis	6 (7.5)	2 (2.9)	8 (5.3)	n.s.
Fibromyalgia	2 (2.5)	10 (7.0)	12 (8.0)	n.s.
Depression	12 (15.0)	20 (28.6)	32 (21.3)	0.0481
Hematological involvement	23 (28.8)	8 (11.4)	31 (20.5)	0.0090
Non-Hodgkin lymphoma	2 (2.5)	0	2 (1.3)	n.s.
Hypergammaglobulinemia	35 (43.8)	2 (2.9)	37 (24.5)	< 0.0001
Positive RF	12 (15.0)	2 (2.9)	14 (9.3)	0.0115
Cryoglobulinemia	4 (5.0)	1 (1.4)	5 (3.3)	n.s.
Symptomatic treatment of pSS	67 (83.7)	58 (84.0)	126 (84.0)	n.s.
Specific treatment of pSS	52 (65.0)	35 (50.7)	88 (58.7)	n.s.
Digestive treatment	33 (41.2)	39 (56.5)	73 (48.7)	n.s.
	mean (sd)			
ESSDAI score	3.5 (4.9)	3.2 (4.8)	3.4 (4.8)	n.s.
ESSPRI score	5.5 (2.1)	6.4 (1.9)	5.9 (2.1)	0.0082

RF rheumatoid factor, *pSS* primary Sjögren's syndrome, *n.s* not significant, *sd* standard deviation

[a]For qualitative variables, a Chi-2 or Fisher's exact test was used to compare different groups of patients (SSA+ patients and seronegative patients). For quantitative variables in a normal distribution, the Student's t-test was used to compare groups of two or more classes; for variables that do not follow a normal distribution, the Wilcoxon signed-rank test or the Kruskal-Wallis test was used to compare groups of two or more classes. The value $p < 0.05$ was considered significant

included standard analgesics ($n = 51$; 34%), specific neuropathic pain treatments ($n = 26$; 17%), and nonsteroidal anti-inflammatory drugs ($n = 13$; 8%). Seventeen percent of the patients ($n = 26$) used antidepressants and 15% ($n = 23$) used benzodiazepines.

Previous digestive disease

Forty-four patients had symptomatic gastroesophageal reflux (29%). Thirteen patients had at least one gastric emptying scintigraphy for clinical signs suggestive of gastroparesis (9%); among them, nine had a confirmed gastroparesis. Of these nine patients, three had mild, three had moderate, and three had severe gastroparesis, according to the fixation rate at 4 h[6]. All of the patients received medical treatment, three patients received botulinum toxin injections, and two underwent endoscopic pylorotomy. Only 7 patients (4.7%) had diabetes mellitus, none of whom had gastroparesis. Another 7 patients had autoimmune hepatitis with 4 cases of primary biliary cholangitis and 3 of sclerosing cholangitis. Twenty-seven cases of gastritis (18%), mostly atrophic, were reported, as well as three cases of pernicious anemia (2%) and one of coeliac disease. Thirty cases of irritable bowel syndrome were documented (20%). Sixteen patients had enteric endoscopic diverticulosis (11%), which was complicated by diverticulitis in five patients. Three cases of dolichocolons were noted. Forty-eight percent of the patients had used at least one treatment for abdominal symptoms in the previous 2 weeks. The most highly represented drug classes were proton pump inhibitors ($n = 45$; 30%), laxatives ($n = 14$; 9%), antispasmodics ($n = 19$; 13%), sodium alginates and/or coals ($n = 11$; 7%), ursodeoxycholic acid ($n = 6$; 4%), prokinetics ($n = 5$; 3%), and anti-diarrheals ($n = 5$; 3%).

Abdominal symptoms

Ninety-five percent of the patients ($n = 143$) suffered from abdominal symptoms (median GSS score = 7.5 ± 5.5 points). The abdominal complaints are shown according to severity in Fig. 1. More than half of the patients had upper abdominal pain, abdominal discomfort, bloating and/or constipation. Several features of pSS were associated with a GSS using a score higher than 10 obtained by supervised discretization (Table 2). There was no correlation between abdominal symptoms and focus score on minor salivary gland biopsy or unstimulated salivary flow.

Regarding the ESSDAI score items, articular involvement was associated with a GSS > 10. Muscular, pulmonary and neurological involvement were more present with a GSS > 10 but not significantly (Table 2).

The total ESSPRI score was correlated with the GSS score (0.48; Rho = 0.5, $p < 0.0001$). The three items of the ESSPRI score were also correlated with a high GSS score (dryness Rho = 0.3, $p = 0.0014$, fatigue Rho = 0.5, $p < 0.0001$ and pain Rho = 0.4, $p < 0.0001$).

Several digestive antecedents were correlated with a high GSS score: hiatal hernia (GSS = 12.4 ± 5.6 vs. 9.0 ± 6.1, $p = 0.007$), gastroesophageal reflux (GSS = 12.3 ± 6.1 vs. 8.7 ± 5.9, $p = 0.001$), gastroparesis (GSS = 15.9 ± 2.5 vs. 9.4 ± 6.1, $p = 0.0032$), atrophic gastritis (GSS = 15.1 ± 4.9 vs. 9.4 ± 6.1, $p = 0.0097$), irritable bowel syndrome (GSS = 13.4 ± 5.8 vs. 8.8 ± 5.9, $p = 0.0002$), at least one previous abdominal surgery (GSS = 13.4 ± 5.8 vs. 8.8 ± 5.9, $p = 0.0440$), and pernicious anemia (GSS = 19.0 ± 8.5 vs. 9.6 ± 6.0, $p = 0.0306$). Use of treatments for gastrointestinal symptoms was correlated with a high GSS (trimebutine [GSS = 15.6 ± 6.5 vs. 9.4 ± 6.0, $p = 0.0047$] and proton pump inhibitors [GSS = 12.4 ± 6.5 vs. 8.6 ± 5.6, $p = 0.0004$]). In addition, a high GSS score was correlated with a higher frequency of endoscopic explorations and gastric emptying scintigraphy (GSS = 14.6 ± 6.1 vs. 9.3 ± 6.0, $p = 0.0037$). No pSS-specific therapy was correlated with a high abdominal symptoms score. Serologic status influenced the overall abdominal score as well as the prevalence of several abdominal symptoms (Table 3). Indeed, the median GSS score was significantly higher in seronegative patients (GSS = 11.8 ± 5.8 vs. 7.9 ± 5.9, $p = 0.02$).

The multivariate analysis of the total GSS score (linear regression) and upper gastrointestinal symptoms (logistic regression) vs. patient characteristics is shown in Table 4. No item was significantly related to reduced abdominal symptoms in the multivariate analysis. The multivariate analysis confirmed the significant association between the GSS total score, ESSPRI score, and seronegativity ($p < 0.01$; Table 4). The fatigue and fever items of the GSS score were associated with seronegativity (OR = 8.45; $p = 0.0152$) and a high ESSPRI score (OR = 1.31; $p < 0.0001$).

Discussion

This study is the first to use the 2016 ACR-EULAR criteria to systematically evaluate the severity of abdominal symptoms in patients with pSS. Abdominal disorders are rarely reported during pSS and are probably underestimated [2]. The reported prevalence varies markedly depending on the pSS diagnostic criteria and the number of patients evaluated. Moreover, studies have typically focused on one type of abdominal involvement [2]. For example, Retamozo reported a 6.2% prevalence of abdominal disorders but evaluated only chronic gastritis, acute pancreatitis, and dysphagia [21]. We found a high frequency of major upper and lower abdominal complaints in patients with pSS.

These symptoms are likely to be responsible for deterioration in the quality of life of pSS patients. Indeed, Krogh

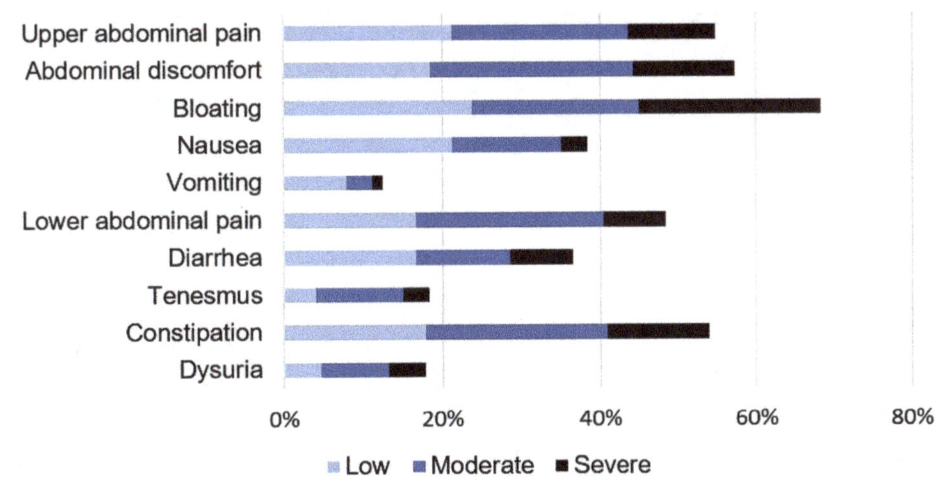

Fig. 1 Severity of abdominal symptoms according to the results of the abdominal symptoms score

Table 2 Association between a GSS and characteristics of pSS

	GSS ≤ 10 (*n* = 85) n (%) or mean (sd)	GSS > 10 (*n* = 63)	*p-value* [a]
GSS	5.2 (2.8)	15.8 (3.5)	< 0.0001
ESSPRI score	16.4 (5.9)	20.1 (5.3)	0.0001
SSA negative status	28 (32.9%)	23 (63.5%)	0.0003
Articular involvement [b]	54 (63.5%)	52 (82.5%)	0.0112
Muscular involvement [b]	33 (38.8%)	34 (54.0%)	0.0672
Pulmonary involvement [b]	6 (7.1%)	10 (15.9%)	0.0877
Neurological involvement [b]	16 (18.8%)	18 (28.6%)	0.1633
Antecedent of gastroparesis	0 (0%)	9 (14.3%)	0.0003
Standard antalgics	21 (24.7%)	28 (44.4%)	0.0116
Neurotropic antalgics	11 (12.9%)	14 (22.2%)	0.1362
Digestive treatment	35 (41.2%)	37 (58.7%)	0.0346

GSS global symptom score, *sd* standard deviation, *pSS* primary Sjögren's syndrome
[a]For quantitative variables in a normal distribution, the Student's t-test was used to compare groups of two or more classes; for variables that do not follow a normal distribution, the Wilcoxon signed-rank test or the Kruskal-Wallis test was used to compare groups of two or more classes
[b]as defined by the ESSDAI score

et al. demonstrated that abdominal complaints were a source of impairment of quality of life for pSS patients [22]. However, the correlation between abdominal complaints and ESSPRI score has not been evaluated [22]. Our study showed a strong association between abdominal symptoms and a high ESSPRI score.

A retrospective Indian study showed clustering of gastrointestinal symptoms and depression/psychiatric symptoms in pSS, but only evaluated irritable bowel syndrome [23]. Although depressive symptoms were the most frequent in seronegative patients with pSS, they were not significantly associated with gastrointestinal symptoms.

Despite their frequency, digestive symptoms are not part of the ESSDAI activity score for pSS. Likewise, the ESSPRI score evaluating the frequent symptoms of pSS did not account for abdominal complaints. Almost half of the patients used treatments for digestive symptoms, which was correlated with a high abdominal score. This suggests that these treatments are ineffective and unsuitable for pSS with digestive involvement. Otherwise, pSS treatments did not influence abdominal symptoms, suggesting both their ineffectiveness and the absence of an exclusive adverse side effect that may explain such symptoms. Therefore, large prospective studies of the pathophysiology of these frequent symptoms are needed.

Table 3 Comparison of GSS symptoms and serological status

	SSA+ (*n* = 80) n (%) or mean (sd)	SSA- (*n* = 70)	Total (*n* = 150)	*p-value* [a]
Upper abdominal symptoms	63 (78.8)	67 (97.1)	131 (87.3)	0.0008
Upper abdominal pain	31 (38.7)	52 (75.4)	84 (56.0)	< 0.0001
Abdominal discomfort	40 (50.0)	47 (68.1)	88 (58.7)	0.0253
Bloating	50 (62.5)	54 (78.3)	105 (70.0)	0.0367
Nausea	25 (31.2)	35 (50.7)	60 (40.0)	0.0157
Vomiting	10 (12.5)	11 (15.9)	21 (14.0)	n.s.
Lower abdominal symptoms	63 (78.8)	59 (85.5)	123 (82.0)	n.s.
Lower abdominal pain	35 (43.7)	39 (56.5)	75 (50.0)	n.s.
Diarrhea	21 (26.2)	35 (50.7)	56 (37.3)	0.0021
Tenesmus	14 (17.5)	13 (18.8)	28 (18.7)	n.s.
Constipation	42 (52.5)	40 (58.0)	82 (54.7)	n.s.
Dysuria	10 (12.5)	19 (27.5)	29 (19.3)	0.0208

sd standard deviation, *GSS* global symptoms score, *n.s* not significant
[a]For quantitative variables in a normal distribution, the Student's t-test was used to compare groups of two or more classes; for variables that do not follow a normal distribution, the Wilcoxon signed-rank test or the Kruskal-Wallis test was used to compare groups of two or more classes. The value $p < 0.05$ was considered significant

Table 4 Multivariate analysis investigating effect of GSS on patient characteristics

GSS total	Coef	95% CI	*p-value* [a]
SSA negative status	2.34	[0.62–4.06]	0.00812
Number of past lower abdominal events	0.74	[0.23–1.25]	0.00499
Antecedent of gastroparesis	4.77	[1.20–8.35]	0.00912
ESSPRI score	0.36	[0.21–0.51]	< 0.0001
Upper abdominal symptoms	OR		
Seronegative status	6.01	[1.52–40.12]	0.0239
Digestive treatment	4.64	[1.37–21.50]	0.0241
ESSPRI score	1.11	[1.02–1.21]	0.0201

Coef coefficient, *CI* confidence interval, *GSS* global symptoms score, *OR* odds ratio
[a]*p*-values for trend are obtained with multivariable linear regression for GSS and logistic regression for upper abdominal symptoms

Dysfunction of the autonomic nervous system plays an important role in the pathogenesis of gastrointestinal manifestations of pSS. Autonomic neuropathy has been described in patients with pSS and is associated with orthostatic hypotension, urinary retention, segmental anhidrosis, and dysfunction of the digestive and urinary systems [24]. Muscarinic receptors M3 are expressed on vascular smooth muscle cells, particularly in the gastrointestinal and genitourinary systems, as well as on exocrine gland cells [25, 26]. In patients with pSS, autoantibodies are directed against muscarinic receptors [25], suggesting these antibodies to be the cause of autonomic neuropathy, which can lead to bladder insufficiency or gastrointestinal disorders [26]. Such autoantibodies were implicated in altered colonic contraction in an ex vivo model [27]. Intravenous immunoglobulin shows promise for the treatment of immunologically induced digestive or urinary disorders. Smith et al. showed that intravenous immunoglobulin neutralized anti-muscarinic M3 receptor antibodies and improved the urinary and diarrhea scores in a patient with pSS [28].

The multivariate analysis showed an association between a high abdominal symptom score and a prior diagnosis of gastroparesis. Gastroparesis is likely to be underdiagnosed in patients with pSS. We found a 69% rate of confirmed gastroparesis among patients who underwent emptying gastric scintigraphy to explore symptoms suggestive of this condition. Few studies have evaluated gastroparesis during pSS [25, 29, 30]. Kovacs et al. reported a 70% rate of scintigraphy-proven gastroparesis in 30 symptomatic patients with pSS [25]. Another study of 28 patients with pSS found a prevalence of 43% for subjective signs of gastroparesis and 29% for gastroparesis confirmed by octanoate breath tests [29]. In a retrospective study of 11 patients with pSS-associated gastroparesis, 82% had bloating and abdominal pain [30]. The relationship between gastroparesis and involvement of the autonomic nervous system in pSS is unclear. Such a relationship is hypothesized based on inhibition of gastric emptying by anti-muscarinic receptor type 3 antibodies [25]. Unfortunately, no study has evaluated the correlation of the level of these antibodies with the gastric emptying time. Our findings suggest the necessity of excluding gastroparesis in the presence of unexplained persistent upper digestive symptoms in a patient with pSS.

This study had several limitations. The GSS is based on a questionnaire that is easy to use in routine practice with patients, but it is a non-validated tool. We did not evaluate abdominal symptoms in a healthy patient cohort. It is a preliminary study mainly to highlight the presence of these symptoms in a cohort of Sjögren's patients and to evaluate their relationship to disease activity (ESSDAI) and to the most frequent symptoms (ESSPRI). This exploratory study included only patients attending a single university hospital center, which could have resulted in selection bias. However, the prevalence of systemic involvement was consistent with the findings of other French pSS studies [31, 32]. The non-interventional study design precluded demonstration of a causal link between digestive symptoms and pSS. Also, we did not systematically investigate digestive symptoms by endoscopy, which may have led to their mis- or under-diagnosis. Regarding the hypothetical link between gastrointestinal involvement and autonomic neuropathy, we did not perform physiological testing, quantitative measurement of autonomic nervous system function, or assays of anti-muscarinic receptor antibodies.

The chief strength of this study was its evaluation of a simple and rapid tool to screen and assess digestive symptoms among a large cohort of pSS patients. The majority of patients with pSS had abdominal complaints that affected their quality of life. Therefore, the questionnaire could enable not only detection but also monitoring of abdominal complaints over time. Furthermore, the questionnaire was capable of diagnosing gastroparesis, a poorly described, potentially debilitating condition associated with pSS.

Conclusion

We detected gastrointestinal symptoms in the majority of patients with pSS. Prospective studies are needed to clarify the relationship between abdominal complaints and depressive disorders and/or fibromyalgia, and investigate the underlying pathophysiological mechanisms.

Acknowledgements

None.

Authors' contributions

Each named author has substantially contributed to the research and/or drafting of the manuscript. The author(s) read and approved the final manuscript.

Author details

[1]Internal Medicine Department, Limoges University Hospital, 16 rue du Professeur Bernard Descottes, 87042 Limoges, France. [2]EA 3842 - Cellular Homeostasis and Diseases, Faculty of Medicine, University of Limoges, 2 rue du Docteur Marcland, 87025 Limoges, France. [3]Gastroenterology Department, Limoges University Hospital, 2 Avenue Martin Luther King, 87042 Limoges, France. [4]BioEM, UMR 7252, CNRS, Limoges, France.

References

1. Qin B, Wang J, Yang Z, Yang M, Ma N, Huang F, et al. Epidemiology of primary Sjögren's syndrome: a systematic review and meta-analysis. Ann Rheum Dis. 2015;74:1983–9.
2. Ebert EC. Gastrointestinal and hepatic manifestations of Sjogren syndrome. J Clin Gastroenterol. 2012;46:25–30.
3. Shiboski CH, Shiboski SC, Seror R, Criswell LA, Labetoulle M, Lietman TM, et al. 2016 American College of Rheumatology/European league against rheumatism classification criteria for primary Sjögren's syndrome: A consensus and data-driven methodology involving three international patient cohorts. Arthritis Rheum. 2017;69:35–45.
4. Seror R, Theander E, Brun JG, Ramos-Casals M, Valim V, Dörner T, et al. Validation of EULAR primary Sjögren's syndrome disease activity (ESSDAI) and patient indexes (ESSPRI). Ann Rheum Dis. 2015;74:859–66.
5. Marie I, Gourcerol G, Leroi AM, Ménard JF, Levesque H, Ducrotté P, et al. Delayed gastric emptying determined using the 13C-octanoic acid breath test in patients with systemic sclerosis. Arthritis Rheum. 2012;64:2346–55.
6. Latella G, Pimpo M, Sottili S, Zippi M, Viscido A, Chiaramonte M, et al. Rifaximin improves symptoms of acquired uncomplicated diverticular disease of the colon. Int J Color Dis. 2003;18:55–62.
7. Di Mario F, Aragona G, Leandro G, Comparato G, Fanigliulo L, Cavallaro LG, et al. Efficacy of mesalazine in the treatment of symptomatic diverticular disease. Dig Dis Sci. 2005;50:581–6.
8. Di Mario F, Stefani N, Dal Bò N, Rugge M, Pilotto A, Cavestro GM, et al. Natural course of functional dyspepsia after helicobacter pylori eradication: a seven-year survey. Dig Dis Sci. 2005;50:2286–9.
9. Marie I, Leroi AM, Gourcerol G, Levesque H, Menard JF, Ducrotte P. Lactose malabsorption in systemic sclerosis. Aliment Pharmacol Ther. 2016;44:1123–33.
10. Gemignani L, Savarino V, Ghio M, Parodi A, Zentilin P, de Bortoli N, et al. Lactulose breath test to assess oro-cecal transit delay and estimate esophageal dysmotility in scleroderma patients. Semin Arthritis Rheum. 2013;42:522–9.
11. Marie I, Ducrotté P, Denis P, Menard JF, Levesque H. Small intestinal bacterial overgrowth in systemic sclerosis. Rheumatology. 2009;48:1314–9.
12. Parodi A, Sessarego M, Greco A, Bazzica M, Filaci G, Setti M, Savarino E, Indiveri F, Savarino V, Ghio M, Parodi A, et al. Small intestinal bacterial overgrowth in patients suffering from scleroderma: clinical effectiveness of its eradication. Am J Gastroenterol. 2008;103:1257–62.
13. Marie I, Antonietti M, Houivet E, Hachulla E, Maunoury V, Bienvenu B, et al. Gastrointestinal mucosal abnormalities using videocapsule endoscopy in systemic sclerosis. Aliment Pharmacol Ther. 2014;40:189–99.
14. Camilleri M, Parkman HP, Shafi MA, Abell TL, Gerson L. American College of Gastroenterology. Clinical guideline: management of gastroparesis. Am J Gastroenterol. 2013;108:18–37.
15. Palsson OS, Whitehead WE, van Tilburg MA, Chang L, Chey W, Crowell MD, et al. Development and validation of the Rome IV diagnostic questionnaire for adults. Gastroenterology. 2016;150:1481–91.
16. Carayon P. Guidelines of the French Society of Digestive Endoscopy: total colonoscopy indications. The Council of the French Society of digestive endoscopy (SFED). Endoscopy. 2000;32:434–5.
17. https://www.has-sante.fr/portail/upload/docs/application/pdf/gastro_endoscopy.pdf.
18. Couturier O, Victor G, Faivre-Chauvet A, Baulieu F, Le Rest C, Bridji B, et al. Guide de bonnes pratiques en scintigraphie de la vidange gastrique. Méd Nucl. 2002;26:211–9.
19. Harrell F. Regression modeling strategies: with applications to linear models, logistic regression, and survival analysis. New York: Springer; 2001.
20. Chai J, Herrmann DN, Stanton M, Barbano RL, Logigian EL. Painful small-fiber neuropathy in Sjogren syndrome. Neurology. 2005;65:925–7.
21. Retamozo S, Acar-Denizli N, Rasmussen A, Horváth IF, Baldini C, Priori R, et al. Systemic manifestations of primary Sjögren's syndrome out of the ESSDAI classification: prevalence and clinical relevance in a large international, multi-ethnic cohort of patients. Clin Exp Rheumatol. 2019;37:97–106.
22. Krogh K, Asmussen K, Stengaard-Pedersen K, Laurberg S, Deleuran BW. Bowel symptoms in patients with primary Sjögren's syndrome. Scand J Rheumatol. 2007;36:407–9.
23. Sandhya P, Jeyaseelan L, Scofield RH, Danda D. Clinical characteristics and outcome of primary Sjogren's syndrome: A large Asian Indian cohort. Open Rheumatol J. 2015;9:36–45.
24. Pavlakis PP, Alexopoulos H, Kosmidis ML, Mamali I, Moutsopoulos HM, Tzioufas AG, et al. Peripheral neuropathies in Sjögren's syndrome: a critical update on clinical features and pathogenetic mechanisms. J Autoimmun. 2012;39:27–33.
25. Kovács L, Papós M, Takács R, Róka R, Csenke Z, Kovács A, et al. Autonomic nervous system dysfunction involving the gastrointestinal and the urinary tracts in primary Sjögren's syndrome. Clin Exp Rheumatol. 2003;21:697–703.
26. Goodman BP, Crepeau A, Dhawan PS, Khoury JA, Harris LA. Spectrum of autonomic nervous system impairment in Sjögren syndrome. Neurologist. 2017;22:127–30.
27. Park K, Haberberger RV, Gordon TP, Jackson MW. Antibodies interfering with the type 3 muscarinic receptor pathway inhibit gastrointestinal motility and cholinergic neurotransmission in Sjögren's syndrome. Arthritis Rheum. 2011; 63:1426–34.
28. Smith AJ, Jackson MW, Wang F, Cavill D, Rischmueller M, Gordon TP. Neutralization of muscarinic receptor autoantibodies by intravenous immunoglobulin in Sjögren syndrome. Hum Immunol. 2005;66:411–6.
29. Hammar O, Ohlsson B, Wollmer P, Mandl T. Impaired gastric emptying in primary Sjogren's syndrome. J Rheumatol. 2010;37:2313–8.
30. Geyl S, Jacques J, Parreau S, Cypierre A, Tabouret T, Gondran G, et al. Gastroparesis may be the cause of unexplained dyspepsia in patients with primary Sjögren syndrome. Rev Med Interne. 2018;39:427–30.
31. Martel C, Gondran G, Launay D, Lalloué F, Palat S, Lambert M, et al. Active immunological profile is associated with systemic Sjögren's syndrome. J Clin Immunol. 2011;31:840–7.
32. Carvajal Alegria G, Guellec D, Mariette X, Gottenberg JE, Dernis E, Dubost JJ, et al. Epidemiology of neurological manifestations in Sjögren's syndrome: data from the French ASSESS cohort. RMD Open. 2016;20:e000179.

3

Correlating cognition and cortical excitability with pain in fibromyalgia

Vikas Kumar Tiwari[1], Srishti Nanda[1], Suvercha Arya[1], Uma Kumar[2], Ratna Sharma[3], Senthil S. Kumaran[4] and Renu Bhatia[1*]

Abstract

Background: Fibromyalgia is a chronic pain disorder characterized by widespread musculoskeletal symptoms, primarily attributed to sensitization of somatosensory system carrying pain. Few reports have investigated the impact of fibromyalgia symptoms on cognition, corticomotor excitability, sleepiness, and the sleep quality — all of which can deteriorate the quality of life in fibromyalgia. However, the existing reports are underpowered and have conflicting directions of findings, limiting their generalizability. Therefore, the present study was designed to compare measures of cognition, corticomotor excitability, sleepiness, and sleep quality using standardized instruments in the recruited patients of fibromyalgia with pain-free controls.

Methods: Diagnosed cases of fibromyalgia were recruited from the Rheumatology department for the cross-sectional, case-control study. Cognition (Mini-Mental State Examination, Stroop color-word task), corticomotor excitability (Resting motor threshold, Motor evoked potential amplitude), daytime sleepiness (Epworth sleepiness scale), and sleep quality (Pittsburgh sleep quality index) were studied according to the standard procedure.

Results: Thirty-four patients of fibromyalgia and 30 pain-free controls were recruited for the study. Patients of fibromyalgia showed decreased cognitive scores ($p = 0.05$), lowered accuracy in Stroop color-word task (for color: 0.02, for word: 0.01), and prolonged reaction time (< 0.01, < 0.01). Excessive daytime sleepiness in patients were found (< 0.01) and worsened sleep quality (< 0.01) were found. Parameters of corticomotor excitability were comparable between patients of fibromyalgia and pain-free controls.

Conclusions: Patients of fibromyalgia made more errors, had significantly increased reaction time for cognitive tasks, marked daytime sleepiness, and impaired quality of sleep. Future treatment strategies may include cognitive deficits and sleep disturbances as an integral part of fibromyalgia management.

Keywords: Fibromyalgia, Chronic Pain, Cognition, Stroop Test, Reaction Time, Sleep, Sleepiness, Cortical Excitability, Evoked Potential, Pain Measurement, Cross-Sectional Studies, Case-Control Studies

Introduction

Fibromyalgia syndrome is a common neurological condition that is characterized by widespread musculoskeletal pain and the presence of typical tender points throughout the body. The prevalence has been estimated to be up to 1.75% in general population [1] and remains one of the common reasons for rheumatological referrals [2]. Despite many decades of research, the diagnosis and treatment of fibromyalgia remains a contentious topic.

At its core, fibromyalgia is characterized by a heightened pain response to non-nociceptive (allodynia) or nociceptive stimuli (hyperalgesia) [3]. In addition to

* Correspondence: renuaiims28@gmail.com; renubhatia@aiims.edu
[1]Pain Research and TMS Laboratory, Department of Physiology, All India Institute of Medical Sciences, New Delhi, India

increased pain, more than 70% of patients of fibromyalgia present a complex symptomatology comprising of fatigue [4], cognitive problems [5, 6], and sleep disturbances [7]. In recognition of their importance, the latest definition of fibromyalgia has undergone major revisions [8, 9]. The driving force of the revision of definition criteria was to broaden the symptom range of patients of fibromyalgia and ease the diagnostic process at the clinical level [10]. From a research point of view, however, the complex symptomatology brings in a few complications: firstly, the symptom profile has become too varied, especially in terms of the nature and extent of co-morbidities; secondly, it can make the management strategy very complicated.

An ongoing experience of pain symptoms is traditionally believed to interfere in the cognitive abilities by limiting the neuronal circuitries available to carry out cognitive functions, especially for attention, psychomotor speed, inhibition, and interference. Thus, a progressive decline in cognitive functions in patients of chronic pain is a logical assumption [11]. Mini-Mental State Examination is a common instrument for assessment of mild cognitive impairments [12]. Stroop test evaluates various components of cognition such as processing speed, selective/task attention, automaticity, and parallel processing [13]. Closely related to musculoskeletal pain is the poor quality of sleep. In fact, self-reported unrefreshed sleep is one of the oldest reported symptoms of fibromyalgia. It is believed that the inability to sleep would lead to daytime excessive sleepiness and easy fatiguability. Several attempts have been made to document cognitive decline [5, 6, 14–19] and disrupted sleep [20–26]; however, the cognitive decline in relation to sleep has not been extensively studied yet.

People with chronic pain often adopt a sedentary lifestyle resulting in a decrease in muscular strength and dysfunction due to the restriction of activities [27, 28]. In addition to myographic changes [29], recent evidence suggests altered structure [30–34] and function [35–37] of the motor system in patients of fibromyalgia. Under laboratory conditions, parameters of corticomotor excitability using transcranial magnetic stimulation can be used to quantify changes in the excitability of corticomotor and corticospinal tracts [38]. Few reports have assessed corticomotor excitability in patients of fibromyalgia [39–42] with conflicting results [43]. The present report is a part of a larger project to investigate the role of putative treatment options for the managmenet of fibromyalgia. However, given the current problem of varied symptomatology, it is imperative to conduct an investigation of the co-morbidities and the relation they share with pain symptoms prior to a clinical trial.

Materials & methods

Study design

It was a cross-sectional case-control study conducted in a tertiary health care centre. Diagnosed patients of fibromyalgia were recruited according to the latest definition, based on 2010/2011 criteria with modifications suggested in 2016, given by the American college of rheumatology [8, 9]. Age- and sex- matched pain-free controls were recruited from following sources: attendees & care-givers of the patients (genetically unrelated), and other hospital staff (unrelated to the study).

Participant recruitment

Right-handed female participants between 18 to 65 years were recruited after taking their medical history. Patients of fibromyalgia and pain-free controls were excluded if they had other chronic diseases such as major psychiatric disorders, autoimmune diseases, rheumatic disease; or were contraindicated to transcranial magnetic stimulation (metallic implants, pacemaker, history of substance abuse, epileptic seizure, head injury or brain surgery, pregnancy, use of antidepressants or anticonvulsants) [44]. All tests were conducted between 09:30 am to 11:30 am in a dedicated assessment laboratory at the same health care centre. The participants were asked to refrain from taking analgesics and other neuro-active substances (caffeine, nicotine, or alcohol) 24 h prior to the investigations. Since hormonal fluctuations could affect these outcomes, the tests were scheduled between the 18th to 23rd days of the menstrual cycle, keeping start of the last menstrual period as the 1st day. Pain characteristics were recorded as intensity of pain (using 11-pt Numerical pain rating scale), number of tender points (using manual palpation), and detailed evaluation of pain perception (using McGill pain questionnaire). Methodological details for pain assessments have been detailed in a recent paper from our group [45].

Cognitive assessment

i) Mini-Mental State Examination; was used to screen mild to moderate impairments in cognitive functions [12]. The vernacular version allows cognitive screening instrument of people of wide literacy and age range [46]. It has 19-items that have a binary response - 'Yes' or 'No'. One mark was given for every correct and zero for an incorrect response resulting in a maximum score of 30. It is a simple bedside test with capacity to examine cognitive functions including attention, registration, orientation, recall, and calculation.
ii) Stroop color-word test; was a cognitive parameter that tests for attention span and task execution [13]. The task was designed and adminstered using

SuperLab software (version 5.1; Cedrus Corporation, Arizona, USA) on the computer screen [47]. The initial phase of the test acclimatized the subjects to the monitor, response keys, pattern of the task. It also helped us evaluate adequate color perception, and comprehension of the word. Congruent stimuli were words that meant the same as the color of the font, for example, RED written in red color. While in the incongruent stimuli, the two aspects were mismatched. The principal of the task is that incongruent stimuli generates conflict that is then modulated and resolved by top-down cognitive control. During the test phase, the congruent stimuli were presented interleaved with incongruent stimuli. Participants were asked to correspond to font color (in one block), or word comprehension (in another block) with instructions displayed before each block. The following parameters were recorded for color-word blocks: (a) Accuracy; percentage of correct responses was calculated as the number of correct responses averaged across three trials; (b) Reaction time; average time taken to respond correctly.

Corticomotor excitability

Participants were made to sit on a chair and asked to relax as much as possible with the arm muscles adequately supported with cushions. Scalp landmarks were used to tentatively determine the most excitable region on the scalp overlying the representative area on the motor cortex for the thumb muscles, also known as the 'motor hotspot'. A figure-of-8 coil (70 mm) transcranial magnetic stimulation (NeuroSoft Neuro-MS/D magnetic stimulator, Ivanovo, Russia; max 4 T) coil was placed such that antero-posteriorly and navigated in small steps to locate the actual 'hotspot' of the motor cortex. The point was marked with a pen to ensure the coil position and orientation throughout the experiment. Biphasic pulses were delivered at an interval of 5–7 s [48–50].

(i) Resting motor threshold; was defined as the minimum stimulus intensity that elicited an evoked potential with a peak-to-peak amplitude of at least 50 μV in at least five out of ten trials, while maintaining quiescence on the electromyography. Values have been expressed as a percentage of maximum stimulator output.

(ii) Motor evoked potential; was identified as the peak-to-peak amplitude elicited by averaging ten consecutive stimuli [51] acquired at 100% resting motor threshold. Acquisition window for each trial had a width of 100 msec pre-stimulus and 200 msec post-stimulus.

Sleepiness

Sleepiness was measured using Epworth sleepiness scale in subjects. The questionnaire comprised of situations commonly encountered in daily life situations and had four responses to each item. The investigator gave a score to the option wherein, '0' implies 'would never doze off', and '3' implies 'high chances of dozing', resulting in scoring ranging from 0 to 24. Total scores of Epworth sleepiness scale were obtained by summing the all the responses. It is well established and validated score in Indian population [52].

Sleep quality

Pittsburgh sleep quality index was used to assess sleep quality and disturbances during the month preceding the evaluation. There were 19 individual items, each with four options, in increasing order of severity. Additionally, various aspects of sleep quality like subjective sleep quality, sleep latency, sleep duration, habitual sleep efficiency, sleep disturbances, use of sleeping medications, and daytime dysfunction have also been reported. Each item is scored on a 0–3 interval scale. The global Pittsburgh sleep quality index score is then calculated by summating the seven component scores, providing an overall score ranging from 0 to 21, where lower scores denote a healthier sleep quality [53]. It also validated in the Indian population with an excellent internal consistency and test-retest reliability [54].

Statistical analysis

Data summary has been presented as the proportions, mean ± standard deviation, or median (q1 – q3). Patients of fibromyalgia and pain-free control groups were compared using Chi-squared goodness-of-fit test, unpaired Student's t-tests, or Mann-Whitney U-rank tests, as appropriate. The effect size has been presented as partial eta squared (η2) and interpretated as: less than or equal to 0.003 as no effect, 0.10 to 0.039 as small effect, 0.060 to 0.110 as intermediate effect, and 0.140 to 0.200 as large effect [56] Spearman's rank test was used for correlation of the independent variables. Strength of association was interpreted as: less than 0.1 as a small association, less or equal to 0.3 as a medium association, less than or equal to 0.5 as a large association [55]. *P*-value less than 0.05 was considered statistically significant, and all tests were performed using GraphPad Prism version 8.00 for Mac OS (GraphPad Software, California US).

Results

Thirty-four patients of fibromyalgia and 30 pain-free controls were recruited for the study, Fig. 1 shows the details of the recruitment. The mean age was 38.6 ± 9.0 with 80% population being urban (all of controls and 21 of patients). Three-fourths of the population belonged to a middle or higher-middle socioeconomic stratum. All participants were literate, with 26% of the subjects being graduates (9 controls and 8 patients) and 29% being post-graduates (11 controls and 8 patients). No differences were found between patients of fibromyalgia and controls. Table 1 shows the sociodemographic features of the participants.

On average, patients of fibromyalgia reported moderate to severe pain 7.4 ± 1.3 (range 5 to 9) on the 11-point Numerical pain rating scale. The time since the onset of symptoms was 6.8 ± 2.9 years. The total score of McGill pain questionnaire was 32.6 ± 5.3 (range 25 to 48). Clinical examination showed that they had an average of 10.5 ± 2.0 tender points (range 8 to 14). The most common sites of tender points were lower back and calf, forearm and elbow regions. Few patients also reported mild headaches intermittently throughout the day; each bout of pain was felt as dull, boring and aching that often caused the patient to feel extremely tired. The symptoms were aggravated by prolonged sitting, emotional distress, and cold weather. Some degree of relief was felt after using analgesic drugs, local pressure or bandage, and sprays were used to reduce the pain.

Cognitive assessment

There was a significant difference in Mini-Mental State Examination scores of patients of fibromyalgia when compared to controls (p value = 0.054, U-statistic = 382.5, z-score = 4.069, η^2 = 0.046, small effect). For the Stroop color-word task, all participants required three familiarity runs before the actual task. There was a significant difference between patients of fibromyalgia and controls in all the four Stroop color-word test parameters. The reaction time for correct answers was prolonged (color: p value < 0.001, U-statistic = 24, z-score = 6.531, η^2 = 0.668, intermediate effect | word: p value < 0.001, U-statistic = 27.5, z-score = 6.484, η^2 = 0.658, intermediate effect), and the percentage of accuracy was lower for participants with fibromyalgia (color: p value < 0.001, U-statistic = 342.5, z-score = 6.531, η^2 = 0.079, intermediate effect | word: p value 0.001, U-statistic = 272.5, z-score = 6.531, η^2 = 0.16, small effect).

Corticomotor excitability

Most participants were able to tolerate the transcranial magnetic stimulation pulses comfortably. Resting motor threshold and motor evoked potential amplitudes p value = 0.111, U-statistic = 395, z-score = 4.069, η^2 = 0.037, small effect) were found to be statistically comparable between patients of fibromyalgia and pain-free controls. Few participants reported mild headache lasting up to 24 h after the test. No transcranial magnetic stimulation-induced adverse effects were noted.

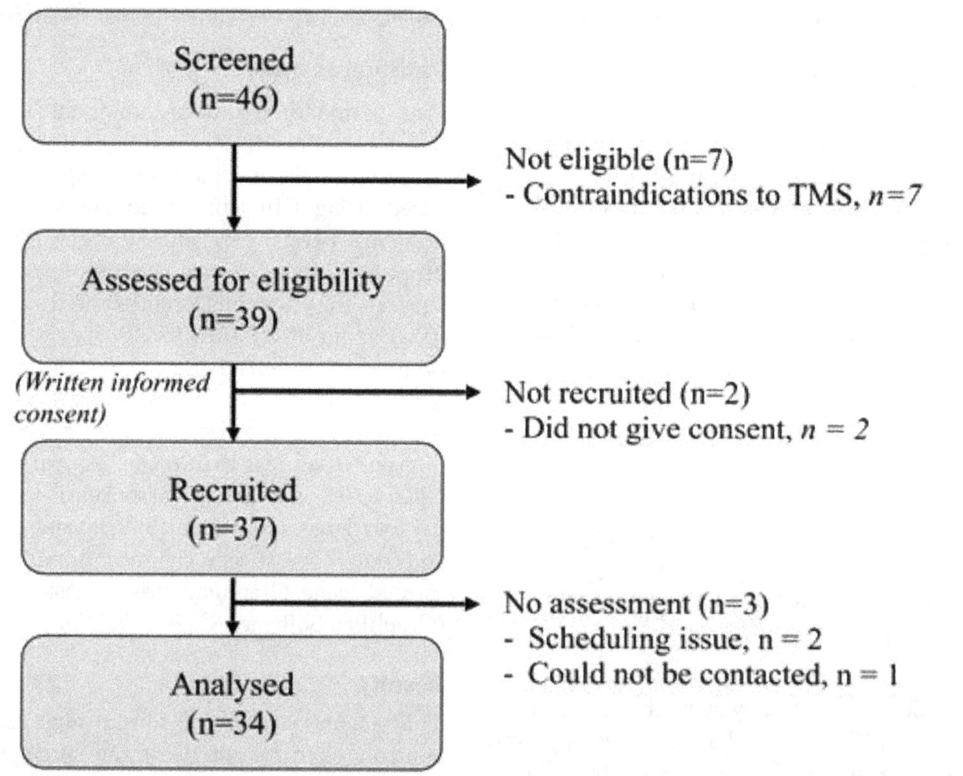

Fig. 1 Strengthening the reporting of observational studies in epidemiology 2007 (STROBE) flow chart. *TMS* Transcranial magnetic stimulation

Table 1 Demographic parameters comparison between patients of fibromyalgia and pain-free controls

Characteristics	Fibromyalgia (n = 34)	Controls (n = 30)	p-value
Age (yr)	40.6 ± 8.7	36.5 ± 9.2	0.050
Weight (kg)	65.6 ± 13.5	64.3 ± 9.9	0.572
Height (cm)	151.8 ± 10.2	154.1 ± 7.8	0.918
BMI (kg/m^2)	28.8 ± 6.7	26.6 ± 5.3	0.155
SBP (mm Hg)	121.5 ± 15.9	119.9 ± 14.9	0.608
DBP (mm Hg)	81.4 ± 10.8	79.2 ± 11.1	0.430
Pulse rate	81.0 ± 11.3	78.5 ± 11.1	0.278
Respiratory rate	20.0 ± 2.1	19.4 ± 2.5	0.209
Geographical location (Urban: rural)	21:13	22:08	0.325

Data were compared using unpaired t-test or Chi-squared goodness-of-fit test, as applicable. Level of significance was set at 5%. Values represented as mean ± standard deviation or as proportions. *BMI* Body mass index, *SBP* Systolic blood pressure, *DBP* Diastolic blood pressure

Sleepiness and sleep quality

There were significant differences in Epworth sleepiness scale scores of fibromyalgia when compared to the controls (p value < 0.001, U-statistic = 207, z-score = 4.069, η^2 = 0.724, intermediate effect). Total scores of the Pittsburgh sleep quality index were significantly different (p value < 0.001, U-statistic = 100.5, z-score = 5.502, η^2 = 0.046, intermediate effect). On comparing the domains, significant differences were found for sleep quality (p value < 0.001, U-statistic = 142, z-score = 4.944, η^2 = 0.474, small effect), latency (p value < 0.001, U-statistic = 22, z-score = 6.558, η^2 = 0.673, intermediate effect), duration (p value < 0.001, U-statistic = 81, z-score = 5.764, η^2 = 0.52, intermediate effect), efficiency (p value < 0.001, U-statistic = 42.5, z-score = 6.282, η^2 = 0.618, intermediate effect), disturbances (p value < 0.001, U-statistic = 60, z-score = 6.047, η^2 = 0.573, small effect), medication (p value < 0.001, U-statistic = 450, z-score = 6.047, η^2 = 0.046, small effect). Only the daytime sleep was comparable for patients of fibromyalgia and controls (p value 0.116, U-statistic = 48, z-score = 6.208, η^2 = 0.604, intermediate effect). Table 2 shows a summary of

Table 2 Parameters of cognition, corticomotor excitability, and sleep parameters compared between participants with fibromyalgia and controls

Characteristics	Fibromyalgia (n = 34)	Pain-free Controls (n = 30)	p-value
MMSE scores	22.5 (15.0, 29.0)	23.0 (19.0, 28.0)	0.054*
Stroop Task			
Color- reaction time (s)	2.9 (1.9, 4.5)	1.4 (0.6, 2.7)	< 0.001*
Word- reaction time (s)	2.9 (2.0, 4.0)	1.6 (0.9, 2.5)	< 0.001*
Color- correct response (%)	60.5 (41.0, 67.0)	63.0 (51.0, 76.0)	0.023*
Word- correct response (%)	55.0 (41.0, 63.0)	59.0 (48.0, 71.0)	0.001*
RMT (% MSO)	52.0 (38.0, 70.0)	55.0 (35.0, 65.0)	0.121
MEP amplitude (uV)	67.0 (55.0, 87.0)	72.7 (56.7, 98.0)	0.111
PSQI scores	12.0 (6.0, 20.0)	3.0 (2.0, 5.0)	< 0.001*
Subjective sleep quality	2.0 (1.0, 3.0)	1.0 (1.0, 2.0)	< 0.001*
Sleep latency	2.0 (1.0, 3.0)	0.0 (0.0, 1.0)	< 0.001*
Sleep duration	2.0 (1.0, 3.0)	1.0 (0.0, 1.0)	< 0.001*
Habitual sleep efficiency	1.0 (0.0, 3.0)	0.0 (0.0, 1.0)	< 0.001*
Sleep disturbances	2.0 (1.0, 3.0)	1.0 (0.0, 1.0)	< 0.001*
Use of sleep medications	0.0 (0.0, 2.0)	0.0 (0.0, 0.0)	0.116
Daytime sleepiness	2.0 (1.0, 3.0)	1.0 (0.0, 1.0)	< 0.001*
ESS scores	7.5 (2.0, 15.0)	3.0 (1.0, 5.0)	< 0.001*

Data were analysed using Mann-Whitney U-rank test. Asterisk(*) shows significance at 5%. Values represented as median (q1 - q3). *MMSE* Total scores of Mini-mental examination scale; *RMT* Resting motor threshold, *MSO* Maximum stimulator output, *MEP* Motor evoked potential, *PSQI* Total scores of Pittsburgh sleep quality index, *ESS* Epworth sleepiness scale

the comparisons between the pain-free controls and patients of fibromyalgia.

Correlation

No significant correlations were found between pain symptoms (intensity, duration, tender points) and other outcome variables (cognition, corticomotor excitability, or sleep). However, total scores of Mini-Mental State Examination showed a negative correlation with the total score of Pittsburgh sleep quality index ($r = -0.37$, $p = 0.029$). Also, reaction time for word task in Stroop color-word task was negatively correlated with sleep duration ($r = -0.36$, $p = 0.038$) and sleep disturbance ($r = -0.35$, $p = 0.045$) components of Pittsburgh sleep quality index. All three associations were medium in strength.

Discussion

The present study was aimed at investigating the pain-induced symptoms of cognition, corticomotor excitability, sleepiness, and sleep quality in the fibromyalgia patients compared to pain-free controls. Cognition and sleep quality were found to be negatively correlated with each other. No differences were found for the parameters of corticomotor excitability.

The Mini-Mental State Examination indicated that patients of fibromyalgia have mild cognitive impairments; also, the participants performed poorly in all parameters of the Stroop Test. The results show that self-reported cognitive decline (the Mini-Mental State Examination scores) are in concordance with the objective test, the Stroop Test. The study is in line with case-control studies [14] and previous meta-analyses of cognitive deficits in fibromyalgia patients [5, 6]. Imaging studies reported that anterior cingulate cortex and dorsolateral prefrontal cortex are among the main areas involved. Decision making and response evaluation are specific domains controlled by dorsal anterior cingulate cortex. These areas are also reported for pain perception and modulation. Anterior cingulate cortex has vital role in various behavioral responses such as processing of attention and anticipation of pain [56]. This activity may correspond to shared neural pain representations that allow deduction of the affective state of the pain and facilitating empathy [57]. Dorsolateral prefrontal cortex has shown activation, when resolving conflicts and catching errors, also it assists in memory and other executive functions, so ultimately affects cognition. Dorsolateral prefrontal cortex is involved in encoding and modulating acute pain perception. Elevated high-frequency oscillatory activities in the dorsolateral prefrontal cortex and orbitofrontal cortex correspond with higher affective pain scores, cognitive, and emotional modulation of pain in fibromyalgia patients. Structural brain changes in patients of fibromyalgia, indexed using voxel-based morphometry, found that central sensitization is correlated with reduced gray matter volume in specific brain regions such as anterior cingulate cortex and prefrontal cortex [32, 33]. Decreased scores in Stroop test indicates that fibromyalgia symptoms could affected the functioning of anterior cingulate cortex and dorsolateral prefrontal cortex.

No significant changes in corticomotor excitability parameters like resting motor threshold and motor evoked potential amplitude were found in patients of fibromyalgia. This is in contradiction to existing literature [39–42]. The discrepancies in the findings may be attributed to pain characteristics such as chronicity of pain. Latest studies have shown that the time since onset of painful disease could influence the changes in the corticomotor excitability [58]. Another source of dissimilarity could be the methodological differences. Salerno et al., [39] defined resting motor threshold as at least 100 μV amplitude in at least 50% of trials, whereas we used 50 μV cut-off as per the latest guidelines for recording corticomotor excitability by International Federation of Clinical Neurophysiology [49]. Another difference was the site of recording taken for our study is the abductor policies brevis, while the earlier studies used first dorsal interossei [39–41] or flexor muscle of forearm [42]. Although it is still unclear if using a different muscle group of the hand recording can contribute to the differences in findings [43] or the differences in the patient cohort being tested is the main cause of discrepancy.

Currently available pharmacotherapy for fibromyalgia includes pregabalin, duloxetine, milnacipran, amitriptyline, cyclobenzaprine and tramadol but remain far from satisfactory [59] In the same way, the present cohort of the patients was also allowed to continue the recommended drug as a part of the standard of care [45] (see supplementary file 1). The rationale is based on the fact that these drugs have demonstrated a moderate-to-large effect size for pain symptoms and somewhat on sleep quality, at least in the short term. Evidence suggests that long-term use of neuro-active drugs may induce cognitive deficits. A decline in cognitive ability has also been found to result in interference in daily activities, low coping, and poorer treatment outcomes. If the evidence can be extended to patients of fibromyalgia , then the current management may compound the issue at hand [59–61]. But cognitive abilities as outcome measures of the randomized controlled trials are currently missing from the literature. Going forward, an ideal treatment strategy must address pain symptoms and, at least to some degree, the associated co-morbidities.

Limitations

The findings of the study only pertain to middle-aged, regularly menstruating females with fibromyalgia who were refractory to standard of care regime. Factors like age and past treatments can affect pain perception, cognition, and sleep quality. Thus, more studies in patients of fibromyalgia are required to see the generalizability of our findings.

Conclusions

The study confirms a decline in cognitive function and sleep quality in patients of fibromyalgia. Most of the current treatments for fibromyalgia may have some effect on pain perception and to some extent, sleep quality. Introducing adjunct therapies that can help overcome issues of refractoriness and cognitive decline may have better outcomes. More research into treatments that address cognitive deficits vis-à-vis pain and other symptoms need to be conducted.

Acknowledgements

The authors acknowledge the contributions of Dr. Danveer Bhadu and Dr. Sandeep for patient recruitment, Dr. Ragini Adhikari for scoring the questionnaires, Dr. Suman Tanwar for helping with the review of literatue, Dr. Vinay Chitturi for helping paradigm design, and Ms. Chaithanya Leon for interpreting the Stroop Test analysis.

Authors' contributions

Study was conceived and designed by RB; proposal writing and ethical clearance was obtained by VKT, SN, and RB; standardization of methodology was done by VKT, RS, SSK, and RB; participant diagnosis was done by UK; recruitment of participants was done by VKT and SA; data was acquired by VKT and SA; data processing done by VKT and SN with help of RS, SSK, and RB; statistical analysis was done by VKT and SN. Data interpretation, manuscript writing, and revision was done by all authors. RB takes responsibility for the correspondence, further queries, and guarantee of the study. All authors(s) read and approved the final manuscript.

Author details

[1]Pain Research and TMS Laboratory, Department of Physiology, All India Institute of Medical Sciences, New Delhi, India. [2]Department of Rheumatology, All India Institute of Medical Sciences, New Delhi, India. [3]Stress and Cognition Electroimaging Laboratory, Department of Physiology, All India Institute of Medical Sciences, New Delhi, India. [4]Department of Nuclear Magnetic Resonance and MRI Facility, All India Institute of Medical Sciences, New Delhi, India.

References

1. Walitt B, Nahin RL, Katz RS, Bergman MJ, Wolfe F. The prevalence and characteristics of fibromyalgia in the 2012 National Health Interview Survey. PLoS One. 2015;10:e0138024.
2. Al-Allaf AW, Dunbar KL, Hallum NS, Nosratzadeh B, Templeton KD, Pullar T. A case-control study examining the role of physical trauma in the onset of fibromyalgia syndrome. Rheumatology. 2002;41:450–3.
3. Üçeyler N, Burgmer M, Friedel E, Greiner W, Petzke F, Sarholz M, et al. Etiology and pathophysiology of fibromyalgia syndrome: updated guidelines 2017, overview of systematic review articles and overview of studies on small fiber neuropathy in FMS subgroups. Schmerz. 2017;31:239–45.
4. Arnold LM, Clauw DJ, McCarberg BH. Improving the recognition and diagnosis of fibromyalgia. Mayo Clin Proc. 2011;86:457–64.
5. Bell T, Trost Z, Buelow MT, Clay O, Younger J, Moore D, et al. Meta-analysis of cognitive performance in fibromyalgia. J Clin Exp Neuropsychol. 2018;40: 698–714.
6. Wu Y-LL, Huang C-JJ, Fang S-CC, Ko L-HH, Tsai P-SS. Cognitive impairment in fibromyalgia: a meta-analysis of case-control studies. Psychosom Med. 2018;80:432–8.
7. Lawson K. Sleep dysfunction in fibromyalgia and therapeutic approach options. OBM Neurobiol. 2020;4:16.
8. Wolfe F, Clauw DJ, Fitzcharles MA, Goldenberg DL, Häuser W, Katz RL, et al. 2016 revisions to the 2010/2011 fibromyalgia diagnostic criteria. Semin Arthritis Rheum. 2016;46:319–29.
9. Wolfe F, Clauw DJ, Fitzcharles MA, Goldenberg DL, Katz RS, Mease P, et al. The American College of Rheumatology preliminary diagnostic criteria for fibromyalgia and measurement of symptom severity. Arthritis Care Res. 2010;62:600–10.
10. Häuser W, Ablin J, Perrot S, Fitzcharles MA. Management of fibromyalgia: key messages from recent evidence-based guidelines. Pol Arch Intern Med. 2017;127:47–56.
11. Hedges D, Farrer TJ, Bigler ED, Hopkins RO, Hedges D, Farrer TJ, et al. Chronic pain and cognition. In: The brain at risk. Basel: Springer International Publishing; 2019. p. 113–24.
12. Folstein MF, Folstein SE, McHugh PR. "Mini-mental status". A practical method for grading the cognitive state of patients for the clinician. J Psychiatr Res. 1975;12:189–98.
13. Stroop JR. Studies of interference in serial verbal reactions. J Exp Psychol. 1935;18:643–62.
14. Rodríguez-Andreu J, Ibez-Bosch R, Portero-Vzquez A, Masramon X, Rejas J, Glvez R. Cognitive impairment in patients with fibromyalgia syndrome as assessed by the mini-mental state examination. BMC Musculoskelet Disord. 2009;10:162.
15. Martinsen S, Flodin P, Berrebi J, Lö fgren M, Bileviciute-Ljungar I, Ingvar M, et al. Fibromyalgia patients had normal distraction related pain inhibition but cognitive impairment reflected in caudate nucleus and hippocampus during the Stroop color word test. PLoS One. 2014;9:e108637.
16. Walteros C, Sánchez-Navarro JP, Muñoz MA, Martínez-Selva JM, Chialvo D, Montoya P. Altered associative learning and emotional decision making in fibromyalgia. J Psychosom Res. 2011;70:294–301.
17. González JL, Mercado F, Barjola P, Carretero I, López-López A, Bullones MA, et al. Generalized hypervigilance in fibromyalgia patients: an experimental analysis with the emotional Stroop paradigm. J Psychosom Res. 2010;69: 279–87.
18. Suhr JA. Neuropsychological impairment in fibromyalgia: relation to depression, fatigue, and pain. J Psychosom Res. 2003;55:321–9.
19. Gelonch O, Garolera M, Valls J, Rosselló L, Pifarré J. Executive function in fibromyalgia: comparing subjective and objective measures. Compr Psychiatry. 2016;66:113–22.
20. Pimentel MJ, Gui MS, Reimão R, Rizzatti-Barbosa CM. Sleep quality and facial pain in fibromyalgia syndrome. J Craniomandib Pract. 2015;33:122–8.
21. Bigatti SM, Hernandez AM, Cronan TA, Rand KL. Sleep disturbances in fibromyalgia syndrome: relationship to pain and depression. Arthritis Care Res. 2008;59:961–7.
22. Mutlu P, Zateri Ç, Zöhra A, Özerdoğan Ö, Mirici AN. Prevalence of obstructive sleep apnea in female patients with fibromyalgia. Saudi Med J. 2020;41:740–5.
23. Choy EHS. The role of sleep in pain and fibromyalgia. Nat Rev Rheumatol. 2015;11:513–20.
24. Keskindag B, Karaaziz M. The association between pain and sleep in fibromyalgia. Saudi Med J. 2017;38:465–75.
25. Jennum P, Drewes AM, Andreasen A, Neilsen DK. Sleep and other symptoms in primary fibromyalgia and in healthy controls. J Rheumatol. 1993;20:1956–9.
26. Wu YL, Chang LY, Lee HC, Fang SC, Tsai PS. Sleep disturbances in fibromyalgiaA meta-analysis of case-control studies. J Psychosom Res. 2017;96:89–97.
27. Nijs J, Daenen L, Cras P, Struyf F, Roussel N, Oostendorp RAB. Nociception affects motor output: a review on sensory-motor interaction with focus on clinical implications. Clin J Pain. 2012;28:175–81.
28. Chang WJ, O'Connell NE, Beckenkamp PR, Alhassani G, Liston MB, Schabrun SM. Altered primary motor cortex structure, organization, and function in chronic pain: a systematic review and meta-analysis. J Pain. 2018;19:341–59.

29. Umay E, Gundogdu I, Ozturk EA. What happens to muscles in fibromyalgia syndrome. Ir J Med Sci. 2020;189:749–56.
30. Martínez E, Aira Z, Buesa I, Aizpurua I, Rada D, Azkue JJ. Embodied pain in fibromyalgia: disturbed somatorepresentations and increased plasticity of the body schema. PLoS One. 2018;13:e0194534.
31. Fallon N, Chiu Y, Nurmikko T, Stancak A. Functional connectivity with the default mode network is altered in fibromyalgia patients. PLoS One. 2016; 11:e0159198.
32. Robinson ME, Craggs JG, Price DD, Perlstein WM, Staud R. Gray matter volumes of pain-related brain areas are decreased in fibromyalgia syndrome. J Pain. 2011;12:436–43.
33. Sundermann B, Dehghan Nayyeri M, Pfleiderer B, Stahlberg K, Jünke L, Baie L, et al. Subtle changes of gray matter volume in fibromyalgia reflect chronic musculoskeletal pain rather than disease-specific effects. Eur J Neurosci. 2019;50:3958–67.
34. Wood PB, Glabus MF, Simpson R, Patterson JC. Changes in gray matter density in fibromyalgia: correlation with dopamine metabolism. J Pain. 2009;10:609–18.
35. Gentile E, Brunetti A, Ricci K, Delussi M, Bevilacqua V, M de T. Mutual interaction between motor cortex activation and pain in fibromyalgia: EEG-fNIRS study. PLoS One. 2020;15:e0228158.
36. Hsiao FJ, Wang SJ, Lin YY, Fuh JL, Ko YC, Wang PN, et al. Altered insula–default mode network connectivity in fibromyalgia: a resting-state magnetoencephalographic study. J Headache Pain. 2017;18:89.
37. Ichesco E, Quintero A, Clauw DJ, Peltier S, Sundgren PM, Gerstner GE, et al. Altered functional connectivity between the insula and the cingulate cortex in patients with temporomandibular disorder: a pilot study. Headache. 2012;18:89.
38. Barker AT, Jalinous R, Freeston IL. Non-invasive magnetic stimulation of human motor cortex. Lancet. 1985;325:1106–7.
39. Salerno A, Thomas E, Olive P, Blotman F, Picot MC, Georgesco M. Motor cortical dysfunction disclosed by single and double magnetic stimulation in patients with fibromyalgia. Clin Neurophysiol. 2000;111:994–1001.
40. Mhalla A, de Andrade DC, Baudic S, Perrot S, Bouhassira D. Alteration of cortical excitability in patients with fibromyalgia. Pain. 2010;149:495–500.
41. Caumo W, Deitos A, Carvalho S, Leite J, Carvalho F, Dussán-Sarria JA, et al. Motor cortex excitability and BDNF levels in chronic musculoskeletal pain according to structural pathology. Front Hum Neurosci. 2016;10:357.
42. Schwenkreis P, Voigt M, Hasenbring M, Tegenthoff M, Vorgerd M, Kley RA. Central mechanisms during fatiguing muscle exercise in muscular dystrophy and fibromyalgia syndrome: a study with transcranial magnetic stimulation. Muscle Nerve. 2011;43:479–84.
43. Parker R, Lewis G, Rice D, Stimulation PM. Is motor cortical excitability altered in people with chronic pain? A systematic review and meta-analysis. Brain Stimul. 2016;9:488–500.
44. Klein MM, Treister R, Raij T, Pascual-Leone A, Park L, Nurmikko T, et al. Transcranial magnetic stimulation of the brain: guidelines for pain treatment research. Pain. 2015;156:1601–14.
45. Tiwari VK, Nanda S, Arya S, Kumar U, Bhatia R. Effect of repetitive transcranial magnetic stimulation in male patients of fibromyalgia. Indian J Rheumatol. 2020;15:134–40.
46. Ganguli M, Ratcliff G, Chandra V, Sharma S, Gilby J, Pandav R, et al. A hindi version of the MMSE: the development of a cognitive screening instrument for a largely illiterate rural elderly population in India. Int J Geriatr Psychiatry. 1995;10:367–77.
47. Algom D, Chajut E. Reclaiming the stroop effect back from control to input-driven attention and perception. Front Psychol. 2019;10:1683.
48. Chipchase L, Schabrun S, Cohen L, Hodges P, Ridding M, Rothwell J, et al. A checklist for assessing the methodological quality of studies using transcranial magnetic stimulation to study the motor system: an international consensus study. Clin Neurophysiol. 2012;123:1698–704.
49. Groppa S, Oliviero A, Eisen A, Quartarone A, Cohen LG, Mall V, et al. A practical guide to diagnostic transcranial magnetic stimulation: report of an IFCN committee. Clin Neurophysiol. 2012;123:858–82.
50. Rossini PM, Rossi S. Transcranial magnetic stimulation: diagnostic, therapeutic, and research potential. Neurology. 2007;68:484–8.
51. Cavaleri R, Schabrun SM, Chipchase LS. The number of stimuli required to reliably assess corticomotor excitability and primary motor cortical representations using transcranial magnetic stimulation (TMS): a systematic review and meta-analysis. Syst Rev. 2017;6:48.
52. Bajpai G, Shukla G, Pandey R, Gupta A, Afsar M, Goyal V, et al. Validation of a modified Hindi version of the Epworth sleepiness scale among a north Indian population. Ann Indian Acad Neurol. 2016;19:499.
53. Buysse DJ, Reynolds CF, Monk TH, Berman SR, Kupfer DJ. The Pittsburgh sleep quality index: a new instrument for psychiatric practice and research. Psychiatry Res. 1989;28:193–213.
54. Manzar MD, Moiz JA, Zannat W, Spence DW, Pandi-Perumal SR, Bahammam AS, et al. Validity of the Pittsburgh sleep quality index in Indian university students. Oman Med J. 2015;30:193–202.
55. Cohen J. Statistical power analysis for the behavioural science. 2nd ed. London: Lawrence Erlbaum Associates, Publishers; 1988.
56. Fuchs PN, Peng YB, Boyette-Davis JA, Uhelski ML. The anterior cingulate cortex and pain processing. Front Integr Neurosci. 2014;8:35.
57. Gougeon V, Gaumond I, Goffaux P, Potvin S, Marchand S. Triggering descending pain inhibition by observing ourselves or a loved-one in pain. Clin J Pain. 2016;32:238–45.
58. Schabrun SM, Christensen SW, Mrachacz-Kersting N, Graven-Nielsen T. Motor cortex reorganization and impaired function in the transition to sustained muscle pain. Cereb Cortex. 2016;26:1878–90.
59. Calandre EP, Rico-Villademoros F, Slim M. Pharmacological treatment of fibromyalgia: is the glass half empty or half full? Pain Manag. 2017;7:5–10.
60. Calandre EP, Rico-Villademoros F, Rodríguez-López CM. Monotherapy or combination therapy for fibromyalgia treatment. Curr Rheumatol Rep. 2012; 14:568–75.
61. Kravitz HM, Katz RS. Fibrofog and fibromyalgia: a narrative review and implications for clinical practice. Rheumatol Int. 2015;35:1115–25.

4

Is rituximab effective for systemic sclerosis?

Marina Maria Vieira de Figueiredo Caldas[1†], Kesley Pablo Morais de Azevedo[2*†], Ana Clara de França Nunes[2], Victor Hugo de Oliveira[2], Isac Davidson Santiago Fernandes Pimenta[2], Isabela Dantas Torres de Araújo[3], Francisco Alves Bezerra Neto[4], Ana Katherine da Silveira Gonçalves de Oliveira[5] and Grasiela Piuvezam[2,6]

Abstract

Background: Systemic sclerosis (SSc) is a clinically complex and challenging disease, that leads to skin fibrosis. Its most frequent complication is interstitial lung disease (ILD), which leads to a worse prognosis. In this situation, cyclophosphamide is considered the gold standard for its treatment, despite the controversies regarding its efficacy and toxicity. However, studies using rituximab (RTX) have shown that this drug may be a promising therapeutic option.

Objectives: This paper objective was to analyze the scientific evidence on the RTX effects on SSc.

Methods: A systematic review (SR) was performed including clinical trials (CTs) on the use of RTX in SSc, published up to May 2020. The studies were identified through systematic searches in bibliographic databases using a predefined search strategy. The following databases were used: PUBMED, SCOPUS, SCIELO, LILACS, SCIENCE DIRECT, WEB OF SCIENCE, COCHRANE, WHOLIS, PAHO and EMBASE. Also, a manual search was performed. The methodological quality of the studies was determined using Jadad scale, Risk of Bias Tool (RoB 2.0) and Risk of Bias in Non-Randomized Studies - of Interventions tool (ROBINS-I). A meta-analysis of the randomized CTs was performed, using Review Manager.

Results: Ten CTs were included in this SR. Of these, three were randomized and seven were non-randomized. Five showed a statistically significant improvement in forced vital capacity (FVC) at some time during follow-up. Regarding the skin, eight studies showed statistically significant improvements according toa the modified Rodnan skin score. The meta-analysis found positive effects of RTX in SSc, with a statistical significance for lung disease.

Conclusion: Rituximab is a promising strategy for the SSc-associated ILD and cutaneous fibrosis treatment.

PROSPERO registration number: CRD42019132018.

Keywords: Systemic sclerosis, Rituximab, Interstitial lung disease, Cutaneous fibrosis, Systematic review

Introduction

Systemic sclerosis (SSc) is an autoimmune connective tissue disease characterized by vascular dysfunction and excessive collagen deposition, resulting in skin fibrosis and internal organs involvement [1–4].

The SSc pathogenesis is not completely understood, but B cell abnormalities are part of this complex disorder [5, 6]. The disease is associated with significant incapacity and mortality [2]. Pulmonary involvement is a common clinical presentation. Dyspnea or cough are late signs, but systematic CT practice shows that about 40–50% of patients have interstitial lung lesions and 10–20% of all patients will develop respiratory failure [7]. Interstitial lung disease (ILD) and pulmonary artery hypertension (PAH) are the two major causes of death in SSc [4,

* Correspondence: kesley@ufrn.edu.br
†Marina Maria Vieira de Figueiredo Caldas and Kesley Pablo Morais de Azevedo contributed equally to this work.
[2]Post-Graduation Program in Public Health (PPGSCol), Federal University of Rio Grande do Norte, Natal, Rio Grande do Norte, Brazil

8–10]. According to the skin involvement degree, there are different clinical presentations, especially limited systemic sclerosis and diffuse systemic sclerosis, with various extents of internal organ damage [1, 2].

Classical immunosuppressants have shown very modest effects and their clinical relevance is uncertain [7]. Methotrexate can be used as treatment for skin manifestations in early diffuse SSc [11]. Treatment for SSc-associated ILD is based on the European League Against Rheumatism (EULAR) recommendations, i.e. the use of cyclophosphamide (CYC) [2, 9, 12, 13]. However, this drug is associated with teratogenicity, gonadal failure, bone marrow suppression and infection [2]. Besides, within the first SSc lung study, the CYC effect decreased a few months after cessation [14]. Mycophenolate mofetil (MMF) has been suggested as an alternative for induction and maintenance of the imunosuppressive treatment and has been shown to stabilize lung function in some studies [14]. Recently, other immune-based, targeted therapies have been investigated. Hematopoietic stem cell transplantation and B cell depletion therapy (CD20) have shown good results [12, 15, 16].

Rituximab (RTX) is a monoclonal chimeric antibody against CD20 that depletes peripheral B cells. It was first approved for indolent non-Hodgkin lymphoma treatment in 1994. Over the last few years, RTX has been used off-label in transplant rejection and immune-mediated diseases such as multiple sclerosis, autoimmune hemolytic anemia, immune thrombocytopenic purpura, and systemic autoimmune rheumatic diseases other than rheumatoid arthritis [11]. Its use in SSc has been proposed because of the growing evidence about the B cells role in SSc [17].

The incapacity and mortality caused by SSc-ILD, the fragility of current therapies and the new evidence supporting treatment with RTX justifies the importance of this review. Therefore, the aim of this study was to analyze the evidence available in experimental studies that evaluated the rituximab effects on the pulmonary and skin function in patients with systemic sclerosis.

Methods

Protocol and registration

This review was conducted in accordance with a study protocol [18] and the Preferred Reporting for Systematic Reviews and Meta-Analyses (PRISMA) guidelines [19]. The protocol was registered in the International Prospective Register of Systematic Reviews (PROSPERO) on 24 July 2019 (CRD42019132018).

Eligibility criteria

Inclusion criteria

Studies that met the following eligibility criteria were included: (P) studies performed on patients with systemic sclerosis, diagnosed using the ACR/EULAR (2013) [20] and/or Leroy classification for SSc [21]; (I) interventions with the use of rituximab; (C) placebo or other treatment; (O) analysis of ILD and pulmonary fibrosis; (S) randomized clinical trials (RCT) and nonrandomized (Non-RCT).

Exclusion criteria

Reviews, case reports, abstracts, thesis and other types of epidemiologic studies were excluded of the Systematic Review.

Information sources and literature search

The search was performed independently by the researchers MMVFC, ACFN, IDSFP and IDTA in the following databases: PUBMED, SCOPUS, SCIELO, LILA CS, SCIENCE DIRECT, WEB OF SCIENCE, COCHRANE, WHOLIS, PAHO and EMBASE, until May 20th, 2020. The search strategy used was: ("RITUXIMAB") AND ("SCLERODERMA SYSTEMIC" OR "SYSTEMIC SCLEROSIS") AND ("CLINICAL TRIAL"). Also, a manual search was performed.

The first selection was focused on the title and abstract, with no limitations on the publication date. The articles were uploaded in Rayyan platform [22] for title and abstract reading. In this stage, all articles that did not directly address the subject of interest were excluded and duplicated titles were removed. Three reviewers (MMVFC, ACFN, IDSFP) did independently this step; doubts were clarified with the aid of a fourth researcher (KPMA).

The articles that met the criteria were directed to a full reading (second stage). After reading the complete articles, the researchers (MMVFC, ACFN, IDSFP) selected the articles to be included in the review. The discrepancies or doubts were resolved under the guidance of a fourth researcher (KPMA).

Data extraction

The following data were extracted from the selected articles: authors, year of publication, study location, type of study, sample size and age, patient characteristics, duration of intervention, therapeutic scheme, follow-up time, main variables and main results.

Two reviewers (MMVFC and IDTA) were responsible for extracting and managing the data independently, which were inserted into an EXCEL® spreadsheet; doubts were clarified with the help of the third researcher (KPMA).

Risk of bias assessment

The methodological quality of the randomized clinical trials was assessed using the Jadad scale. The Jadad scale consists of five questions that assess three factors:

randomization, blinding and withdrawals and dropouts description [23]. For the risk of bias assessment, the risk of bias tool (RoB 2.0) was applied in the randomized clinical trials. The risk of bias tool assessed the adequate random sequence generation, allocation concealment, participant and staff blinding, blinding outcome assessment, selective reporting, and other sources of bias. Regarding the classification, the risk of bias was assessed as low, high or unclear [24].

Non-RCTs were evaluated by the "Risk of Bias in Non-Randomized Studies - of Interventions" tool (ROBINS-I) [25]. Domains can be classified as [1]: low risk of bias [2]; moderate risk of bias [3]; serious risk of bias [4]; critical risk of bias; and [5] no information. Three researchers (KPMA, VHOS and ACFN) independently assessed the methodological quality of the studies (RCTs and Non-RCTs) and the differences were resolved with the help of the fourth researcher (GP).

Data analysis and synthesis

The means and standard deviations of the pre and post-intervention evaluations were extracted. With these values the variation delta (△) and the variation standard deviations were calculated for the intervention and control groups. In the descriptive analysis, the results were presented by means of standardized mean differences (SMD) between the groups (intervention and control). Then, the assessment of heterogeneity was calculated using the chi-square and I^2 statistical tests. To calculate the total effect size of the studies, the random effects model was applied. All analyses were performed using Review Manager 5.3 [26].

Results

A total of 2790 articles were generated through the database first search. After duplicates were removed, the new total was 1784 articles. These were screened using the titles and abstracts. The full texts of the remaining 23 articles were then assessed for eligibility. Thirteen articles were excluded because they did not fulfill the eligibility criteria or did not answer the research question. Through manual search, only one article was included. Figure 1 shows the PRISMA flowchart.

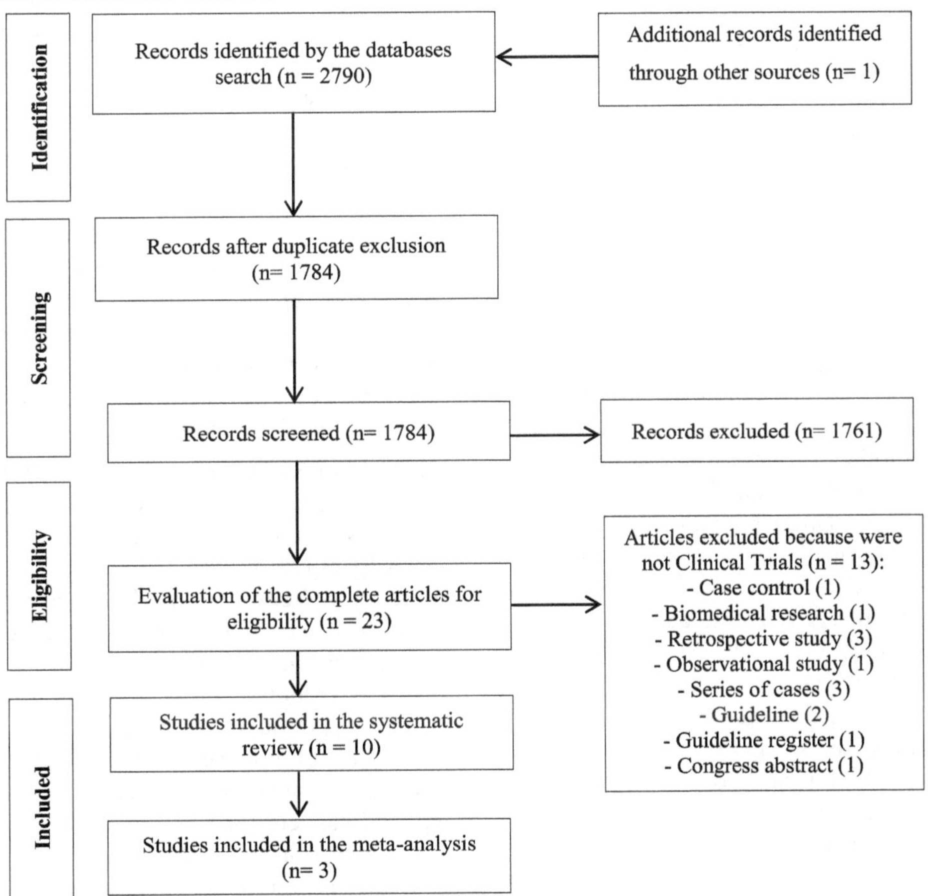

Fig. 1 Selection of manuscripts for the systematic review

In total, 10 articles met the inclusion criteria. Of these studies, three were RCTs [17, 27, 28] and seven were Non-RCTs [5, 12, 16, 29–32]. Patients were confirmed to have SSc based on ACR/EULAR and/or LeRoy criteria.

RCTs

The total number of SSc patients included was 90. The studies were performed in Netherlands, Greece and India. Sample sizes ranged from 14 to 60 patients. The ages ranged from 32.3 to 68.5 years. Most of the patients were female (85.4%). The follow up time ranged from 6 months to 2 years (Table 1).

Regarding lung fibrosis assessments and the treatment response follow-up, all three articles used FVC pulmonary function tests and lungs diffusing capacity for carbon monoxide. Only Boonstra et al. (2017) and Daoussis et al. (2010) used high resolution computed tomography. Daoussis et al. (2010) also used forced expiratory volume in one second (FEV1). For the cutaneous fibrosis evaluation, the studies used the modified Rodnan skin score (mRSS) and histological assessment of skin fibrosis.

About the pulmonary fibrosis tomographic evaluation, Boonstra et al. (2017) used the Goh criteria for analysis, showing a change in the lung tissue affected percentage by comparing the initial analysis and the evaluation at 12 months: – 1.6% in the RTX group and + 2.8% in the placebo group ($p = 0.28$). Daoussis et al. (2010), using the score proposed by Warrick et al. (1991), reported that CT scores were identical at baseline and at 24 weeks in all patients in the RTX group; a non-statistically significant increase was reported in the control group [33].

About the adverse events, Boonstra et al. (2017) reported one death (placebo group) due to disease progression, and Sircar et al. (2018) reported two deaths: one patient developed severe pulmonary arterial hypertension 5 months after the completion of the trial (in RTX group) and another patient, in control group, developed scleroderma renal crises and died 3 months after the sixth dose of CYC. However, pulmonary infection, breast carcinoma, abnormal cervical histology leading to hysterectomy, anemia due to severe menstruation, pancytopenia and digital ulcers were the adverse events related to RTX groups. Two studies reported mild reactions to the RTX [27, 28].

The Jadad scale was used to assess the quality of the randomized controlled trials. This score consists of five questions that assess three factors: randomization, blinding, and the withdrawals and dropouts description. After the evaluation, it was observed that all three articles obtained 3 points and that the main problems were related to blinding (Table 2). Regarding the evaluation of the risk of bias from RCTs, Table 3 presents the assessments of the two articles for all Rob 2.0 domains.

Analyzing the risk of bias, the study by Boonstra et al. (2017) [27] and the one by Sircar et al. (2018) [28] had a low risk of bias. On the other hand, in the research carried out by Daoussis et al. (2010) [17] some concerns were observed in the randomization process and in the deviations from the intended interventions (Table 3).

Characteristics and study designs are available on Tables 1 below.

NRCTs

The total number of SSc patients included was 128. The studies were performed in several locations: three studies in Belgium, two in Italy, one in Greece and one in the USA. Sample sizes ranged from 8 to 51 patients. The ages ranged from 28.3 to 69 years. Most of the patients were female (64.4%). The follow up time ranged from 24 weeks to 86 months (Table 4).

Regarding lung fibrosis assessments and the treatment response follow-up, all articles used FVC pulmonary function tests, lungs diffusing capacity carbon monoxide and high-resolution computed tomography. Some articles also used total pulmonary capacity and forced expiratory volume in one second (FEV1). For the cutaneous fibrosis evaluation, most articles used the modified Rodnan skin score (mRSS) and/or biopsy and immunohistochemical analysis.

Regarding the tomographic evaluation of pulmonary fibrosis, Bosello et al. (2015) used the criteria proposed by Kazerooni et al. [34], with no significant change in the tomographic scores. Lafyatis et al. (2009) and Melsens et al. (2017) concluded that patients did not show new lesions or lung disease progression on CT. Smith et al. (2010), Smith et al. (2013) and Bosello et al. (2010) did not report the results of tomographic lung analyses performed on their patients. Data on the evolution of mRSS and FVC can be found in Table 4.

Four Non-RCTs reported deaths. The study by Bosello et al. (2015) reported two deaths (cardiovascular involvement). Smith et al. (2013) reported one death from sepsis (port vein catheter infection after coronary bypass surgery). Melsens et al. (2017) reported one death due to sepsis (central venous catheter infection after coronary bypass) and one death from pancreatic cancer. Five deaths were noted in the RTX group of the study performed by Daoussis et al. (2017): three of respiratory failure, one of lung cancer and one died while sleeping.

Regarding serious adverse events, there were some types of cancers (breast, prostate and pancreas), herpes zoster infection, ulcer infections, respiratory infections, dental abscess, fever without an infectious focus, coronary bypass, secondary infection, urinary infection, hospitalizations for hyperventilation and renal crisis from scleroderma.

Table 1 Summary of randomized clinical trial data according to author, country, sample characterization, RTX scheme and follow-up, adverse events and main results

Author (year)	Country	Randomization	Sample (Total / RTX / Control)	Age (Min-Max/ Mean + /– SD)	Female sex (%)	Follow-up	RTX scheme	AE	Outcomes					Tomographic analysis	Jadad score
Sircar et al. (2018)	India	Yes	60/ 30/ 30	CG: 36.50 ± 9,73 RTX: 34.67 ± 8.13	83	6 months	Two RTX pulses of 1000 mg at 0 and 15 days i.v, and 1000 mg of RTX after 6 months as maintenance therapy	Yes		Skin - mRSS		Lung - FVC (%)		No	3
									Time	Control group	RTX group	Control group	RTX group		
									Start	23.83 ± 9.28	21.77 ± 9.86	59.25 ± 12.96	61.30 ± 11.28		
									6 months	18.33 ± 7.69 (+)	12.10 ± 10.14 (+)	58.06 ± 111.23	67.52 ± 13.59		
Boonstra et al. (2017)	Netherlands	Yes	16/ 8/ 8	CG: 36.6 ± 4.3 RTX: 44.5 ± 5.6	87.5	2 years	1000 mg, two infusions, two weeks apart, and one 1000 mg RTX consolidation treatment once, after 6 months	Yes		Skin - mRSS		Lung - FVC (%)		Yes	**3**
									Time	Control group	RTX group	Control group	RTX group		
									Start	14.0 ± 3.8	16.4 ± 4.4	92.0 ± 6.1	97.9 ± 6.6		
									12 months (Δ)	- 1.8	- 3.6	+ 0.3	+ 4.7		
									24 months (Δ)	- 1.9	- 5.3	- 1.4	+ 4.0		
Daoussis et al. (2010)	Greece	Yes	14/ 8/ 6	CG: 47.7–68.5/ 56 RTX: 41.0–66.5/ 53	85.7	1 year	Two cycles of RTX. Each cycle consisted of four infusions of 375 mg per m^2 of body area, once a week, repeated after 6 months	Yes		Skin - mRSS		Lung - FVC (%)		Yes	**3**
									Time	Control group	RTX group	Control group	RTX group		
									Start	11.5 ± 2.16	13.5 ± 6.9	86.0 ± 19.6	68.1 ± 19.7		
									12 months	9.7 ± 3.4	8.4 ± 6.5 (+)	81.7 ± 20.7	75.6 ± 19.7 (+)		

*** Data not reported in article; (+) statistically significant**

Table 2 Methodological design evaluation of the RCTs according to the JADAD scale (2005), classified in descending order

	Was the study described as randomized?	Was the randomization method appropriate?	Was the study described asblinding?	Was the blinding method appropriate?	Was there a withdrawals and dropouts description?	Total score
Sircar et al. (2018)	1	1	0	0	1	3
Boonstra et al. (2017)	1	0	1	0	1	**3**
Daoussis et al. (2010)	1	1	0	0	1	**3**

Regarding the evaluation of the risk of bias from NRCTs, Table 5 presents the assessments of the studies evaluated by ROBINS-I. It was observed that 3 studies had a low risk of bias [30–32], 3 critical bias [12, 16, 29] and 1 serious bias [5]. It is worth noting that the most problematic domains in the evaluations were related to confounding and missing data (Table 5).

Meta-analysis of the effects of rituximab on the lung and skin

In the meta-analysis, the three RCTs were included and the results are presented for pulmonary and skin outcomes after the follow-up period (6 to 12 months). The data described in Fig. 2 point to a positive and significant effect on lung function with the rituximab use (SMD 0.66 (Forced Vital Capacity - FVC); 95% CI 0.23 to 1.09; $p = 0.003$). In this analysis, low heterogeneity was found ($I^2 = 0\%$; $p = 0.69$).

Regarding the skin outcome, although we did not detect any significant difference between the experimental and control group, favorable results were observed for the rituximab use with a skin fibrosis reduction (SMD −0.40 (modified Rodnan skin score - mRSS); 95% CI −0.92 to 0.11; $p = 0.12$). Heterogeneity was classified as moderate ($I^2 = 43\%$; $p = 0.28$) (Fig. 3).

Discussion

This SR verified that, for SSc-associated ILD, the RTX use led to, in most cases, a non-statistically significant improvement. However, the results obtained in the meta-analysis point to a positive effect of the rituximab use on the lung function and skin fibrosis in patients with systemic sclerosis, but the significant effect was detected only for the pulmonary outcome. The results of this meta-analysis may have been influenced by the small sample size. Besides, the studies in this SR revealed a small number of clinical trials with few included subjects, the absence of blinding, disparate RTX therapeutic schemes and the use of several different parameters to evaluate the treatment response.

Following the EULAR recommendations, two studies guided the treatment of SSc-associated ILD with CYC and were classified by the Jadad score as having high quality [13, 23]. The two articles included in the EULAR protocol obtained the maximum score (5 points) in addition to good methodological quality, as they were randomized, double-blind, placebo-controlled and multicentric studies. Tashkin et al. (2006) reported that one year of oral CYC treatment resulted in a slight but significant improvement in FVC and total lung capacity [35]. Conversely, Hoyles et al. (2006) found no significant improvement in FVC and computed tomography in the CYC group [36].

Comparing these studies with those included in this systematic review, it can be noted that, in most of the studies, FVC was used as the primary endpoint with computed tomography of the chest as a secondary analysis. The RCTs included in our meta-analysis have lower scores in Jadad (3 points) and have some frailty on evaluation of risk of bias in ROB 2.

Regarding cutaneous involvement in SSc, this SR found that the use of RTX led to, in eight of the ten studies, a statistically significant improvement at some point during follow-up [5, 12, 16, 17, 30–32]. In the

Table 3 Risk of bias in RCTs (Rob 2.0)

	Randomization process	Intended interventions deviations	Missing outcome data	Outcome measurement	Reported result selection	Overall bias
Sircar et al. (2018	Low	Low	Low	Low	Low	Low
Boonstra et al. (2017)	Low	Low	Low	Low	Low	Low
Daoussis et al. (2010)	Some concerns	Some concerns	Low	Low	Low	Some concerns

Table 4 Summary of non-randomized clinical trial data according to author, country, sample characterization, RTX scheme and follow-up, adverse events and main results

Author (year)	Country	Sample (Total / RTX / Control)	Age (Min-Max/ Mean +/– SD)	Female sex (%)	Follow-up	RTX scheme	AE	Outcomes					Tomographic analysis
Daoussis et al. 2017	Greece	51/ 33/ 18	CG: 52.11 ± 16.10 RTX: 54.3 ± 14.33	80.39	7 years	Two or more RTX cycles. Each cycle consisted of four infusions of 375 mg per m^2 of body area, once a week, repeated every 6 months.	Yes		Skin - mRSS		Lung - FVC (%)		Yes
								Time	Control group	RTX group	Control group	RTX group	
								Start	17.78 ± 9.48	14.72 ± 10.52	77.72 ± 18.29	80.6 ± 21.21	
								12 months	15.78 ± 9.89	8.83 ± 7.83 (+)	77.18 ± 19.25	83.02 ± 19.05	
								24 months	13.72 ± 9.67 (+)	5.93 ± 5.15 (+)	77.59 ± 19.45	86.9 ± 20.56 (+)	
								36 months	15.53 ± 9.53(+)	4.53 ± 5.29 (+)		*	
								48 months	13.64 ± 8.56(+)	5.37 ± 8.34 (+)		*	
								7 years	*	*	61.11 ± 15.73 (+)	91.69 ± 14.81	
Bosello et al. 2015	Italy	20/20/0	RTX: 41.4 ± 13.1	85	86 months	1000 mg, two infusions, two weeks apart.	Yes	Time	Skin - mRSS		Lung - FVC (%)		Yes
								Start	22.3 ± 9.5		87.4 ± 19.5		
								6 months	14.4 ± 8.4(+)		89.0 ± 17.		
								12 months	11.2 ± 7.5(+)		90.7 ± 17.9 (+)		
								24 months	9.95 ± 6.0(+)		89.9 ± 21.2		
								36 months	8.1 ± 5.2(+)		94.0 ± 16.1		
								48 months	9.8 ± 7.2(+)		95.6 ± 20.7		
Lafyatis et al. 2009	USA	15/15/0	RTX: 32.0–57.0/ 45.8	86.66	1 year	1000 mg, two infusions, two weeks apart.	Yes	Time	Skin - mRSS		Lung - FVC (%)		Yes
								Start	20.6 ± 4.4		89.2 ± 10.8		
								6 months	20.2 ± 5.5		92.7 ± 10.3		
								12 months	21.1 ± 5.2		*		

Table 4 Summary of non-randomized clinical trial data according to author, country, sample characterization, RTX scheme and follow-up, adverse events and main results *(Continued)*

Author (year)	Country	Sample (Total / RTX / Control)	Age (Min-Max/ Mean +/− SD)	Female sex (%)	Follow-up	RTX scheme	AE	Outcomes			Tomographic analysis
Melsens et al. 2017	Belgium	17/17/0	RTX: 36.0–69.0/ 51.0	35,3	2 years	1000 mg, two infusions, two weeks apart and 1000 mg, two infusions, two weeks apart, after 6 months.	Yes	Time	Skin - mRSS	Lung - FVC (%)	Yes
								Start	25.5 ± 6.0	93.5 ± 11.3	
								3 months	18.6 ± 6.5 (+)	90.7 ± 11.6	
								6 months	14.6 ± 6.2 (+)	93.3 ± 13.4	
								12 months	10.7 ± 3.5 (+)	95.6 ± 13.5	
								15 months	9.7 ± 3.5(+)	98.0 ± 13.7 (+)	
								18 months	9.8 ± 3.8(+)	95.0 ± 15.4	
								24 months	12.6 ± 5.1(+)	90.5 ± 16.3	
Smith et al. 2010	Belgium	8/8/0	RTX: 49.0–57.0	37.5	24 weeks	1000 mg, two infusions, two weeks apart.	Yes	Time	Skin - mRSS	Lung - FVC (%)	Yes
								Start	24.8 ± 3.4	83.9 ± 8.1	
								12 weeks	19.4 ± 5.4(+)	81.0 ± 17.7	
								24 weeks	14.3 ± 3.5(+)	77.0 ± 9.8	
Smith et al. 2013	Belgium	8/8/0	RTX: 49.0–69.0/ 38.0	37,5	2 years	1000 mg, two infusions, two weeks apart and 1000 mg, two infusions, two weeks apart, after 6 months.	Yes	Time	Skin - mRSS	Lung - FVC (%)	Yes
								Start	24.8 ± 3.4	92.8 ± 8.6	
								3 months	19.4 ± 5.4(+)	88.5 ± 12.9	
								6 months	14.3 ± 3.5(+)	88.3 ± 9.3	
								12 months	10.8 ± 4.6(+)	89.2 ± 13.7	
								15 months	10.0 ± 2.6(+)	94.4 ± 10.1	
								18 months	10.8 ± 2.6(+)	89.8 ± 12.0	
								24 months	13.6 ± 5.6(+)	84.7 ± 13.3 (+)	

Table 4 Summary of non-randomized clinical trial data according to author, country, sample characterization, RTX scheme and follow-up, adverse events and main results *(Continued)*

Author (year)	Country	Sample (Total / RTX / Control)	Age (Min-Max/ Mean +/− SD)	Female sex (%)	Follow-up	RTX scheme	AE	Outcomes			Tomographic analysis
Bosello et al. 2010	Italy	9/9/0	RTX: 40.9 ± 11.1	88,9	3 years	1000 mg, two infusions, two weeks apart.	Yes	Time	Skin - mRSS	Lung - FVC (%)	Yes
								Start	21.1 ± 9.0	91.6 ± 20.7	
								3 months	15.2 ± 6.0	*	
								6 months	12.0 ± 6.1(+)	*	
								12 months	7.0 ± 4.0	*	
								18 months	7.0 ± 3.5	*	
								24 months	5.0 ± 2.0	*	
								36 months	4.0 ± 1.4	96.8 ± 18.9	

* Data not reported in article; (+) statistically significant

Table 5 Risk of bias in Non-RCTs (ROBINS-I)

	Confounding	Particpants selection	Interventions classification	Intended interventions deviations	Missing data	Outcomes measurement	Reported results classification	Overall judgment
Daoussis et al. (2017)	Serious	Low	Low	Low	Critical	Low	Low	Critical
Bosello et al. (2015)	Critical	Low	Low	Low	Low	Low	Low	Critical
Lafyatis et al. (2009)	Critical	Low	Low	Low	Low	Low	Low	Critical
Melsens et al. (2017)	Low	Low	Low	Low	Low	Low	Low	Low
Smith et al. (2010)	Low	Low	Low	Low	Low	Low	Low	Low
Smith et al. (2013)	Low	Low	Low	Low	Low	Low	Low	Low
Bosello et al. (2010)	Serious	Low	Low	Low	Low	Low	Low	Serious

meta-analysis, although we did not detect any significant difference in relation to the control group, favorable results were observed for the rituximab use in skin fibrosis reduction. The studies included in the meta-analysis used different RTX schemes, have lower scores in Jadad (3 points) and have some frailty on the risk of bias evaluation in ROB 2.

According to the EULAR recommendations for SSc cutaneous fibrosis, methotrexate (MTX) is indicated as the gold standard for treatment, based on two studies indicating that this drug improves the modified Rodnan skin score (mRSS), but the effects on other organs have not been established [37, 38]. The studies were rated with scores 3 and 5 on the Jadad scale and were randomized, used a placebo in the control group and assessed the mRSS.

Van Den Hoogen et al. (1996) concluded that a greater number of SSc patients responded favorably to MTX compared to placebo [37]. The results of Pope et al. (2001) showed a favorable trend with the MTX use over placebo, but the differences between groups were considered subtle [38]. However, despite the EULAR recommendations for the MTX use, it is important to point out that, from the patient safety point of view, the use of this drug can cause liver toxicity, pancytopenia, teratogenesis and lung injury [39].

The main adverse events associated with the RTX use in SSc were mild infusion reactions, besides sepsis, urinary tract, pulmonary, herpes zoster and cardiovascular involvement. In addition, four studies reported deaths [12, 16, 28, 30, 32].

Infusion-related reactions (IRRs) are common, especially when no premedication is given. Infections are the most prevalent side effect next to IRRs [11]. However, severe infusion reactions occur in approximately 10% of patients. In most cases adverse events are reversible by interruption of RTX in addition to supportive care, but severe consequences of infusion reactions have been reported, including pulmonary and cardiovascular events [40].

Regarding the malignancy risk, no elevations in solid tumor or lymphoma rates have been observed in patients using RTX, except for patients with T cell deficiency in HIV infection [40]. From this perspective, the pattern of AEs of the RTX use in these diseases is like that found in this SR, using RTX in SSc.

As a chronic disease with different types of presentation, SSc symptoms significantly disrupt daily activities and diminish quality of life [41, 42]. The major complaints are the classic skin hardening that restricts everyday activities, especially manual ones, and the substantial symptom burden [43]. Fatigue, pain and depressive

	Experimental			Control				Std. Mean Difference
Study or Subgroup	Mean	SD	Total	Mean	SD	Total	Weight	IV, Random, 95% CI
Boonstra et al. (2017)	0.6	4.4	8	-0.4	2.3	8	18.8%	0.27 [-0.72, 1.26]
Daoussis et al. (2010)	7.5	15.27	8	-4.33	15.63	6	15.0%	0.72 [-0.39, 1.82]
Sircar et al. (2018)	6.22	9.86	30	-1.19	9.5	30	66.2%	0.76 [0.23, 1.28]
Total (95% CI)			**46**			**44**	**100.0%**	**0.66 [0.23, 1.09]**

Heterogeneity: Tau² = 0.00; Chi² = 0.74, df = 2 (P = 0.69); I² = 0%
Test for overall effect: Z = 3.02 (P = 0.003)

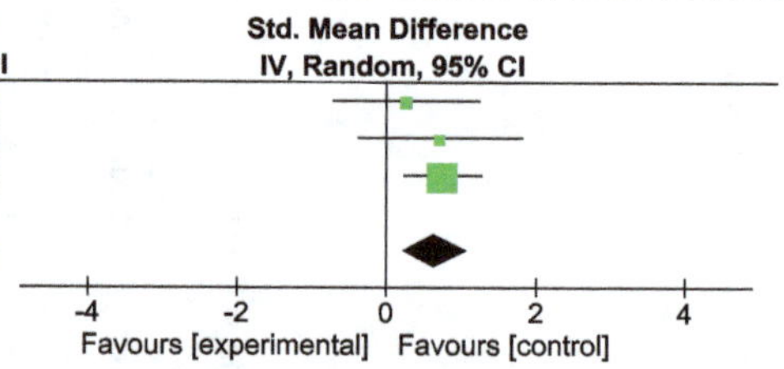

Fig. 2 Effects of Rituximab – Lung (FVC) (RCTs)

Study or Subgroup	Experimental Mean	SD	Total	Control Mean	SD	Total	Weight	Std. Mean Difference IV, Random, 95% CI
Sircar et al. (2018)	-9.67	7.75	30	-5.5	6.73	30	58.4%	-0.57 [-1.08, -0.05]
Daoussis et al. (2010)	-5.13	5.16	8	-1.84	2.42	6	18.8%	-0.73 [-1.83, 0.38]
Boonstra et al. (2017)	-1.4	3.1	8	-2.7	5.5	8	22.8%	0.28 [-0.71, 1.26]
Total (95% CI)			**46**			**44**	**100.0%**	**-0.40 [-0.92, 0.11]**

Heterogeneity: Tau² = 0.05; Chi² = 2.51, df = 2 (P = 0.28); I² = 20%
Test for overall effect: Z = 1.55 (P = 0.12)

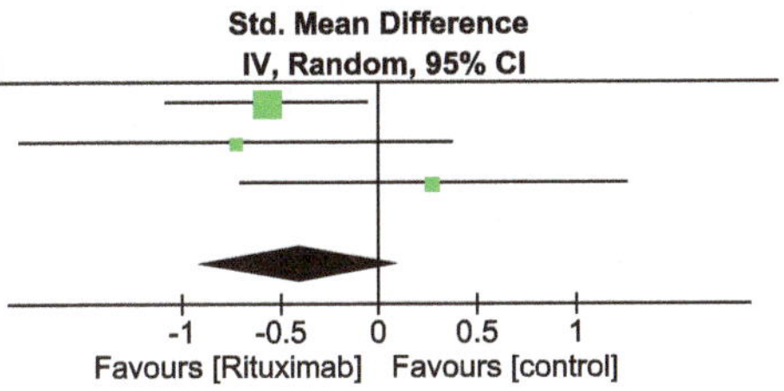

Fig. 3 Effects of Rituximab - Skin (RCTs)

symptoms are also common. Other complaints include unpredictable disease course, especially the diffuse form, and internal organs ailments [44]. Because SSc is diagnosed in early to middle age and has no cure, individuals with SSc face many years of managing the manifestations of a complex and progressive condition [45]. Thus, the improvement of parameters related to skin and pulmonary function may bring greater comfort and quality of life to patients with systemic sclerosis, relieving their main complaints.

The main difficulties in conducting this study were that most of the selected articles were not controlled clinical trials (NRCT), the disparate RTX therapeutic regimens and the use of several different parameters to evaluate the treatment response.

A recent systematic review with meta-analysis, performed by Tang at al. (2020), analyzed the improvement in cutaneous fibrosis and pulmonary function associated to the RTX use, similar to our study, however, the focus was on the safety and efficacy profile of Rituximab in SSc patients, as well as adverse events. Besides that, they did not include only clinical trials and used a different strategy to analyze risk of bias and the methodological quality of RCTs and NRCTs (the Newcastle – Ottawa scale) [46].

Tang et al. showed a long-term improvement in the modified Rodnan skin score (mRSS). Pulmonary function (using Forced Vital Capacity – FVC – and Diffusing Capacity of the Lungs for Carbon Monoxide – DLCO) remained stable. The ΔmRSS was: 7.00 at 6 months, 9.70 at 12 months, and 10.93 at 24 months. The ΔFVC: – 0.69 at 6 months, – 2.62 at 12 months, and – 0.67 at 24 months. ΔDLCO was: – 2.39 at 6 months, – 3.28 at 12 months, and – 0.79 at 24 months. The rate of Rituximab-related adverse events was 12% [46]. Thus, our review aims to ratify these results, bringing more accurate data in the meta-analysis, since it addressed only RCTs and provided guidance and recommendations for new studies.

Conclusion

Rituximab is a drug that has been causing growing interest in the scientific community as an important alternative for the sclerosis treatment and should be widely studied. Analyzing the results presented in our review, we can conclude that rituximab represents a promising strategy for the treatment of ILD and cutaneous fibrosis associated with SSc. The meta-analysis of the three RCTs identified that RTX use had a positive effect both on pulmonary function and on improving skin changes in patients with systemic sclerosis, with a significant difference for the lung outcome. However, studies with good methodological quality and larger sample must be performed to a more effective conclusion. The present study recommends that randomized, double-blind, crossover, multicenter trials should be performed, with an appropriate sample number and a well-defined follow-up time. Moreover, these trials should standardize the RTX and control group therapeutic regimens and the clinical methods of assessing the disease and treatment response. These studies will demonstrate the RTX behavior in the systemic sclerosis treatment, so that clinical decisions regarding its use in SSc are well-supported and patients can benefit from this new therapeutic option.

Abbreviations

SSc: Systemic sclerosis; ILD: Interstitial lung disease; RTX: Rituximab; SR: Systematic review; CTs: Clinical trials; PAH: Pulmonary artery hypertension; EULAR: European League Against Rheumatism; CYC: Cyclophosphamide; MMF: Mycophenolate mofetil; CD20: Hematopoietic stem cell transplantation and B cell depletion therapy; PRISMA: Preferred Reporting for Systematic Reviews and Meta-Analyses; SMD: Standardized mean differences; RCT: Randomized clinical trials; FVC: Forced vital capacity; mRSS: Rodnan skin score; MTX: Methotrexate

Acknowledgements

Not applicable.

Authors' contributions

Writing of the scientific paper: Marina Caldas, Kesley Azevedo. Research: All. Research in the area of treatment of RTX: Francisco Neto, Ana Katherine. Metodology: Marina Caldas, Kesley Azevedo, Victor Hugo, Ana Clara Nunes, Isac Davidson, Isabela Dantas, Grasiela Piuvezam. Data analysis: Kesley Azevedo. Reading and Final Revision of the Text: All. Project administration: Francisco Neto, Grasiela Piuvezam. The author(s) read and approved the final manuscript.

Author details

[1]Medicine Student, Federal University of Rio Grande do Norte, Natal, Rio Grande do Norte, Brazil. [2]Post-Graduation Program in Public Health (PPGS

Col), Federal University of Rio Grande do Norte, Natal, Rio Grande do Norte, Brazil. [3]Post-Graduation Program in Dental Sciences, Federal University of Rio Grande do Norte, Natal, Rio Grande do Norte, Brazil. [4]Department of Clinical Medicine, Federal University of Rio Grande do Norte, Natal, Rio Grande do Norte, Brazil. [5]Department of Tocoginecology, Post-Graduation Program in Health Sciences, Federal University of Rio Grande do Norte, Natal, Rio Grande do Norte, Brazil. [6]Department of Public Health, Post-Graduation Program in Public Health (PPGSCol), Federal University of Rio Grande do Norte, Natal, Rio Grande do Norte, Brazil.

References

1. Barnes J, Mayes MD. Epidemiology of systemic sclerosis: incidence, prevalence, survival, risk factors, malignancy, and environmental triggers. Curr Opin Rheumatol. 2012;24(2):165–70.
2. Pellar RE, Pope JE. Evidence-based management of systemic sclerosis: navigating recommendations and guidelines. Semin Arthritis Rheum [Internet]. 2017;46(6):767–74 Available from: https://www.scopus.com/inward/record.uri?eid=2-s2.0-85009495497&doi=10.1016%2Fj.semarthrit.2016.12.003&partnerID=40&md5=5bcdb25b18503678add9e44831c471d4.
3. Mouthon L, Bérezné A, Guillevin L, Valeyre D. Therapeutic options for systemic sclerosis related interstitial lung diseases. Respir Med. 2010; 104(SUPPL. 1):S59–69.
4. Bussone G, Mouthon L. Interstitial lung disease in systemic sclerosis. Autoimmun Rev. 2011;10(5):248–55.
5. Bosello S, De Santis M, Lama G, Spanò C, Angelucci C, Tolusso B, et al. B cell depletion in diffuse progressive systemic sclerosis: safety, skin score modification and IL-6 modulation in an up to thirty-six months follow-up open-label trial. Arthritis Res Ther [Internet]. 2010 [cited 2018 Jan 8];12(2): R54. Available from: http://arthritis-research.biomedcentral.com/articles/ https://doi.org/10.1186/ar2965
6. Pittman N, Rawn SM, Wang M, Masetto A, Beattie KA, Larché M. Treatment of small intestinal bacterial overgrowth in systemic sclerosis: a systematic review. Rheumatology. 2018;57(10):1802–11.
7. Allanore Y. Avancées thérapeutiques dans l'atteinte interstitielle pulmonaire au cours de la sclérodermie systémique. Rev du Rhum Monogr 2018;85(3): 165–170. doi:https://doi.org/https://doi.org/10.1016/j.monrhu.2018.02.003.
8. Hax V, Bredemeier M, Didonet Moro AL, Pavan TR, Vieira MV, Pitrez EH, et al. Clinical algorithms for the diagnosis and prognosis of interstitial lung disease in systemic sclerosis. Semin Arthritis Rheum [Internet] 2017;47(2):228–234. Available from: http://dx.doi.org/https://doi.org/10.1016/j.semarthrit.2017.03.019
9. Desbois AC, Cacoub P. Systemic sclerosis: an update in 2016. Autoimmun Rev. 2016;15(5):417–26.
10. Volkmann ER, Tashkin DP, Sim M, Li N, Goldmuntz E, Keyes-Elstein L, et al. Short-term progression of interstitial lung disease in systemic sclerosis predicts long-term survival in two independent clinical trial cohorts. Ann Rheum Dis. 2018:122–30.
11. Berghen N, Vulsteke J, Westhovens R, et al. Rituximab in systemic autoimmune rheumatic diseases : indications and practical use practical use. Acta Clin Belg. 2018;00(00):1–8. https://doi.org/10.1080/17843286.2018.1521904.
12. Daoussis D, Melissaropoulos K, Sakellaropoulos G, Antonopoulos I, Markatseli TE, Simopoulou T, et al. A multicenter, open-label, comparative study of B-cell depletion therapy with rituximab for systemic sclerosis-associated interstitial lung disease. Semin Arthritis Rheum [Internet]. 2017;46(5):625–31 Available from: https://www.scopus.com/inward/record.uri?eid=2-s2.0-85006271564&doi=10.1016%2Fj.semarthrit.2016.10.003&partnerID=40&md5=157c14914cef5ccd551dd3500113b555.
13. Kowal-Bielecka O, Fransen J, Avouac J, Becker M, Kulak A, Allanore Y, et al. Update of EULAR recommendations for the treatment of systemic sclerosis. Ann Rheum Dis. 2017;76(8):1327–39.
14. Adler S, Huscher D, Siegert E, et al. Systemic sclerosis associated interstitial lung disease - individualized immunosuppressive therapy and course of lung function: Results of the EUSTAR group. *Arthritis Res Ther.* 2018;20(1). doi:https://doi.org/10.1186/s13075-018-1517-z
15. Daoussis D, Tsamandas A, Antonopoulos I, Filippopoulou A, Papachristou DJ, Papachristou NI, et al. B cell depletion therapy upregulates Dkk-1 skin expression in patientswith systemic sclerosis: association with enhanced resolution of skinfibrosis. Arthritis Res Ther. 2016;18.
16. Bosello SL, De Luca G, Rucco M, Berardi G, Falcione M, Danza FM, et al. Long-term efficacy of B cell depletion therapy on lung and skin involvement in diffuse systemic sclerosis. Semin Arthritis Rheum [Internet]. 2015;44(4):428–436. Available from: http://dx.doi.org/https://doi.org/10.1016/j.semarthrit.2014.09.002
17. Daoussis D, Liossis SNC, Tsamandas AC, Kalogeropoulou C, Kazantzi A, Sirinian C, et al. Experience with rituximab in scleroderma: results from a 1-year, proof-of-principle study. Rheumatology. 2010;49(2):271–80.
18. Caldas MMV de F, Neto FAB, Azevedo KPM de, Pimenta IDSF, Oliveira AKDSG De, Piuvezam G. Rituximab in systemic sclerosis: A protocol for systematic review. *Medicine (Baltimore).* 2019;98(38). https://journals.lww.com/md-journal/Fulltext/2019/09200/Rituximab_in_systemic_sclerosis__A_protocol_for.18.aspx.
19. Moher D, Liberati A, Tetzlaff J, et al. Preferred reporting items for systematic reviews and meta-analyses: the PRISMA statement (Chinese edition). J Chinese Integr Med. 2009;7(9):889–96. https://doi.org/10.3736/jcim20090918.
20. Hoogen F Van Den, Khanna D, Fransen J, et al. Arthritis & Rheumatism 2013 Classification Criteria for Systemic Sclerosis. 2013;65(11):2737–2747. doi: https://doi.org/10.1002/art.38098.
21. LeRoy EC, Medsger TAJ. Criteria for the classification of early systemic sclerosis. J Rheumatol. 2001;28(7):1573–6.
22. Ouzzani M, Hammady H, Fedorowicz Z, Elmagarmid A. Rayyan-a web and mobile app for systematic reviews. Syst Rev. 2016;5(1):210. https://doi.org/10.1186/s13643-016-0384-4.
23. Stephen H. Halpern MJD. Jadad scale for reporting randomized controlled trials Many. Evidence-based Obstet Anesth [Internet]. 2005;237–8. Available from: http://onlinelibrary.wiley.com/doi/https://doi.org/10.1002/9780470988343.app1/pdf
24. Higgins JPT, Altman DG, Gøtzsche PC, et al. The Cochrane Collaboration's tool for assessing risk of bias in randomised trials. BMJ. 2011;343. https://doi.org/10.1136/bmj.d5928.
25. Sterne JAC, Hernán MA, Reeves BC, et al. ROBINS-I: a tool for assessing risk of bias in non-randomised studies of interventions. BMJ. 2016;355. https://doi.org/10.1136/bmj.i4919.
26. Review Manager (RevMan) [Computer program]. Version 5.3. Copenhagen: The Nordic Cochrane Centre, The Cochrane Collaboration, 2014.
27. Boonstra M, Meijs J, Dorjée AL, et al. Rituximab in early systemic sclerosis. RMD Open. 2017;3:e000384. https://doi.org/10.1136/rmdopen-2016-000384.
28. Sircar G, Goswami RP, Sircar D, Ghosh A, Ghosh P. Intravenous cyclophosphamide vs rituximab for the treatment of early diffuse scleroderma lung disease: Open label, randomized, controlled trial. Rheumatol (United Kingdom) [Internet]. 2018;57(12):2106–13. Available from: https://www.scopus.com/inward/record.uri?eid=2-s2.0-85057264332&doi=10.1093%2Frheumatology%2Fkey213&partnerID=40&md5=efd115c63c163b9bb928cc2218de7e64
29. Lafyatis R, Kissin E, York M, Farina G, Viger K, Fritzler MJ, et al. B cell depletion with rituximab in patients with diffuse cutaneous systemic sclerosis. Arthritis Rheum. 2009;60(2):578–83.
30. Melsens K, Vandecasteele E, Deschepper E, Badot V, Blockmans D, Brusselle G, et al. Two years follow-up of an open-label pilot study of treatment with rituximab in patients with early diffuse cutaneous systemic sclerosis. Acta Clin Belg [Internet]. 2017 11 [cited 2018 Jan 8];1–7. Available from: https://www.tandfonline.com/doi/full/https://doi.org/10.1080/17843286.2017.1372244
31. Smith V, Van Praet JT, Vandooren B, Van der Cruyssen B, Naeyaert J-M, Decuman S, et al. Rituximab in diffuse cutaneous systemic sclerosis: an open-label clinical and histopathological study. Ann Rheum Dis [Internet]. 2010 Jan Jan;69(1):193–7. [cited 2018 Jan 8];69(1):193–7. Available from: http://ard.bmj.com/cgi/doi/https://doi.org/10.1136/ard.2008.095463
32. Smith V, Piette Y, Van Praet JT, Decuman S, Deschepper E, Elewaut D, et al. Two-year results of an open pilot study of a 2-treatment course with rituximab in patients with early systemic sclerosis with diffuse skin involvement. J Rheumatol. 2013;40(1):52–7.
33. Warrick JH, Bhalla M, Schabel SI, Silver RM. High resolution computed tomography in early scleroderma lung disease. J Rheumatol [Internet]. 1991; 18(10):1520–8 Available from: http://europepmc.org/abstract/MED/1765976.
34. Kazerooni EA, Martinez FJ, Flint A, Jamadar DA, Gross BH, Spizarny DL, et al. Thin-section CT obtained at 10-mm increments versus limited three-level thin-section CT for idiopathic pulmonary fibrosis: correlation with pathologic scoring. AJR Am J Roentgenol. 1997;169:977–83.
35. Tashkin DP, Elashoff R, Clements PJ, Goldin J, Roth MD, Furst DE, et al. Cyclophosphamide versus placebo in scleroderma lung disease. N Engl J Med [Internet] 2006;354(25):2655–2666. Available from: http://www.nejm.org/doi/abs/https://doi.org/10.1056/NEJMoa055120
36. Hoyles RK, Ellis RW, Wellsbury J, Lees B, Newlands P, Goh NSL, et al. A multicenter, prospective, randomized, double-blind, placebo-controlled trial of corticosteroids and intravenous cyclophosphamide followed by oral

azathioprine for the treatment of pulmonary fibrosis in scleroderma. Arthritis Rheum. 2006;54(12):3962–70.
37. Van den Hoogen FH, Boerbooms AM, Swaak AJ, et al. Comparison of methotrexate with placebo in the treatment of systemic sclerosis: a 24 week randomized double-blind trial, followed by a 24 week observational trial. Br J Rheumatol. 1996;35(4):364–72 Available from: http://cochranelibrary-wiley.com/o/cochrane/clcentral/articles/651/CN-00124651/frame.html.
38. Pope JE, Bellamy N, Seibold JR, Baron M, Ellman M, Carette S, et al. A randomized, controlled trial of methotrexate versus placebo in early diffuse scleroderma. Arthritis Rheum. 2001;44(6):1351–8.
39. Lateef O, Shakoor N, Balk RA. Methotrexate pulmonary toxicity. Expert Opin Drug Saf. 2005;4(4):723–30.
40. Cvetković RS, Perry CM. Rituximab: a review of its use in non-Hodgkin's lymphoma and chronic lymphocytic leukaemia. Drugs. 2006;66(6):791–820.
41. Bassel M, Hudson M, Taillefer SS, Schieir O, Baron M, Thombs BD. Frequency and impact of symptoms experienced by patients with systemic sclerosis: results from a Canadian national survey. Rheumatology. 2011;50:762–7.
42. Sandusky SB, McGuire L, Smith MT, Wigley FM, Haythornthwaite JA. Fatigue: An overlooked determinant of physical function in scleroderma. Rheumatology. 2009;48:165–9.
43. Murphy SL, Kratz AL, Whibley D, Poole JL, Khanna D. Fatigue and its association with social participation, functioning, and quality of life in systemic sclerosis. Arthritis Care Res. 2019;1:1–22.
44. Sierakowska M, Doroszkiewicz H, Sierakowska J, et al. Factors associated with quality of life in systemic sclerosis: a cross-sectional study. Qual Life Res. 2019;28(12):3347–54. https://doi.org/10.1007/s11136-019-02284-9.
45. Schnitzer M, Hudson M, Baron M, Steele R. Disability in systemic sclerosis-a longitudinal observational study. J Rheumatol. 2010;38:685–92.
46. Tang R, Yu J, Shi Y, et al. Safety and efficacy of rituximab in systemic sclerosis : a systematic review and meta-analysis. Int Immunopharmacol. 2020;83(87):106389. https://doi.org/10.1016/j.intimp.2020.106389.

5

The relevance of anti-Jo-1 autoantibodies in patients with definite dermatomyositis

Vanessa Posener de Andrade[1], Fernando Henrique Carlos De Souza[1], Gustavo Luiz Behrens Pinto[1] and Samuel Katsuyuki Shinjo[1,2]*

Abstract

Background: To assess the prevalence and clinical relevance of anti-Jo-1 autoantibodies in a representative sample of patients with definite dermatomyositis (DM).

Methods: This retrospective cohort study took place from 2005 to 2020 and assessed 118 adult patients from a tertiary center who were diagnosed with definite DM. A commercial kit was used to detect anti-Jo-1 autoantibodies.

Results: The presence of anti-Jo-1 autoantibodies was observed in 10 out of 118 (8.5%) patients with definite DM. The following variables were comparable between individuals with and without anti-Jo-1 autoantibodies: age at diagnosis, sex, ethnicity, disease duration, follow-up period, recurrence rate, complete clinical response, death rate, and cancer incidence. There was no difference in clinical features between groups, except for an increased prevalence of "mechanic's hands," joint involvement, and lung disease, as well as a reduced occurrence of skin findings in patients positive for anti-Jo-1 autoantibodies. No anti-Jo-1-positive patients went into remission; they required greater use of glucocorticoids and immunosuppressive drugs.

Conclusions: Anti-Jo-1 positivity was found in 8.5% of patients with definite DM. This autoantibody was associated with an antisynthetase syndrome phenotype and might predict clinical outcomes in patients with definite DM.

Keywords: Autoantibodies, Dermatomyositis, Inflammatory myopathies, Myositis

Introduction

Dermatomyositis (DM) is a systemic autoimmune disease whose cardinal features include classical cutaneous findings and mostly proximal muscle weakness affecting the limbs [1–3].

The classical cutaneous manifestations of DM are Gottron's papules and heliotrope rash, but other findings such as digital ulcers, photosensitivity, calcinosis cutis, the "shawl" and "V-neck" signs, cuticular hypertrophy, periungueal erythema, and "mechanic's hands" might be present [4]. In addition, extramuscular manifestations such cardiac, gastrointestinal, joint, and lung involvement might occur [5, 6]. DM therefore has a broad spectrum of phenotypical presentations.

A variety of autoantibodies have been described in DM patients, who have myositis-associated or myositis-specific autoantibodies [6–14]. Myositis-specific autoantibodies include anti-Mi-2, anti-TIF1-γ, anti-NXP-2, anti-MDA-5, anti-SAE, and anti-aminoacyl-tRNA synthetase [6–14]. These autoantibodies are associated with different clinical phenotypes of systemic autoimmune myopathies, making them potentially useful as prognostic markers and predictors of clinical response to drug therapy [6–14].

Among anti-aminoacyl-tRNA synthetase autoantibodies, anti-Jo-1 is most commonly found in systemic autoimmune myopathies [6, 7, 9, 13]. Anti-Jo-1 positivity in DM ranges from 5 to 20% [6, 7, 9, 13] and is linked to

* Correspondence: samuel.shinjo@usp.br
[1]Division of Rheumatology, Faculdade de Medicina FMUSP, Universidade de Sao Paulo, Sao Paulo, SP, Brazil
[2]Disciplina de Reumatologia, Faculdade de Medicina, Universidade de Sao Paulo, Av. Dr. Arnaldo, 455, 3º andar, sala 3184 - Cerqueira César, CEP: 01246-903, Sao Paulo, Brazil

the occurrence of joint involvement [9, 11–14], interstitial lung disease [10, 12–17], Raynaud's phenomenon [13, 14], myositis [9, 16], and "mechanic's hands" [6, 9, 10, 13]. However, those variables were investigated in samples comprising patients with different subtypes of systemic autoimmune myopathies, including overlap syndromes [5, 8–16]. In addition, even when only DM cases were evaluated, samples were small [10, 11, 14], or the Bohan and Peter criteria [1, 2], which are restricted to muscle involvement and a narrow number of skin manifestations, were used for diagnosis. These limitations preclude an overall assessment of the relevance of anti-Jo-1 autoantibodies concerning the potential clinical features of DM.

Therefore, this study was aimed at describing the prevalence of anti-Jo-1 positivity in a representative sample of patients with definite DM and assessing the potential associations of anti-Jo-1 positivity with clinical, laboratory, and therapeutic characteristics, remission and relapse rates, and prognosis.

Patients and methods

This was a single-center, retrospective cohort study that took place from 2005 to 2020 and involved adult patients diagnosed with definite DM according to the Bohan and Peter classification criteria [1, 2], as well as the European League Against Rheumatism/American College of Rheumatology (EULAR/ACR) 2017 criteria [3]. To be included, patients had to present with pathognomonic skin rashes, as well as muscle involvement (objective muscle weakness in the upper and/or lower limbs accompanied by elevated serum creatine phosphokinase or aldolase levels). The following ancillary tests were also considered: an electromyography and nerve conduction studies suggesting an isolated myopathic process and/or a muscle biopsy suggesting an inflammatory myopathy.

Patients with clinically amyopathic DM (CADM), cancer-associated myositis, overlap syndromes as well as those with anti-OJ, anti-EJ, anti-PL-7, anti-PL-12, anti-SRP, anti-Ku, or anti-PM/Scl autoantibodies were excluded.

The following data were collected from electronic medical records containing previously parameterized and standardized information:

- General characteristics: age at diagnosis, sex, ethnicity, disease duration, and outpatient follow-up period;
- Initial and cumulative clinical manifestations: constitutional symptoms (weight loss and fever), Gottron's papules, Gottron's sign, heliotrope rash, facial erythema, Raynaud phenomenon, "shawl" sign, "V-neck" sign, cutaneous vasculitis, digital ulcers, calcinosis cutis, periungueal erythema, "mechanic's hands," dysphagia, joint involvement (arthralgia or arthritis), and lung involvement (dyspnea and chest high-resolution computed tomography - CT - imaging showing incipient interstitial lung disease, ground-glass opacities, and pulmonary fibrosis). All patients with respiratory symptoms underwent chest CT scans.
- Laboratory data: maximum serum creatine phosphokinase (reference range: 32–294 U/L) and aldolase (reference range: 1.0–7.5 U/L) levels during outpatient follow-up; blood samples collected at the beginning of the investigation of disease activity were assayed for myositis-specific (anti-Jo-1, -OJ, -EJ, -PL-7, -PL-12, -SRP, and -Mi-2) and myositis-associated (anti-Ro-52, -Ku, and -PM/Scl) autoantibodies. Myositis Profile Euroline blood test kits (Euroimmun, Germany) were used to detect the above-mentioned autoantibodies, and samples were processed as per manufacturer's instructions. The assessment of results was based on a predetermined method described elsewhere [6]. The indirect immunofluorescence assay on HEp-2 cells was used for the detection of antinuclear antibodies.

The following data were also collected at the last follow-up appointment and/or at the end of outpatient follow-up:

- Disease in remission: no evidence of disease activity for at least 6 months with no drug therapy for DM;
- Complete clinical response: no evidence of disease activity for at least 6 months with drug therapy for DM;
- Disease relapse: recurrence of clinical (muscle and/or skin manifestations) and/or laboratory findings (elevated muscle enzymes creatine phosphokinase and aldolase) with no explanation other than disease activity;
- Drug therapy (glucocorticoids and immunosuppressants or immunomodulators);
- Occurrence of death or diagnosis of neoplasia during the follow-up period.

Statistical analysis

The Kolmogorov-Smirnov test was used to assess the distribution of continuous variables. Results are presented as means ± standard deviations (SD) for continuous variables and as frequencies (%) for categorical variables. Medians and interquartile ranges (75th - 25th) were calculated for continuous variables with non-normal distribution. Student's t-test or Mann-Whitney U test were used for continuous variables, and the chi-square test or Fisher's exact test were used for categorical variables in order to compare patients with and without of anti-Jo-1 autoantibodies. Odds ratios (OR) and 95% confidence intervals (CI) were estimated by a logistic regression model that was used to evaluate the association between anti-Jo-1 positivity and relevant co-variates with statistical significance in the univariate analysis. We adopted P values < 0.05 to indicate statistical significance. SPSS Statistics, version 15.0 (Chicago, USA), was used for all analyses performed.

Results

In the present study, 152 DM patients were evaluated. Of these, 7 patients had CADM, 12 patients had cancer-associated myositis, 2 patients had overlap syndromes, and 13 patients had anti-OJ, anti-EJ, anti-PL-7, anti-PL-12, anti-SRP, anti-Ku, or anti-PM/Scl autoantibodies. These patients were excluded and, therefore, 118 patients with definite DM were finally analyzed.

Anti-Jo-1 autoantibodies were detected in 10 out of 118 (8.5%) patients with definite DM. Table 1 shows the general characteristics of DM patients with and without anti-Jo-1 autoantibodies.

A significantly increased prevalence of "mechanic'S hands," as well as joint and lung involvements, and a reduced prevalence of facial erythema, "shawl" sign, and "V-neck" sign were found among patients positive for anti-Jo-1 autoantibodies compared to anti-Jo-1-negative patients (Table 1).

No patients with anti-Jo-1 autoantibodies had vasculitides, digital ulcers, or calcinosis cutis (Table 1).

Regarding treatment, current use of glucocorticoids (prednisone) and immunosuppressive drugs (particularly mycophenolate mofetil) was significantly more prevalent among anti-Jo-1-positive patients compared to those without this autoantibody (Table 2).

Relapse rates, complete clinical response, and death were also comparable between the two groups. No anti-Jo-1-positive patients achieved disease remission or had active disease at the end of follow-up (Table 2).

In addition, all patients with anti-Jo-1 autoantibodies continued to be regularly followed up, unlike anti-Jo-1-negative patients (Table 2).

All significant variables shown in Tables 1 and 2 were strongly associated with anti-Jo-1 autoantibody positivity (Table 3).

Discussion

In the present study, anti-Jo-1 positivity was observed in 8.5% of patients with definite DM, and it was associated with "mechanic's hands," as well as joint and lung involvement.

In contrast, anti-Jo-1-positive patients exhibited a decreased frequency of skin manifestations such as facial erythema, "shawl" sign, and "V-neck" sign compared to anti-Jo-1-negative patients.

The frequency of anti-Jo-1 positivity ranges from 5 to 20% in the literature [6, 7, 9, 10, 13], and such wide variation occurs because of the different ethnic groups evaluated, which included Indians [10], Europeans [13], Brazilians [6], and cohorts comprising patients from multiple ethnicities [9]. In the present study, the prevalence of anti-Jo-1 positivity was 8.5% in Brazilian patients, which is within the range found in the literature. However, unlike other published research [9, 10, 12–14, 16], the presence of anti-Jo-1 autoantibodies was evaluated in a sample comprising only patients with DM in the present study. Moreover, only patients exclusively with definite DM were included, and patients with possible or probable DM, according to both the EULAR/ACR 2017 [3] and the Bohan and Peter criteria [1, 2], were excluded. Patients with clinically amyopathic DM, myositis associated with neoplasia or other systemic autoimmune disorders, and patients with other myositis-specific (e.g., anti-OJ, -EJ, -PL-7, and -PL-12) or myositis-associated (e.g., anti-Ku and anti-PM/Scl) autoantibodies were also excluded. Although this was a retrospective study, patient data were collected from records containing previously parameterized and standardized information, including that of interest to the present study.

Although the manifestations of DM are primarily cutaneous and muscular, we observed a significant prevalence of joint involvement in our cohort. We also identified a strong association between anti-Jo-1 positivity and the occurrence of joint involvement in our sample. This association has also been found in other studies. For instance, in a large European cohort [13] comprising 1637 patients with probable or definite DM, or polymyositis (PM) according to the Bohan and Peter criteria [1, 2], arthritis was strongly associated with anti-Jo-1 positivity. In addition, in a study by Ohashi et al. [11], japanese patients with systemic autoimmune myopathies and anti-Jo-1 positivity frequently presented with joint symptoms. Such an association between arthralgia or arthritis and anti-Jo-1 positivity has also been observed among patients with multiple types of idiopathic inflammatory myopathies [9, 12, 14]. Thus, a marked influence of anti-Jo-1 autoantibodies on the phenotype of patients with DM and joint involvement can be inferred.

The cutaneous lesions known as "mechanic's hands," classically associated with antisynthetase syndrome, are characterized by hyperkeratosis, scaling, and fissuring affecting the phalanges of the hands [4]. The correlation between anti-Jo-1 autoantibodies and "mechanic's hands" has been described for Indian and Japanese patients with systemic autoimmune myopathies [10, 12]. In a meta-analysis of 27 studies that included 3487 patients with idiopathic inflammatory myopathies, Lega et al. [9] observed that the frequency of "mechanic's hands"

Table 1 General features of patients with dermatomyositis with versus without anti-Jo-1 autoantibodies

	Anti-Jo-1 (+) (*n* = 10)	Anti-Jo-1 (−) (*n* = 108)	*P* value
Age at diagnosis (years)	46.5 ± 16.4	43.9 ± 15.6	0.638
Sex: female	5 (50.0)	77 (71.3)	0.171
Ethnicity: white	9 (90.0)	86 (79.6)	0.684
Disease duration (years)	5.0 [1.8–8.0]	7.0 [4.0–12.0]	0.093
Duration of follow-up (months)	36.6 [18.8–95.6]	56.0 [27.5–85.5]	0.804
Constitutional symptoms (baseline)	9 (90.0)	77 (71.3)	0.283
Cumulative manifestations			
Cutaneous involvement			
Gottron papules	10 (100.0)	108 (100.0)	> 0.999
Gottron sign	10 (100.0)	108 (100.0)	> 0.999
Heliotrope eruption	10 (100.0)	108 (100.0)	> 0.999
Facial erythema	5 (50.0)	88 (81.5)	0.034
Raynaud phenomenon	8 (80.0)	62 (57.4)	0.312
"V-neck" sign	3 (30.0)	71 (65.7)	0.044
"Shawl" sign	4 (40.0)	54 (50.0)	0.036
Vasculitis	0	37 (34.3)	–
Digital ulcers	0	31 (28.7)	–
Periungual erythema	7 (70.0)	84 (77.8)	0.694
"Mechanic's hands"	7 (70.0)	13 (12.0)	< 0.001
Calcinosis cutis	0	7 (65.0)	–
Joint involvement	8 (80.0)	34 (31.5)	0.004
Lung involvement	10 (100.0)	33 (30.6)	< 0.001
Dyspnea	8 (80.0)	30 (28.7)	0.002
Incipient interstitial lung disease	10 (100.0)	28 (25.9)	< 0.001
Pulmonary fibrosis	1 (10.0)	4 (3.7)	0.363
Ground-glass opacities	6 (60.0)	7 (6.5)	< 0.001
Laboratory findings			
Antinuclear antibodies	9 (90.0)	81 (75.0)	> 0.999
Anti-Mi-2	0	12 (11.1)	–
Anti-Ro-52	2 (20.0)	22 (20.4)	> 0.999
Maximum creatine kinase levels (U/L)	4522 [2173–13,500]	2208 [253–8394]	0.118
Maximum aldolase levels (U/L)	50 [20.6–74.8]	28.1 [9.0–90.5]	0.617

Data are shown as means ± standard deviations, medians [interquartile ranges], or number of patients (%)

increased by about 50% among patients with anti-Jo-1 autoantibodies compared to patients positive for other anti-aminoacyl-tRNA synthetase autoantibodies. Anti-Jo-1 positivity was also associated with an increased frequency of "mechanic's hands" among DM patients in the present study. This finding is also corroborated by Srivastava et al. [10], who found that patients with antisynthetase antibodies as a group and those with anti-Jo-1 antibodies alone had significantly more "mechanics' hands," while this association was not noted with other non-Jo-1 antisynthetase autoantibodies.

As for the other DM skin lesions, we observed a reduced prevalence of facial erythema, "shawl" sign, and "V-neck" sign, and no digital ulcers or calcinosis cutis among our anti-Jo-1-positive patients. Thus, this autoantibody might act as a protective factor against these cutaneous manifestations; however, further research is needed to investigate this hypothesis.

Interstitial lung disease is associated with increased morbidity and mortality in patients with idiopathic inflammatory myopathies [18, 19]. We observed a strong association between anti-Jo-1 autoantibodies and lung involvement, including clinical (dyspnea) and

Table 2 Current treatment, relapsing, disease status, death, neoplasia, and follow-up of patients with dermatomyositis

	Anti-Jo-1 (+) ($n = 10$)	Anti-Jo-1 (−) ($n = 108$)	*P* value
Treatment			
Prednisone			
Current use	7 (70.0)	32 (29.6)	0.015
Current dose (mg/day)	15 [5–40]	10 [5–40]	0.788
Immunosuppressive drugs	10 (100.0)	63 (58.3)	0.013
Methotrexate	3 (30.0)	27 (25.0)	0.715
Azathioprine	1 (10.0)	22 (20.4)	0.684
Mycophenolate mofetil	5 (50.0)	14 (13.0)	0.010
Cyclosporine	1 (10.0)	6 (5.6)	0.471
Leflunomide	1 (10.0)	7 (6.5)	0.519
Intravenous immunoglobulin	1 (10.0)	1 (0.9)	0.163
Rituximab	2 (20.0)	11 (10.2)	0.307
Disease relapse	7 (70.0)	56 (51.9)	0.508
Current disease status			
Disease remission	0	38 (35.2)	–
Complete clinical response	2 (20.0)	32 (29.6)	0.722
Disease activity	0	10 (9.3)	–
Death	1 (10.0)	9 (8.3)	> 0.999
Neoplasia	0	0	–
Follow-up	10 (100.0)	58 (53.7)	0.005

Data are shown as medians [interquartile ranges] or number of patients (%)

radiographic abnormalities on high-resolution CT imaging suggestive of interstitial lung disease. Anti-Jo-1 positivity is indeed associated with interstitial lung disease as defined by imaging findings alone [6] or together with abnormal pulmonary function testing [10, 12–17]. In our cohort, not all patients underwent pulmonary function testing, and therefore we did not include those data in the present study. However, previous research [6, 10, 12–17] has examined heterogeneous samples of patients with systemic autoimmune myopathies, and also has included cases of probable DM or PM, defined according to the Bohan and Peter criteria [1, 2] as well as overlap syndromes [10, 16]. Furthermore, no additional analysis to exclude potential cases of antisynthetase syndrome [10, 12, 13, 15, 17], which might also affect the lungs [20–22], has been performed.

Table 3 Univariate analysis of relevant variables in anti-Jo-1-positive patients

	OR	95% CI
Facial erythema	0.37	0.18–0.77
"V-neck" sign	0.48	0.30–0.78
"Shawl" sign	0.83	0.47–1.43
"Mechanic's hands"	5.82	3.0–11.16
Joint involvement	2.92	1.68–3.85
Lung involvement	3.27	2.46–4.35
Dyspnea	2.88	1.87–4.45
Incipient interstitial lung disease	3.86	2.80–5.31
Ground-glass opacities	9.26	3.85–22.25
Prednisone (current use)	2.36	1.43–3.89
Mycophenolate mofetil	3.86	1.75–8.49
Follow-up	1.86	1.56–2.22

CI confidence interval, *OR* odds ratio

We also found that anti-Jo-1 positivity was associated with lung involvement in patients with definite DM. We excluded patients who were positive for other anti-aminoacyl-tRNA synthetase autoantibodies, anti-Ku, and anti-PM/Scl to avoid biasing the interpretation of our data, as they are also associated with lung involvement [20, 23, 24].

As for other autoantibodies, anti-Ro-52 is a myositis-associated antibody and is commonly related to anti-Jo-1 positivity [6, 9, 16, 25]. The co-occurrence of anti-Ro-52 and anti-Jo-1 positivity was reported by Marie et al. [25] to be prevalent in patients with systemic autoimmune myopathies, suggesting that the simultaneous presence of these autoantibodies is associated with an increased risk of severe interstitial lung disease, more severe myositis, joint involvement, and neoplasia in patients older than 50 years. A potential explanation for the fact that anti-Ro-52 positivity was not associated with the occurrence of anti-Jo-1 autoantibodies in the present study is the small size of our sample.

Anti-Mi-2 positivity is known to be associated with the classical DM skin findings [25–27], to be a protective factor for lung involvement [25, 26], and a marker of high rates of remission [26] and response to glucocorticoid therapy [25, 26]. No anti-Jo-1-positive patients in our sample were found to be positive for anti-Mi-2 autoantibodies, which reaffirms the reports in the literature suggesting myositis-specific antibodies are mutually exclusive [25].

Concerning treatment, patients with anti-Jo-1 autoantibodies were found to be more frequently on glucocorticoids and immunosuppressive drugs when compared to those negative for this autoantibody. Consequently, no anti-Jo-1-positive patients had achieved disease remission at the time of their last medical evaluation, whereas one third of those negative for this autoantibody had gone into clinical remission. Patients in remission are referred to follow-up at primary or secondary care facilities as per our local protocol, which is why approximately half of the anti-Jo-1-negative DM patients had not been receiving follow-up treatment at the time.

No cases of neoplasia were observed during follow-up, but 10% of patients died, with no difference between the groups. Relapse rates were also similar between groups.

As a major limitation of our study, we had a small number of patients with anti-Jo-1 autoantibodies, and so our results should be interpreted with caution. Moreover, since this is a retrospective study, we did not have complete data available, such as serum levels of creatine phosphokinase and aldolase at disease onset or diagnosis or serum levels of the other muscle enzymes (aspartate aminotransferase, alanine aminotransferase, lactic dehydrogenase).

Conclusions

Anti-Jo-1 autoantibodies were detected in 8.5% of DM patients and were correlated with an increased frequency of lung and joint involvement as well as "mechanic's hands," resembling the clinical presentation of antisynthetase syndrome. In contrast, anti-Jo-1 positivity was not correlated with cutaneous manifestations such as the "shawl" sign, "V-neck" sign, vasculitides, and digital ulcers. Anti-Jo-1 autoantibodies were not found to affect relapse rates, but no anti-Jo-1-positive patients went into remission, so they continued to require regular outpatient follow-up. Our study emphasizes the relevant role of anti-Jo-1 autoantibodies in the phenotypical characterization of patients with definite DM, as well as in disease progression, by excluding an important confounder present in other research, which is the inclusion of patients with collagen diseases and different systemic autoimmune myopathies, in addition to patients with antisynthetase syndrome itself. Our data also favor the tendency to characterize DM patients into more homogenous groups according to their phenotypical presentation related to myositis-specific antibodies.

Abbreviations

ACR: American College of Rheumatology; CADM: Clinically amyopathic dermatomyositis; CT: Computed tomography; DM: Dermatomyositis; EULAR: European League Against Rheumatism

Acknowledgments

Not applicable.

Authors' contributions

All authors contributed equally to write and review the manuscript. The author(s) read and approved the final manuscript.

References

1. Bohan A, Peter JB. Polymyositis and dermatomyositis (first of two parts). N Engl J Med. 1975;292:344–7.
2. Bohan A, Peter JB. Polymyositis and dermatomyositis (second of two parts). N Engl J Med. 1975;292:403–7.
3. Lundberg IE, Tjärnlund A, Bottai M, Werth VP, Pilkington C, de Visser M, International Myositis Classification Criteria Project Consortium, the Euromyositis Register, and the Juvenile Dermatomyositis Cohort Biomarker Study and Repository (UK and Ireland), et al. 2017 European league against rheumatism/American college of rheumatology classification criteria for adult and juvenile idiopathic inflammatory myopathies and their major subgroups. Arthritis Rheumatol. 2017;69:2271–82.
4. Muro Y, Sugiura K, Akiyama M. Cutaneous manifestations in dermatomyositis: key clinical and serological features: a comprehensive review. Clinic Rev Allerg Immunol. 2016;51:293–302.
5. Souza FH, Barros TB, Levy-Neto M, Shinjo SK. Adult dermatomyositis: experience of a Brazilian tertiary care center. Rev Bras Reumatol. 2012;37: 264–7.
6. Cruellas MG, Viana VS, Levy-Neto M, Souza FH, Shinjo SK. Myositis-specific and myositis-associated autoantibody profiles and their clinical associations in a large series of patients with polymyositis and dermatomyositis. Clinics. 2013;68:909–14.
7. Wolstencroft PW, Fiorentino DF. Dermatomyositis clinical and pathological phenotypes associated with myositis-specific autoantibodies. Curr Rheumatol Rep. 2018;20:28.
8. Alenzi FM. Myositis specific autoantibodies: a clinical perspective. Open Access Rheumatol. 2020;12:9–14.
9. Lega JC, Fabien N, Reynaud Q, Durieu I, Durupt S, Dutertre M, et al. The clinical phenotype associated with myositis-specific and associated autoantibodies: a meta-analysis revisiting the so-called antisynthetase syndrome. Autoimmun Rev. 2014;13:883–91.
10. Srivastava P, Dwivedi S, Misra R. Myositis-specific and myositis-associated autoantibodies in Indian patients with inflammatory myositis. Rheumatol Int. 2016;36:935–43.
11. Ohashi K, Sada KE, Nakai Y, Matsushima S, Asano Y, Hayashi K, et al. Cluster analysis using anti-aminoacyl-tRNA synthetases and SS-A/Ro52 antibodies in patients with polymyositis/dermatomyositis. J Clin Rheumatol. 2019;25:246–51.
12. Yamasaki Y, Satoh M, Mizushima M, Okazaki T, Nagafuchi H, Ooka S, et al. Clinical subsets associated with different anti-aminoacyl transfer RNA synthetase antibodies and their association with coexisting anti-Ro52. Mod Rheumatol. 2016;26:403–9.
13. Betteridge Z, Tansley S, Shaddick G, Chinoy H, Cooper RG, New RP, et al. Frequency, mutual exclusivity and clinical associations of myositis autoantibodies in a combined European cohort of idiopathic inflammatory myopathy patients. J Autoimmun. 2019;101:48–55.
14. Mielnik P, Wiesik-Szewczyk E, Olesinska M, Chwalinska-Sadowska H, Zabek J. Clinical features and prognosis of patients with idiopathic inflammatory myopathies and anti-Jo-1 antibodies. Autoimmunity. 2006;39:243 7.

15. Zhang L, Wu G, Gao D, Liu G, Pan L, Ni L, et al. Factors associated with interstitial lung disease in patients with polymyositis and dermatomyositis: a systematic review and meta-analysis. PLoS One. 2016;11:e0155381.
16. Hamaguchi Y, Fujimoto M, Matsushita T, Kaji K, Komura K, Hasegawa M, et al. Common and distinct clinical features in adult patients with anti-aminoacyl-tRNA synthetase antibodies: heterogeneity within the syndrome. PLoS One. 2013;8:e60442.
17. Li S, Ge Y, Yang H, Wang T, Zheng X, Peng Q, et al. The spectrum and clinical significance of myositis-specific autoantibodies in Chinese patients with idiopathic inflammatory myopathies. Clin Rheumatol. 2019;38:2171–9.
18. Marie I, Haltron PY, Dominique S, Cherin P, Mouthron L, Menard JF. Short term and long term outcomes of interstitial lung disease in polymyositis and dermatomyositis: a series of 107 patients. Arthritis Rheum. 2011;63:3439–47.
19. Johnson C, Pinal-Fernandez I, Parikh R, Paik J, Albayda J, et al. Assessment of mortality in autoimmune myositis with and without associated interstitial lung disease. Lung. 2016;194:733–7.
20. Souza FH, Cruellas MG, Levy-Neto M, Shinjo SK. Anti-synthetase syndrome: anti-PL-7, anti-PL-12 and anti-EJ. Rev Bras Reumatol. 2013;53:352–7.
21. Baccaro ACCD, Behrens Pinto GL, Carboni RCS, Shinjo SK. The clinical manifestations at the onset of antisynthetase syndrome: a chameleon with multiple faces. Reumatismo. 2020;72:86–72.
22. Cavagna L, Trallero-Araguás E, Meloni F, Cavazzana I, Rojas-Serrano J, Feist E, et al. Influence of antisynthetase antibodies specificities on antisynthetase syndrome clinical spectrum time course. J Clin Med. 2019;8:2013.
23. Alves SP, Silva MG, Borges IBP, Shinjo SK. Patients with pure dematomositis/polymyositis and anti-PM/Scl autoantibody resembling anti-synthetase syndrome. MedicalExpress. 2018;8:mo18002.
24. Yamasaki Y, Yamada H, Nozaki T, Akaogi J, Nichols C, Lyons R, et al. Unusually high frequency of autoantibodies to PL-7 associated with milder muscle disease in Japanese patients with polymyositis/dermatomyositis. Arthritis Rheum. 2006;54:2004–9.
25. Marie I, Hatron PY, Dominique S, Cherin P, Mouthon L, Menard JF, et al. Short-term and long-term outcome of anti-Jo1-positive patients with anti-Ro52 antibody. Semin Arthritis Rheum. 2012;41:890–9.
26. Hamaguchi Y, Kuwana M, Hoshino K, Hasegawa M, Kaji K, Matsushita T, et al. Clinical correlations with dermatomyositis-specific autoantibodies in adult Japanese patients with dermatomyositis: a multicenter cross-sectional study. Arch Dermatol. 2011;147:391–8.
27. Dos Passos Carvalho MIC, Shinjo SK. Frequency and clinical relevance of anti-Mi-2 autoantibody in adult Brazilian patients with dermatomyositis. Adv Rheumatol. 2019;59:27.

6

High YKL-40 serum levels and its expression in the muscle tissues of patients with antisynthetase syndrome

Renata Casseb de Souza Carboni, Gustavo Luiz Behrens Pinto and Samuel Katsuyuki Shinjo*

Abstract

Background: The protein chitinase-3-like-1 (YKL-40) is rarely analyzed in patients with myositis. Therefore, we aimed to evaluate YKL-40 serum levels; correlate them with laboratory and clinical parameters, disease status, and treatment schemes; and analyze the YKL-40 expression in the muscle tissues of patients with antisynthetase syndrome (ASSD).

Methods: This cross-sectional single-center study included 64 adult patients with ASSD who were age-, gender-, and ethnicity-matched to 64 healthy control individuals. Their YKL-40 serum levels were analyzed using the Enzyme-Linked Immunosorbent Assay (ELISA) kit method, while YKL-40 expression in muscle tissues was analyzed using an immunohistochemical technique. Disease status was assessed using the International Myositis Assessment and Clinical Studies Group (IMACS) set scores.

Results: The patients' mean age was 44.8 ± 11.8 years, and median disease duration was 1.5 (0.0–4.0) years. These patients were predominantly female (82.8%) and Caucasian (73.4%). Most patients had stable disease. The median YKL-40 serum level was significantly higher in patients with ASSD when compared to the healthy individuals: 538.4 (363.4–853.1) pg/mL versus 270.0 (201.8–451.9) pg/mL, respectively; $P < 0.001$. However, YKL-40 serum levels did not correlate with any clinical, laboratory, disease status, or therapeutic parameters ($P > 0.050$), except tumor necrosis factor alpha (TNF-α) serum levels (Spearman's correlation, $rho = 0.382$; $P = 0.007$). YKL-40 was highly expressed by inflammatory cells found in muscle biopsy specimens.

Conclusions: High YKL-40 serum levels were observed in patients with ASSD and correlated positively with TNF-α serum levels. Moreover, YKL-40 was expressed by the inflammatory cells of the muscle tissue.

Keywords: Antisynthetase syndrome, Chitinase, Inflammatory myopathy, Muscle biopsy, Myositis

Introduction

Antisynthetase syndrome (ASSD) is a rare systemic autoimmune myopathy characterized by muscle, joint, and pulmonary involvement, as well as by the presence of fever, "mechanic's hands," and Raynaud's phenomenon [1–4]. In the laboratory, the ASSD is characterized by the presence of anti-aminoacyl-tRNA synthetase autoantibodies, such as anti-Jo-1 [1, 2].

* Correspondence: samuel.shinjo@usp.br
Division of Rheumatology, Faculdade de Medicina FMUSP, Universidade de Sao Paulo, Av. Dr. Arnaldo, 455, 3° andar, sala 3184 - Cerqueira César. CEP: 01246-903, Sao Paulo, Brazil

The protein chitinase-3-like-1 (YKL-40) is a glycoprotein secreted by inflammatory cells, including macrophages and neutrophils [5, 6]. YKL-40 is associated with several physiological processes, such as inflammation, cell proliferation, angiogenesis, tissue fibrosis, and tissue remodeling [7]. YKL-40 also participates in a wide range of inflammatory responses, also stimulating the production of pro-inflammatory cytokines (e.g., IL-6, IL-18, and tumor necrosis factor alpha [TNF-α]), which are capable of increasing YKL-40 serum levels as a feedback mechanism [8, 9].

High YKL-40 serum levels have been described in osteoarthritis [10] and in several systemic autoimmune diseases, such as rheumatoid arthritis [11–14], giant cell arteritis [15], systemic sclerosis [16, 17], Takayasu's arteritis [18], and systemic autoimmune myopathies [19–21].

In rheumatoid arthritis, YKL-40 serum levels are not only increased but also correlate positively with the disease activity [11–13]. However, YKL-40 is not associated with radiographic progression or predictive values for disease remission [14]. In patients with systemic sclerosis, YKL-40 serum levels correlate mainly with joint involvement [16], lung involvement (fibrosis or reduction in the diffusing capacity for carbon monoxide [DLCO]), digital articular deformities through cutaneous retraction, and reduced patient survival [17]. High YKL-40 serum levels are also described in patients with dermatomyositis and polymyositis, correlating with the disease activity and severity and with pulmonary involvement [19–21].

However, no studies have assessed YKL-40 serum levels exclusively in patients with ASSD, which was the primary motivation for this study. We aimed to correlate YKL-40 serum levels with clinical and laboratory parameters, disease status, and therapeutic schemes, as well as to analyze the YKL-40 expression in muscle tissue specimens from patients with ASSD.

Patients and methods

This cross-sectional single-center study took place from 2017 to 2019 and included 66 adult patients with ASSD followed up at the outgoing clinic of our service. All patients fulfilled the modified ASSD criteria classification proposed by Connors et al. [1], but with modifications to increase its specificity, including the presence of at least two of the following three manifestations: muscle, joint, and lung involvement; and in addition to persistent fever; Raynaud's phenomenon; "mechanic's hands;" and the presence of serum anti-aminoacyl-tRNA synthetase autoantibody.

Muscle involvement was defined as the presence of progressive and proximal limb muscle weakness, increased serum levels of muscle enzymes, such as creatine phosphokinase (CPK), myopathic pattern on electroneuromyography, and muscle biopsy compatible with inflammatory myopathy. Joint involvement was defined as non-deforming and non-erosive arthritis or arthralgia. Additionally, as part of the internal protocol of our service, patients underwent computed tomography (CT) chest scans at disease onset and during follow-up. In this study, lung involvement was defined as the presence of incipient pneumopathy, pulmonary nodules, ground-glass opacities with or without bronchiectasis, and pulmonary fibrosis (e.g., honeycombing areas).

A commercially available line blot test kit (Myositis Profile Euroline Blot test kit, Euroimmun, Lübeck, Germany) was used to identify anti-aminoacyl-tRNA synthetase autoantibodies (anti-Jo-1, anti-EJ, anti-OJ, anti-PL-7, anti-PL-12, and anti-Ro-52). The assessment was performed according to previously established methods [22]. The immunological patterns evaluated were antinuclear antibodies (ANA) detected by an indirect immunofluorescence technique on HEp-2 cells.

We excluded pregnant patients and those with other systemic autoimmune diseases (overlap syndrome), chronic or acute infection, neoplasia-associated myositis, and uncontrolled and serious comorbidities (e.g., liver disease, nephropathy, and heart disease). Observing the internal protocol of our service, a screening for neoplasms and other lung diseases was performed in all cases of myopathies.

The following pre-standard and pre-parameterized data were collected from the patients' interviews: demographic information (current age, gender, ethnicity), clinical information (disease duration; muscle, pulmonary, and joint involvement; Raynaud's phenomenon; presence of fever; and "mechanic's hands"), laboratory findings (serum levels of CPK, lactate dehydrogenase, aspartate aminotransferase, alanine aminotransferase), disease status, treatment (immunosuppressive, immunomodulatory, and glucocorticoid therapies), and comorbidities. Moreover, on the interview day, blood samples (20 mL) were taken for laboratory analysis after an eight-hour fasting.

Current clinical and laboratory disease status was assessed by applying the following questionnaires and International Myositis Assessment & Clinical Studies Group (IMACS) scores: Myositis Disease Activity Assessment Visual Analogue Scales (MYOACT) [23, 24], Manual Muscle Testing (MMT-8) [25], overall disease assessment by a physician and by the patient using a visual analogue scale (VAS) [26], and the Health Assessment Quality (HAQ) [27].

Pulmonary assessment was performed using chest CT images. The following parameters were investigated: incipient pneumopathy, ground-glass opacities with or without bronchiectasis, pulmonary nodules, and pulmonary fibrosis (honeycombing areas) [1, 28, 29]. All chest CT images were analyzed independently by the two authors of the present study, who are experienced in connective tissue diseases (RCSC and GLBP). In case of disagreement between them, the images were discussed with radiology groups from our institute.

Chest CT images obtained during a period ranging from six months before to six months after the patients' participation were included in this study. When possible, the pulmonary assessment was supplemented by a pulmonary function test that considered the forced expiratory volume in one second (FEV1), forced vital capacity (FVC), FEV1/FVC ratio, and DLCO.

The patients with ASSD were gender-, age-, and ethnicity-matched to healthy control individuals (patients' relatives or employees of our service) selected for convenience. All laboratory tests were performed on the control group, and they were asked to answer all interview questions, except those related to the disease data.

For the cytokine assessment, the material was centrifuged at 3000 rpm for 10 min immediately after blood collection (< 30 min), and the sera were aliquoted and stored at − 80 °C for further cytokine analysis. The YKL-40 quantification was performed using a specific kit (Human CHI3L1 ELISA kit, RayBiotech, USA) and processed following the manufacturer's protocol. The interferon gamma (IFN-γ) and TNF-α tests were performed using the LUMINEX 100/200x xMAP technology (Millipore, USA), as described elsewhere [30].

Additionally, the YKL-40 expression and location were assessed in muscle tissues of three patients with ASSD, whose biopsies were taken from the vastus lateralis muscle upon diagnosis. Sequential 5-μm thick frozen sections were first stained by hematoxylin-eosin and, then, immunohistochemistry was performed. For immunohistochemical analysis, monoclonal antibodies (CD4, CD8, CD68, and YKL-40: Abcam, USA) were used. Frozen specimens were fixed for 10 min in acetone at 4 °C. Endogenous peroxidase was blocked using 1% H_2O_2 in absolute methanol three times for 10 min. After rinsing the specimens in phosphate buffered saline (PBS) (0.01 M, pH 7.4) for five minutes, these were incubated in fetal serum in a wet chamber for one hour at 37 °C. Primary antibodies were diluted in PBS and albumin from 1% bovine serum was applied in wet chamber at 37 °C overnight. Next, slides were washed in PBS and a secondary mouse biotinylated solution (StreptABComplex/HRP) was applied for 30 min at 37 °C and rinsed in PBS. Then, the prepared StreptABComplex/HRP complex was applied and incubated for 30 min at 37 °C. After rinsing in PBS and incubation, the reactions were visualized using a solution of chromogenic substrate (3,3′-diaminobenzidine tetrahydrochloride) for peroxidase. After a final rinse, hematoxylin counterstaining was performed. The slides were then mounted and covered with an aqueous-based mounting medium. All muscle specimens were prepared at the same time as a batch. Human amygdala was used as a positive control, while a muscle specimen from a patient with ASSD, but whose biopsy results were normal (without infiltrate inflammation), was used as a negative control. Inflammatory cell phenotyping (CD4, CD8, CD68, and YKL-40) was analyzed in the endomysium, perimysium, and pericapillary (endomysium and perimysium) areas in 10 fields (200x magnification).

For statistical analysis, the Kolmogorov-Smirnov test was used to assess each parameter distribution. The clinical and demographic characteristics were expressed as mean ± standard deviation (SD), for continuous variables, or as frequencies and percentages (%), for categorical variables. The median (interquartile 25th to 75th) was calculated for continuous variables that did not have a normal distribution. Comparisons between patient and control parameters were made using the Mann-Whitney test and Student *t*-test for continuous variables, while the Fisher's exact test or chi-square test were used to assess categorical variables. Spearman's correlation was used for analyzing the correlation (*rho*) between continuous variables and YKL-40 values. Values between 0 and ± 0.333 were considered weak; values between ± 0.333 and ± 0.666 were considered moderate; and those between ±0.666 and ± 1.000 were considered strong." The relation between YKL-40 values and other variables (identified as the presence or absence of a certain characteristics) was performed using the Student *t*-test. To analyze the factors that together influence YKL-40, a multiple regression was performed considering all variables with *P* value < 0.10 as explanatory and the value of YKL-40 as dependent. A value of $P < 0.05$ was adopted to indicate statistical significance. All analyses were performed using the statistical software SPSS version 22.0 (Chicago, IL, USA).

Results

Sixty-six patients with ASSD were initially included in the present study. Two patients were excluded, one due to overlap and the other due to neoplasia-associated myositis. No patients had acute or chronic infection, were pregnant, or had severe and decompensated comorbidities. Therefore, 64 patients with ASSD were evaluated and age-, gender-, and ethnicity-matched to 64 healthy controls (Fig. 1).

The mean age of the 64 patients with ASSD and of the 64 control individuals was 44.8 ± 11.8 years and 42.6 ± 10.4 years, respectively ($P = 0.278$), with a predominance of females (82.8% versus 82.8%, $P > 0.999$), and Caucasians (73.4% versus 73.4%, $P > 0.999$) in both groups. The median ASSD disease duration was 1.5 (0.0–4.0) years.

The initial and cumulative clinical manifestations, autoantibody panels, and comorbidities of patients with ASSD are shown in Table 1.

The current disease status of patients with ASSD at the time of inclusion in this study, lung parameters, and treatments are shown in Table 2.

YKL-40 serum levels were significantly higher in patients with ASSD when compared to the control group: 538.4 (363.4–853.1) pg/mL versus 270.0 (201.8–451.9) pg/mL, respectively; $P < 0.001$ (Table 2). Additionally, a significant increase in TNF-α levels was observed in patients with ASSD compared to the control group: 48.4 (31.0–66.3) pg/mL versus 39.6 (29.3–49.0) pg/mL; $P =$

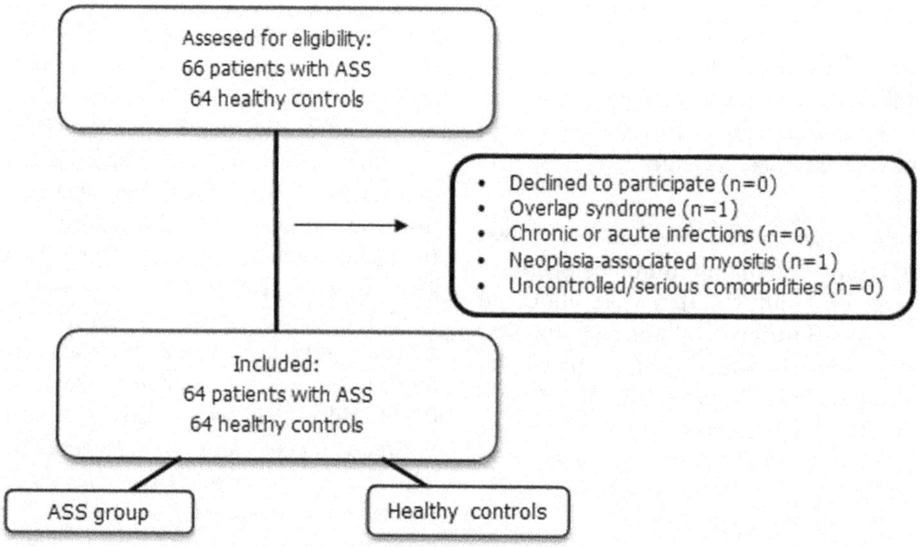

Fig. 1 Study flowchart. ASSD: antisynthetase syndrome

Table 1 Cumulative clinical manifestations, autoantibody panels, initial creatine phosphokinase serum levels, and comorbidities of the patients with antisynthetase syndrome

Antisynthetase syndrome	n = 64
Cumulative clinical manifestations	
Muscle involvement	61 (95.3)
Joint involvement	59 (92.2)
Lung involvement	57 (89.1)
Ground-glass	46 (71.9)
Incipient pneumopathy	40 (62.5)
Pulmonary fibrosis	14 (21.9)
Pulmonary nodules	11 (17.2)
"Mechanic's hands"	57 (89.1)
Raynaud's phenomenon	50 (78.1)
Fever	46 (71.9)
Autoantibody panels	
Antinuclear factor	52 (81.3)
Anti-Ro-52	28 (43.8)
Anti-tRNA aminoacyl transferase	64 (100.0)
Anti-Jo-1	52 (81.3)
Anti-PL-12, anti-PL-7 or anti-EJ	12 (18.7)
Anti-OJ	0
Initial creatine phosphokinase (U/L)	3015 (632–8463)
Comorbidities	
Systemic arterial hypertension	22 (34.4)
Diabetes mellitus	12 (18.8)
Hypothyroidism	3 (4.7)
Acute myocardial infarction	3 (4.7)
Stroke	1 (1.6)

Data are expressed as mean ± standard deviation (SD); median (interquartile 25th - 75th) or frequency (%)

0.011. IFN-γ serum levels were comparable in both groups.

Concerning demographic, clinical, laboratory, treatament, and comorbidity parameters, YKL-40 serum levels had correlation with patients' age (*rho* = 0.294; P = 0.040), TNF-α (*rho* = 0.382; P = 0.007), and current use of prednisone ($P < 0.047$) - Tables 3 and 4. However, in multivariate analysis, only TNF-α levels had significant factor to predict the YKL-40 values (Table 5).

Concerning the immunohistochemical analysis, YKL-40 was expressed by inflammatory cells. Figure 2 shows a muscle biopsy specimen from a patient with ASSD.

Discussion

To the best of our knowledge, this study is the first to show the relevance of YKL-40 in patients with ASSD. High YKL-40 serum levels were observed in patients with ASSD and correlated positively with TNF-α serum levels. Besides, YKL-40 was expressed by inflammatory cells in muscle tissues.

Although ASSD is a rare disease, this study employed strict inclusion criteria to increase the specificity in the selection of the involved patients. In this context, a significant sample was included and paired by age, gender, and ethnicity with healthy individuals, thus allowing for greater accuracy in comparative outcomes. Finally, information on patients was based on parameterized and pre-standardized data to ensure reliable study data.

High YKL-40 expression is described in the pathogenesis of a number of diseases, and its utility as a biomarker has been the subject of several studies [8–18]. Biologically, YKL-40 can stimulate angiogenesis and a wide range of responses, such as inflammation, tissue

Table 2 Demographic, current disease status, pulmonary involvement, treatment, and the cytokines serum levels of the patients with antisynthetase syndrome. Laboratory profiles of the control group

	ASSD (n = 64)	Control (n = 64)	P
IMACS set scores			
MMT-8 (0–80)	78 (71–80)	–	
Patient' VAS (0–10)	4.0 (2.0–6.0)	–	
Physician' VAS (0–10)	3.0 (0.0–5.0)	–	
MYOACT (0–60)	4.0 (0.5–2.5)	–	
HAQ (0.00–3.00)	0.67 (0.13–1.38)	–	
CPK (U/L)	208 (98–597)	106 (78–161)	< 0.001
LDH (U/L)	352 (243–590)	346 (312–345)	0.937
AST (U/L)	24 (17–37)	20 (16–23)	0.009
ALT (U/L)	24 (16–57)	18 (13–25)	0.030
Lung involvements			
Ground-glass	46 (71.9)	–	
Incipient pneumopathy	40 (62.5)	–	
Pulmonary fibrosis	14 (21.9)	–	
Pulmonary nodules	11 (17.2)	–	
FVC (% predict), n = 39	62.5 (48.0–73.5)	–	
FEV1 (% predicted), n = 39	64 (49–77)	–	
FEV1/FVC ratio, n = 39	0.90 (0.93–1.08)	–	
$DLCO_2$ (% predicted), n = 39	61.0 (37.8–73.0)	–	
Treatment			
Prednisone			
Current use	46 (71.9)	–	
Dose (mg/day)	10 (0–40)	–	
Immunosuppressive drugs	47 (73.4)	–	
Azathioprine	23 (35.9)	–	
Mycophenolate mofetil	11 (17.2)	–	
Methotrexate	14 (21.9)	–	
Antimalarial	4 (6.3)	–	
Leflunomide	2 (3.1)	–	
Cyclosporine	3 (4.7)	–	
Cyclophosphamide	1 (1.7)	–	
Rituximab	16 (25.0)	–	
Cytokines			
YKL-40 (pg/mL)	538.4 (363.4–853.1)	270.0 (201.8–451.9)	< 0.001
IFNγ (pg/mL)	0.02 (0.00–1.89)	0.02 (0.00–0.17)	0.876
TNFα (pg/mL)	48.4 (31.0–66.3)	39.6 (29.3–49.0)	0.011

Data are expressed as mean ± standard deviation (SD); median (interquartile 25th - 75th) or frequency (%)
ALT alanine aminotransferase; *ASSD* antisynthetase syndrome; *AST* aspartate aminotransferase; *CPK* creatine phosphokinase; *$DLCO_2$* diffusion of carbon dioxide; *FEV1* forced expiratory volume in one second; *FVC* forced vital capacity; *HAQ* Health Assessment Questionnaire; *IFN* interferon; IMACS: International Myositis Assessment and Clinical Studies Group; *LDH* lactate dehydrogenase; *MMT-8* Manual Muscle Testing; *MYOACT* Myositis Disease Activity Assessment Visual Analogue Scales; *TNF* tumor necrosis factor; *VAS* Visual Analog Scale; *YKL* chitinase-3-like-1 protein

remodeling, and allergic reactions. These responses are often mediated by other cytokines (e.g., IL-6, IL-18, and TNF-α), which can regulate the YKL-40 secretion [8, 9].

YKL-40 is seldom described in studies regarding systemic autoimmune myopathies [19–21]. In this context, Hozumi et al. [19] showed high YKL-40 serum levels in

Table 3 Correlation between YKL-40 serum levels and continuous variables (demographic, clinical, laboratory and lung parameters, and disease status) of the patients with antisynthetase syndrome

	rho	*P*
Demographic data		
Age	0.294	0.040
Clinical parameters		
Fever	0.070	0.631
Raynaud phenomenon	0.144	0.324
"Mechanic's hands"	−0.045	0.757
Muscle involvement	−0.219	0.131
Joint involvement	−0.190	0.192
Laboratory parameters		
TNF-α level	0.382	0.007
IFN-γ level	0.125	0.395
Lung involvement		
FVC (% predict)	0.018	0.930
FEV1 (% predicted)	0.089	0.667
FEV1/FVC ratio	−0.066	0.758
$DLCO_2$ (% predicted)	0.533	0.091
Disease status		
MMT-8	0.037	0.801
Patient' VAS	−0.173	0.239
Physician' VAS	−0.234	0.110
MYOACT	−0.077	0.614
HAQ	0.166	0.266
Creatine phosphokinase	0.131	0.371
Lactate dehydrogenase	0.138	0.460
Aspartate aminotransferase	0.033	0.854
Alanine aminotransferase	0.034	0.866
Treatment		
Prednisone: dose (mg/day)	0.217	0.139

$DLCO_2$ diffusion of carbon dioxide; *FEV1* forced expiratory volume in one second; *FVC* forced vital capacity; *HAQ* Health Assessment Questionnaire; *IFN* interferon; *MMT-8* Manual Muscle Testing; *MYOACT* Myositis Disease Activity Assessment Visual Analogue Scales; *TNF* tumor necrosis factor; *VAS* Visual Analog Scale

patients with dermatomyositis and polymyositis with associated interstitial lung disease, and YKL-40 serum levels were associated with a worse prognosis. Furthermore, the authors correlated YKL-40 levels negatively with DLCO and arterial oxygen pressure (PaO_2), finding a high expression of YKL-40 in alveolar macrophages and bronchial epithelial cells. Notably, the authors found that 42% of their patients had positive anti-aminoacyl-tRNA synthetase autoantibodies. Therefore, they might have included patients with ASSD and not necessarily pure dermatomyositis and polymyositis cases with associated interstitial lung disease. Additionally, patients with neoplasm associated myositis were included.

Gao et al. [20] also observed high YKL-40 serum levels in patients with dermatomyositis and polymyositis, which correlated positively with interstitial lung disease and with the disease activity and severity evaluated via MYOACT, C-reactive protein, ferritin, and erythrocyte sedimentation rates. However, the authors did not analyze anti-aminoacyl-tRNA synthetase autoantibodies in their patients.

Jiang et al. [21] observed a positive correlation between YKL-40 serum levels and patients with clinically amyopathic dermatomyositis and positive anti-MDA-5, especially in those with severe interstitial lung disease.

In our study, high YKL-40 serum levels were also observed in patients with ASSD. However, YKL-40 did not correlate with any clinical and laboratory parameters, disease status, or therapeutic schemes. There was also no correlation with any pulmonary parameters (e.g., patient's lung symptoms, chest CT images, and pulmonary function tests). Since this was a cross-sectional analysis, a prospective analysis of these parameters would be interesting.

To analyze disease status, Hozumi et al. [19] used variables such as ferritin, KL-6 (Krebs von den Lungen-6), SP-D (surfactant protein-D), PaO_2, and DLCO, while Jiang et al. [21] used ferritin, CPK, T CD3+ cell count, C-reactive protein, FVC, and DLCO. In contrast, we used the IMACS set scores, which validated instruments for clinical evaluation in systemic autoimmune myopathies [23–27].

Unlike limited studies regarding YKL-40 in myositis, a limitation of our study was the fact that we did not specifically analyze the YKL-40 expression in lung biopsy specimens. Nonetheless, the YKL-40 expression analyzed in muscle specimens reinforces the hypothesis that YKL-40 expression is systemic, not being limited to lung involvement.

YKL-40 can be expressed and secreted by various types of cells, including macrophages, neutrophils, and chondrocytes. Its expression is regulated by several cytokines, which mediate the proliferation, tissue remodeling, and production of other inflammatory mediators. In ASSD and systemic autoimmune inflammatory disease, the elevated YKL-40 serum levels might derive come from systemic inflammatory cells or local cells (e.g., blood, muscle, skin, lungs). This was the first study to demonstrate the increased expression of YKL-40 in the inflammatory cells of muscle tissue obtained from a patient with ASSD.

As previously mentioned, YKL-40 is regulated by various pro-inflammatory cytokines [8, 9]; therefore, we assessed the TNF-α and IFN-γ serum levels.

Table 4 Relation between YKL-40 serum levels and others variables (demographic, clinical, laboratory and lung parameters, disease status, and comorbidities) of the patients with antisynthetase syndrome

	Group 1		Group 2		*P* value
	n	Mean ± SD	n	Mean ± SD	
Demographic data					
Gender (female)	53	628.5 ± 363.6	11	691.3 ± 461.0	0.658
Ethnicity (Caucasian)	47	572.5 ± 316.7	17	793.2 ± 468.2	0.111
Clinical parameters					
Fever	18	579.4 ± 343.8	46	664.3 ± 394.0	0.484
Raynaud phenomenon	14	536.6 ± 361.8	50	677.4 ± 382.7	0.255
"Mechanic's hands"	7	658.6 ± 334.6	57	637 ± 389.2	0.891
Muscle involvement	3	980.2 ± 178.7	61	625.6 ± 379.2	0.198
Joint involvement	5	973.5 ± 602.1	59	610.4 ± 347.5	0.066
Laboratory parameters					
Antinuclear factor	12	685.7 ± 303.5	52	628.4 ± 398.4	0.674
Anti-Ro-52	35	663.9 ± 406.5	28	638.5 ± 348.0	0.818
Anti-Jo-1	11	728.4 ± 455.9	53	617.4 ± 359.7	0.414
Anti-PL-7	60	619.1 ± 377.6	4	876.1 ± 351.5	0.197
Anti-PL-12	60	627.2 ± 360.9	4	784.8 ± 595.5	0.431
Anti-EJ	61	653.7 ± 380.8	3	320.4 ± 52.2	0.227
Lung involvement					
Ground-glass	18	658.2 ± 348.1	46	634.2 ± 392.6	0.851
Incipient pneumopathy	24	695.9 ± 387.1	40	607.6 ± 376.4	0.437
Pulmonary fibrosis	50	586.2 ± 335.7	14	826.2 ± 471.8	0.063
Treatment					
Prednisone (current use)	17	483.3 ± 222.6	46	684.2 ± 406.3	0.047
Immunosuppressives/biologicals					
Azathioprine	43	618.9 ± 354.7	21	676.5 ± 425.2	0.613
Mycophenolate mofetil	54	648.4 ± 383.8	10	603.1 ± 375.2	0.750
Methotrexate	52	606.3 ± 338.1	12	790.3 ± 521.9	0.337
Antimalarial	61	645.3 ± 385.8	3	516.7 ± 91.7	0.643
Leflunomide	62	642.1 ± 382.5	2	544.0 ± 0	0.801
Cyclosporine	62	650.8 ± 381.1	2	388.7 ± 272.8	0.343
Cyclophosphamide	63	644.0 ± 381.8	1	451.9 ± 0	0.621
Rituximab	48	690.0 ± 364.8	16	537.0 ± 397.9	0.188
Comorbidities					
Systemic arterial hypertension	42	590.4 ± 379.9	22	742.5 ± 366.9	0.190
Diabetes mellitus	52	645.1 ± 395.0	12	610.0 ± 283.2	0.823
Hypothyroidism	61	628.0 ± 381.0	3	922.5 ± 205.8	0.286
Acute myocardial infarction	61	641.6 ± 382.6	3	567.2 ± 0	0.848
Stroke	63	645.2 ± 381.0	1	391.6 ± 0	0.513

SD standard deviation

High TNF-α serum levels were observed in patients with ASSD, similar to what occurs in other systemic autoimmune myopathies [31, 32]. TNF-α can induce YKL-40 production [8]. These data corroborated our study, in which a positive correlation was found between YKL-40 and TNF-α serum levels.

Although IFN-γ is involved in the ASSD pathophysiology, we did not find high cytokine serum levels in the

Table 5 Multivariate analysis

	Coefficient	Standard error	Lower CI (95%)	Upper CI (95%)	*P* value
(Constant)	374.3	105.6	161.6	587.0	0.001
TNF α level	5.4	1.8	1.7	9.0	0.005

$R^2 = 0.163$
CI confidence interval

present study. IFN-γ has a transient effect, being quickly cleared in the bloodstream [31, 33]. Therefore, it is difficult to detect. In the pathophysiology of systemic autoimmune myopathies, the participation of Th1 and Th2 cells is described as follows: IFN-γ is produced by initially present Th1 cells and, then, Th1 cells regulate Th2 cells using other inflammatory cytokines, including YKL-40 [34, 35].

The present study had some limitations. First, spirometry was not performed in all patients because of various internal circumstances, such as patients with difficulty in performing spirometry (dyspnea) and lack of available spirometry equipment at patient selection, even with these tests being carried out only in a later phase of the ASSD diagnosis and treatment (> six months). Second, the degree of dyspnea, six-minute walking distance, and

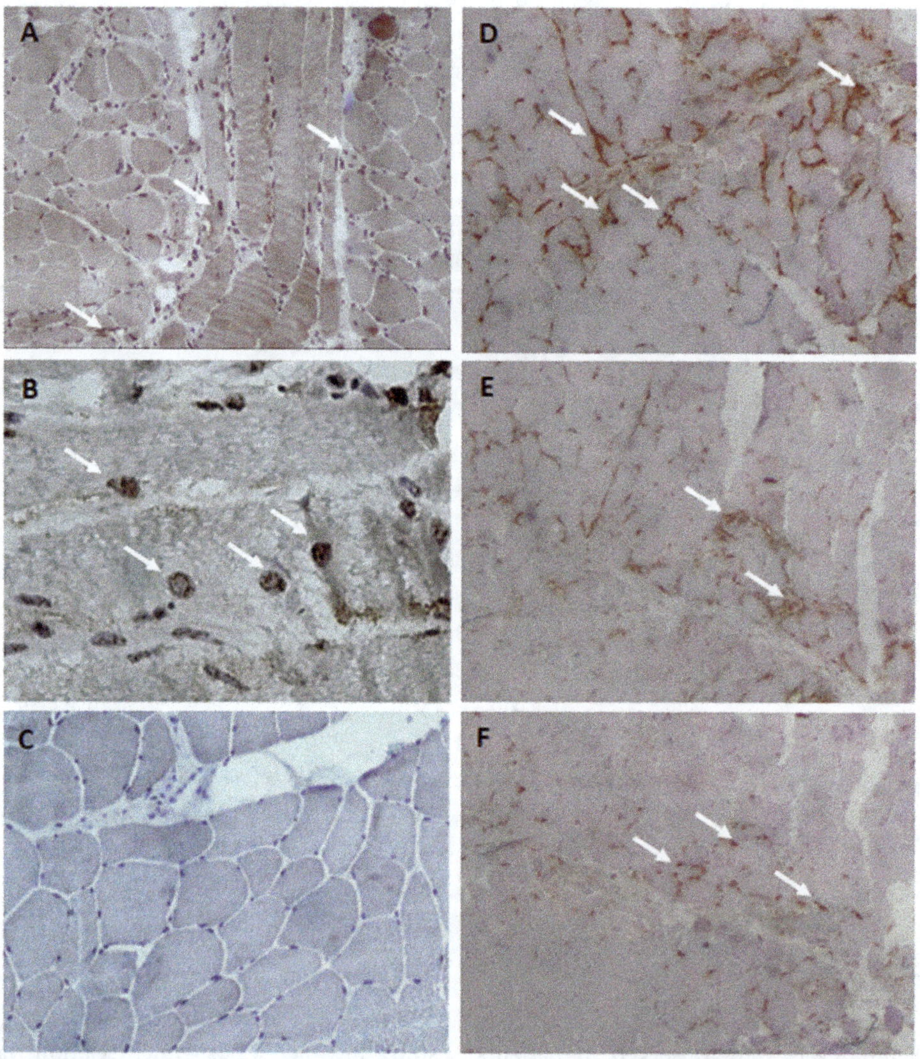

Fig. 2 Expression of YKL-40 in a muscle specimen from a patient with antisynthetase syndrome. Positive immunohistochemistry reaction of (**A**) YKL-40, (**B**) YKL-40*; (**D**) CD68, (**E**) CD4, and (**F**) CD8. Magnification is 200x or 400x*. As a negative control of YKL-40 (**C**), a specimen from a patient with antisynthetase syndrome, but without infiltrate inflammation

oxygen saturation were not analyzed. Third, the analysis of pneumopathy in CT was only descriptive, since there is no criterion in sytemic autoimmune myopathies that quantifies the degree of lung involvement.

Conclusions

This study showed high YKL-40 serum levels in patients with ASSD, and these correlated positively with TNF-α serum levels. Although other studies have shown the expression of YKL-40 in lungs of patients with various systemic autoimmune myopathies, we have shown high YKL-40 levels in inflammatory muscle tissue cells.

Abbreviations

ALT: Alanine aminotransferase; ANA: Antinuclear antibodies; ASSD: Antisynthetase syndrome; AST: Aspartate aminotransferase; CO: Carbon monoxide; CPK: Creatine phosphokinase; CT: Computed tomography; FEV1: Forced expiratory volume in one second; FVC: Forced vital capacity; HAQ: Health Assessment Quality; HE: Hematoxylin-eosin; IMACS: International Myositis Assessment and Clinical Studies Group; LDH: Lactate dehydrogenase; MMT: Manual Muscle Testing; MYOACT: Myositis Disease Activity Assessment Visual Analogue Scales; PBS: Phosphate buffered saline; *Rho*: Correlation; TNF: Tumor necrosis factor; VAS: Visual analogue scale; YKL-40: Protein chitinase-3-like-1

Acknowledgments

Not applicable.

Authors' contributions

All authors contributed equally to write and review the manuscript. The author(s) read and approved the final manuscript.

References

1. Connors GR, Christopher-Stine L, Oddis CV, Danoff SK. Interstitial lung disease associated with the idiopathic inflammatory myopathies: what progress has been made in the past 35 years? Chest. 2010;138(6):1464–74. https://doi.org/10.1378/chest.10-0180.
2. Cavagna L, Trallero-Araguás E, Meloni F, Cavazzana I, Rojas-Serrano J, Feist E, et al. Influence of antisynthetase antibodies specificities on antisynthetase syndrome clinical spectrum time course. J Clin Med. 2019;8(11):2013. https://doi.org/10.3390/jcm8112013.
3. Shinjo SK, Levy-Neto M. Anti-Jo-1 antisynthetase syndrome. Rev Bras Reumatol. 2010;50(5):492–500. https://doi.org/10.1590/S0482-5004201 0000500003.
4. González-Gay MA, Montecucco C, Selva-O'Callaghan A, Trallero-Aragua E, Molberg O, Andersson H, et al. Timing of onset affects arthritis presentation pattern in antisyntethase syndrome. Clin Exp Rheumatol. 2018;36(1):44–9.
5. Hakala BE, White C, Recklies AD. Human cartilage gp-39, a major secretory product of articular chondrocytes and synovial cells, is a mammalian member of a chitinase protein family. J Biol Chem. 1993;268(34):25803–10. https://doi.org/10.1016/S0021-9258(19)74461-5.
6. De Ceuninck F, Gaufillier S, Bonnaud A, Sabatini M, Lesur C, Pastoureau P. YKL-40 (cartilage gp-39) induces proliferative events in cultured chondrocytes and synoviocytes and increases glycosaminoglycan synthesis in chondrocytes. Biochem Biophys Res Commun. 2001;285(4):926–31. https://doi.org/10.1006/bbrc.2001.5253.
7. Lee CG, Da Silva CA, Dela Cruz CS, Ahangari F, Ma B, Kang MJ, et al. Role of chitin and chitinase/chitinase-like proteins in inflammation, tissue remodeling, and injury. Annu Rev Physiol. 2011;73(1):479–501. https://doi.org/10.1146/annurev-physiol-012110-142250
8. Prakash M, Bodas M, Prakash D, Nawani N, Khetmalas M, Mandal A, et al. Diverse pathological implications of YKL-40: answers may lie in 'outside-in' signaling. Cell Signal. 2013;25(7):1567–73. https://doi.org/10.1016/j.cellsig.2 013.03.016.
9. Kazakova MH, Batalov AZ, Mateva NG, Sarafian VS. YKL-40 and cytokines-a new diagnostic constellation in rheumatoid arthritis? Folia Med. 2017;59(1): 37–42. https://doi.org/10.1515/folmed-2017-0013.
10. Huang K, Wu LD. YKL-40: a potential biomarker for osteoarthritis. J Int Med Res. 2009;37(1):18–24. https://doi.org/10.1177/147323000903700102.
11. Johansen JS, Stoltenberg M, Hansen M, Florescu A, Horslev-Petersen K, Lorenzen I, et al. Serum YKL-40 concentrations in patients with rheumatoid arthritis: relation to disease activity. Rheumatology (Oxford). 1999;38(7):618–26. https://doi.org/10.1093/rheumatology/38.7.618.
12. Jafari-Nakhjavani MR, Ghorbanihaghjo A, Bagherzadeh-Nobari B, Malek-Mahdavi A, Rashtchizadeh N. Serum YKL-40 levels and disease characteristics in patients with rheumatoid arthritis. Caspian J Int Med. 2019; 10:92–7.
13. Väänänen T, Vuolteenaho K, Kautiainen H, Nieminen R, Mottonen T, Hannonen P, et al. NEO-RACo Study Group. Glycoprotein YKL-40: A potential biomarker of disease activity in rheumatoid arthritis during intensive treatment with csDMARDs and infliximab. Evidence from the randomised controlled NEO-RACo trial. PLoS One. 2017;12:e0183294.
14. Peltomaa R, Paimela L, Harvey S, Helve T, Leirisalo-Repo M. Increased level of YKL-40 in sera from patients with early rheumatoid arthritis: a new marker for disease activity. Rheumatol Int. 2001;20(5):192–6. https://doi.org/1 0.1007/s002960100115.
15. Johansen JS, Baslund B, Garbarsch C, Hansen M, Stoltenberg M, Lorenzen I, et al. YKL-40 in giant cells and macrophages from patients with giant cell arteritis. Arthritis Rheum. 1999;42(12):2624–30. https://doi.org/10.1002/1529-0131(199912)42:12<2624::AID-ANR17>3.0.CO;2-K.
16. Montagna GL, D'Angelo S, Valentini G. Cross-sectional evaluation of YKL-40 serum concentrations in patients with systemic sclerosis. Relationship with clinical and serological aspects of disease. Rheumatolology. 2003;30:2147–51.
17. Nordenbaek C, Johansen JS, Halberg P, Wiik A, Garbarsch C, Ullman S, et al. High serum levels of YKL-40 in patients with systemic sclerosis are associated with pulmonary involvement. Scand J Rheumatol. 2005;34(4): 293–7. https://doi.org/10.1080/03009740510018598.
18. Sun Y, Kong X, Wu S, Ma L, Yan Y, Lv P, et al. YKL-40 as a new biomarker of disease activity in Takayasu arteritis. Int J Cardiol. 2019;293:231–7. https://doi.org/10.1016/j.ijcard.2019.06.058.
19. Hozumi H, Fujisawa T, Enomoto N, Nakashima R, Enomoto Y, Suzuki Y, et al. Clinical utility of YKL-40 in polymyositis/dermatomyositis-associated interstitial lung disease. J Rheumatol. 2017;44(9):1394–401. https://doi.org/1 0.3899/jrheum.170373.
20. Gao MZ, Wei YY, Xu QW, Ji R, Han Z-J, Jian T-W, et al. Elevated serum YKL-40 correlates with clinical characteristics in patients with polymyositis or dermatomyositis. Ann Clin Biochem. 2019;56(1):95–9. https://doi.org/10.11 77/0004563218786979.
21. Jiang L, Wang Y, Peng Q, Shu X, Wang G, Wu X, et al. Serum YKL-40 level is associated with severity of interstitial lung disease and poor prognosis in dermatomyositis with anti-MDA5 antibody. Clin Rheumatol. 2019;38(6): 1655–63. https://doi.org/10.1007/s10067-019-04457-w.
22. Cruellas MG, Viana V dos S, Levy-Neto M, FHC DS, Shinjo SK. Myositis-specific and myositis-associated autoantibody profiles and their clinical associations in a large series of patients with polymyositis and dermatomyositis. Clinics. 2013;68:909–14.
23. Rider LG, Giannini EH, Harris-Love M, Joe G, Isenberg D, Pilkington C, et al. International myositis assessment and clinical studies group. Defining clinical improvement in adult and juvenile myositis. J Rheumatol. 2003;30(3): 603–17.
24. Rider LG, Feldman BM, Perez MD, Rennebohm RM, Lindsley CB, Zemel LS, et al. Development of validated disease activity and damage indices for the juvenile idiopathic inflammatory myopathies: I. physician, parent, and patient global assessments. Juvenile dermatomyositis disease activity collaborative study group. Arthritis Rheum. 1997;40(11):1976–83. https://doi.org/10.1002/art.1780401109.
25. Harris-Love MO, Shrader JA, Koziol D, Pahlajani N, Jain M, Smith M, et al. Distribution and severity of weakness among patients with polymyositis, dermatomyositis, and juvenile dermatomyositis. Rheumatology (Oxford). 2009;48(2):134–9. https://doi.org/10.1093/rheumatology/ken441

26. Miller FW, Rider GL, Chung YL, et al. International Myositis Outcome Assessment Collaborative Study Group. Proposed preliminary core set measures for disease outcome assessment in adult and juvenile idiopathic inflammatory myopathies. Rheumatology (Oxford). 2001;40:1262–73.
27. Bruce B, Fries JF. The Stanford health assessment questionnaire: dimensions and practical applications. Health Qual Life Outcomes. 2003;1(1):20. https://doi.org/10.1186/1477-7525-1-20.
28. Waseda Y, Johkoh T, Egashira R, Sumikawa H, Saeki K, Watanabe S, et al. Antisynthetase syndrome: pulmonary computed tomography findings of adult patients with antibodies to aminoacyl-tRNA synthetases. Eur J Radiol. 2016;85(8):1421–6. https://doi.org/10.1016/j.ejrad.2016.05.012.
29. Debray MP, Borie R, Revel MP, Naccache J-M, Khalil A, Toper C, et al. Interstitial lung disease in anti-synthetase syndrome: initial and follow-up CT findings. Eur J Radiol. 2015;84(3):516–23. https://doi.org/10.1016/j.ejrad.2014.11.026.
30. Sada KE, Yamasaki Y, Maruyama M, Sugiyama H, Yamamura M, Maeshima Y, et al. Altered levels of adipocytokines in association with insulin resistance in patients with systemic lupus erythematosus. J Rheumatol. 2006;33(8):1545–52.
31. Salomonsson S, Lundberg IE. Cytokines in idiopathic inflammatory myopathies. Autoimmunity. 2006;39(3):177–90. https://doi.org/10.1080/08916930600622256.
32. Lundberg I, Brengman JM, Engel AG. Analysis of cytokine expression in muscle in inflammatory myopathies, Duchenne dystrophy, and non-weak controls. J Neuroimmunol. 1995;63(1):9–16. https://doi.org/10.1016/0165-5728(95)00122-0.
33. Gallay L, Mouchiroud G, Chazaud B. Interferon-signature in idiopathic inflammatory myopathies. Curr Opin Rheumatol. 2019;31(6):634–42. https://doi.org/10.1097/BOR.0000000000000653.
34. Hou C, Baba-Amer Y, Bencze M, Relaix F, Authier FJ. The effect of interferon-gamma on skeletal muscle cell biology. Med Sci. 2018;34:35–8.
35. Isoda K, Kotani T, Takeuchi T, Kiboshi T, Hata K, Ishida T, et al. Comparison of long-term prognosis and relapse of dermatomyositis complicated with interstitial pneumonia according to autoantibodies: anti-aminoacyl tRNA synthetase antibodies versus antimelanoma differentiation-associated gene 5 antibody. Rheumatol Int. 2017;37(8):1335–40. https://doi.org/10.1007/s00296-017-3729-y

7

Risk factors for losing hepatitis B virus surface antibody in patients with HBV surface antigen negative/surface antibody positive serostatus receiving biologic disease-modifying anti-rheumatic drugs

Ming-Hui Hung[1], Ya-Chih Tien[1] and Ying-Ming Chiu[2*]

Abstract

Background: Hepatitis B virus (HBV) reactivation consequent to immunosuppressive therapy is an increasingly prevalent problem with serious clinical implications. Treatment with biologic agents conduces to the loss of protective antibody to HBV surface antigen (anti-HBs), which significantly increases the risk of HBV reactivation. Hence, we investigated the risk factors for losing anti-HBs in patients with rheumatic diseases and HBV surface antigen negative/anti-HBs positive (HBsAg−/anti-HBs+) serostatus during treatment with biologic disease-modifying anti-rheumatic drugs (DMARDs).

Methods: Using a nested case-control design, we prospectively enrolled patients with rheumatoid arthritis, ankylosing spondylitis, psoriatic arthritis/psoriasis, or juvenile idiopathic arthritis, who were treated with biologic DMARDs at Changhua Christian Hospital, Taiwan, from January 2013 to June 2019 and had HBsAg−/anti-HBs+ serostatus; the analytic sample excluded all patients with HBsAg+ or anti-HBs− serostatus. Anti-HBs titers were monitored 6-monthly and cases were defined as anti-HBs < 10 mIU/ml during follow-up. Cases were matched one-to-all with controls with anti-HBs ≥ 10 mIU/ml on the same ascertainment date and equivalent durations of biologic DMARDs treatment (control patients could be resampled and could also become cases during follow-up). Between-group characteristics were compared and risk factors for anti-HBs loss were investigated by conditional logistic regression analyses.

(Continued on next page)

* Correspondence: ymcgreen@yahoo.com.tw
[2]Department of Allergy, Immunology, and Rheumatology, Tungs' Taichung MetroHarbor Hospital, 699, Sec. 8, Taiwan Blvd., Taichung City 43503, Taiwan

(Continued from previous page)

Results: Among 294 eligible patients, 23 cases were matched with 311 controls. The incidence of anti-HBs loss was ~ 2.7%/person-year during biologic DMARDs treatment. Besides lower baseline anti-HBs titer (risk ratio 0.93, 95% CI 0.89–0.97), cases were significantly more likely than controls to have diabetes mellitus (risk ratio 4.76, 95% CI 1.48–15.30) and chronic kidney disease (risk ratio 14.00, 95% CI 2.22–88.23) in univariate analysis. Risk factors remaining significantly associated with anti-HBs loss in multivariate analysis were lower baseline anti-HBs titer (adjusted risk ratio 0.93, 95% CI 0.88–0.97) and chronic kidney disease (adjusted risk ratio 45.68, 95% CI 2.39–871.5).

Conclusions: Besides lower baseline anti-HBs titer, chronic kidney disease also strongly predicts future anti-HBs negativity in patients with HBsAg−/anti-HBs+ serostatus who receive biologic DMARDs to treat rheumatic diseases. Patients with low anti-HBs titer (≤ 100 mIU/ml) and/or chronic kidney disease should be monitored during biologic DMARDs therapy, to enable timely prophylaxis to preempt potential HBV reactivation.

Keywords: Hepatitis B virus (HBV), HBV surface-antigen negative/surface antibody positive (HBsAg−/anti-HBs+), Rheumatic diseases, Biologic disease-modifying anti-rheumatic drug (DMARD), Anti-HBs loss, Chronic kidney disease

Background

Hepatitis B virus (HBV) infection is a global public health concern [1]. Morbid HBV reactivation is characterized by viral replication and the recurrence of active necro-inflammatory liver disease, which may presage severe hepatitis or even death [1–6]. Rising prevalence of cancer and autoimmune diseases and more frequent use of chemotherapeutic or immunosuppressive treatment strategies, have made HBV reactivation consequent to such therapies an exigent problem [1–5]. Iatrogenic HBV reactivation is best known in HBV surface-antigen carriers (HBsAg+), and comprehensive guidelines cover this high-risk group [1–8]. Recently, attention has increasingly focused on patients who are HBsAg-negative with antibodies against HBV core-antigen or surface-antigen (HBsAg−/anti-HBc+ or anti-HBs+), among whom baseline HBV DNA and anti-HBs negative (anti-HBs−) serostatus are known risk factors for HBV reactivation [9–13].

Although serum HBV DNA is a defining characteristic of HBV reactivation [1–4], it does not inevitably progress to morbid viremia but may manifest transiently without symptoms, especially whilst anti-HBs serostatus remains positive [5, 6, 10–12]. On the other hand, anti-HBs loss consequent to immunosuppressive treatment of patients with HBsAg−/anti-HBc+ serostatus significantly increases the risk of progression from clinically silent to symptomatic HBV reactivation [9, 10, 12, 13]. Previous studies have shown that anti-HBs can decline to seronegative during immunosuppressive therapies, especially in patients with a low baseline anti-HBs titer [11, 14], but none have systematically investigated whether there are other predisposing factors.

In this context, especially given burgeoning use of tumor necrosis factor inhibitors (anti-TNF) and other biologic disease-modifying anti-rheumatic drugs (DMARDs) to treat autoimmune diseases, and elevated HBV reactivation rates in this setting [2, 4, 5], it is imperative to further elucidate risk factors for anti-HBs loss. To this end, we prospectively studied patients with HBsAg−/anti-HBc+ serostatus during/after biologic DMARDs therapy for rheumatic diseases.

Methods

Study subjects

The study sample comprised patients at Changhua Christian Hospital, Taiwan, with rheumatoid arthritis, ankylosing spondylitis, psoriasis, psoriatic arthritis, or juvenile idiopathic arthritis, who were treated with biologic DMARDs from January 2013 to June 2019. Only patients with HBsAg−/anti-HBs+ serostatus were included and all with HBsAg+ or HBsAg−/anti-HBs− serostatus were excluded (Fig. 1). All study subjects fulfilled international diagnostic criteria for these diseases and were treated according to Taiwan Rheumatology Association guidelines for screening and management of viral hepatitis [15].

Hepatitis B serologic testing and HBV DNA

HBV serology and DNA assays were done every 6 months according to Taiwan Rheumatology Association recommendations [15]. HBV assays included serum HBsAg, anti-HBs and anti-HBc, measured by Architect i2000SR chemiluminescent microparticle immunoassay (Abbott Laboratories, Abbot Park, Illinois, USA). HBV immunization history of people with anti-HBs+/anti-HBc− serostatus was not ascertained.

Anti-HBs titer < 10 mIU/ml was defined as seronegative. Low anti-HBs titer was defined as 10–100 mIU/ml, based on evidence of significantly increased likelihood of anti-HBs loss and detectable HBV DNA at anti-HBs titers below 100 mIU/ml and protection against HBV reactivation above this threshold [11, 14]. Serum HBV DNA viral load was quantified by Abbott RealTime HBV (Abbott Laboratories, Abbott Park, Illinois, USA), with a minimal sensitivity of 10 IU/ml. HBV DNA titer ≥ 10 mIU/ml was defined as

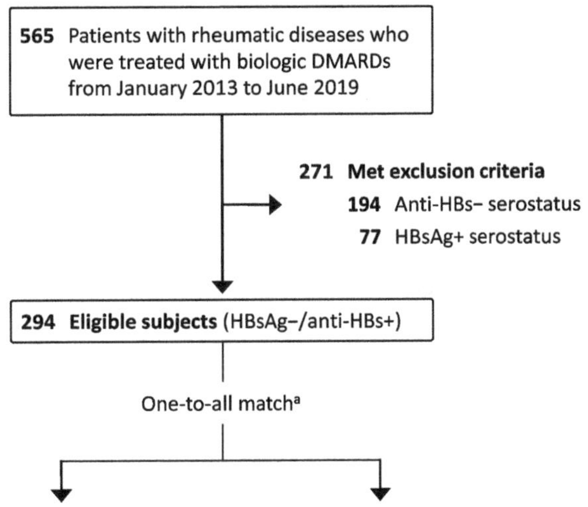

Rheumatic disease type	Cases (anti-HBs <10 mIU/ml)	Controls (anti-HBs ≥10 mIU/ml)[b]
Any	**23**	**311**
Rheumatoid arthritis	13	155
Ankylosing spondylitis	5	100
Psoriatic arthritis/psoriasis	4	52
Juvenile idiopathic arthritis	1	4

[b]Anti-HBs >10 mIU/ml on the case ascertainment date and equivalent biologic DMARD treatment duration.

Fig. 1 Case-control selection flow chart. DMARDs, disease-modifying anti-rheumatic drugs; HBV, hepatitis B virus; DNA, deoxyribonucleic acid; anti-HBs, HBV surface antibody; HBsAg, HBV surface-antigen; mIU, million International Units. [a]One patient could serve as a control repeatedly during follow-up and control subjects could become cases during the study

detectable viral load [11], while the criteria defining clinical HBV reactivation at any serial 6-monthly follow-up check, were HBV replication ≥ 2 log increase from baseline or a new appearance of HBV DNA to ≥ 100 IU/ml in people with previously stable or undetectable levels [1].

Covariate information

Baseline data included: age, sex, type of rheumatic disease (rheumatoid arthritis, ankylosing spondylitis, psoriatic arthritis/psoriasis, juvenile idiopathic arthritis), accumulated doses of conventional DMARDs (prednisolone, hydroxychloroquine, sulfasalazine, methotrexate, leflunomide, cyclosporine) and biologic DMARDs (etanercept, adalimumab, golimumab, ustekinumab, secukinumab, tocilizumab, rituximab, abatacept, tofacitinib). Chronic kidney disease was defined as estimated glomerular filtration rate < 60 ml/min/ 1.73 m^2. Chronic liver disease status was determined from medical charts or hepatic ultrasound results and included cirrhosis, fatty liver, and "parenchymal liver disease", which is a term used in Taiwan, to denote ultrasound findings intermediate between "normal" and "cirrhosis", based on sonographic evaluation criteria for liver surface, liver parenchyma, hepatic vessels, and spleen size [16].

Nested case-control design

We used a nested case-control design, which enables efficient analysis of time-dependent exposures on rare outcomes where only a limited sample from a larger population is practical, without compromising statistical power [17–19]. Unlike conventional cohort studies, which compare cases versus controls from a fully enumerated population, a nested case-control design identifies occurrences of events of interest in a defined sub-population and matches these with a specified number of control subjects drawn from the same sub-sample, but who were not yet affected by the same event when it occurred in their corresponding case [18, 19]. This design means that controls can become cases later during follow-up and that each patient may serve as a control repeatedly (though at different times); thus, cases are compared with controls from the same patient sample, which lessens the likelihood of selection bias [17–20].

The first prescription of a biologic DMARD defined the start point. Cases were defined upon occurrences of serum anti-HBs titer < 10 mIU/ml during follow-up, with the date when anti-HBs loss was ascertained designated the event date. Each case was matched one-to-all with subjects whose serum HBsAb titer was ≥ 10 mIU/ml on the respective case ascertainment date and who had an equivalent duration of biologic DMARDs treatment.

Data analysis and statistics

All analyses were done using nonparametric statistical software (LogXact 11, Cytel Software Corp, Cambridge, MA, USA) with penalized maximum likelihood to remove first-order bias. A p-value < 0.05 for two-sided tests was considered statistically significant. Continuous variables were expressed as means plus/minus standard deviation or mean [range], categorical variables as numbers (percentages). Conditional logistic regression analysis was used to estimate risk ratios and 95% confidence intervals for loss of anti-HBs; putative associated factors included age, sex, type of rheumatic disease, conventional DMARDs, biologic DMARDs (anti-TNF or others), comorbidity, and baseline anti-HBs titer.

Results

Demographic characteristics and clinical status

The analytic samples drawn from 294 patients with HBsAg–/anti-HBs+ serostatus at baseline, comprised 23 cases and 311 matched controls (Fig. 1); Table 1 shows their demographic and clinical characteristics. Mean age and rheumatic disease types were similar between case and control groups. No patients with HBsAg–/anti-HBs+ serostatus had detectable HBV DNA at enrolment. Compared with controls, cases had lower baseline serum anti-HBs titers, more prevalent comorbidities (including hepatitis C virus infection, chronic liver disease, diabetes mellitus, chronic kidney disease), and relatively higher accumulated doses of sulfasalazine, leflunomide, and prednisolone. Most people in both groups used anti-TNF agents (etanercept, adalimumab, golimumab). No study subjects were kidney transplant recipients.

Incidence of anti-HBs loss and associated risk factors

The incidence rate of anti-HBs loss in 294 patients with HBsAg–/anti-HBs+ serostatus during biologic DMARDs treatment was 23/852 person-years: ~ 2.7%/person-year.

Table 2 shows risk factors associated with loss of anti-HBs in univariate and multivariate conditional logistic regression analyses. Besides lower baseline anti-HBs titer (risk ratio 0.93, 95% CI 0.89–0.97), cases were significantly more likely than controls to have diabetes mellitus (risk ratio 4.76, 95% CI 1.48–15.30) and chronic kidney disease (risk ratio 14.00, 95% CI 2.22–88.23) in the univariate analysis. However, the only factors remaining significant in the multivariate model, were lower baseline serum anti-HBs titer (adjusted risk ratio 0.93, 95% CI 0.88–0.97) and chronic kidney disease (adjusted risk ratio 45.68, 95% CI 2.39–871.5).

Clinical features and outcomes of subjects with anti-HBs loss

Thirteen cases had rheumatoid arthritis (Table 3). All cases' baseline anti-HBs titers were low (≤ 100 mIU/ml), mean 22.6. Fourteen were prescribed anti-TNF agents: four etanercept, six adalimumab, and four golimumab. Three were prescribed tofacitinib. Two cases each were prescribed ustekinumab or tocilizumab, while one each received abatacept or rituximab.

No cases (nor anti-HBs+ controls) had clinical HBV reactivation during follow-up (852 person-years), and no cases developed alanine transaminase elevation, or received any anti-viral treatment during median follow-up of 30 months (range 0–77) after anti-HBs loss. Only one of the 16/23 cases whose serum HBV DNA was monitored after anti-HBs loss ever had a detectable viral load (Table 3), which was observed only once, with no recurrence as of August 2020.

Discussion

We believe this to be the first report of risk factors associated with loss of anti-HBs in rheumatic patients during biologic DMARDs therapy, after controlling for putative risk factors. We discovered that besides lower baseline anti-HBs titer, chronic kidney disease independently predicts anti-HBs loss.

Our finding that lower pretreatment anti-HBs titer (≤ 100 mIU/ml) is a risk factor for loss of anti-HBs, is consistent with a study of rituximab-based therapy for lymphoma [14]. Moreover, baseline anti-HBs positivity was protective against HBV reactivation among patients with HBsAg–/anti-HBc+ serostatus who received immunosuppressive or biologic agents [9–14]. Therefore, our results suggest that anti-HBs may be lost during/after immunosuppressive/biologic therapy, especially in people with a low baseline titer, with consequently elevated risk of HBV reactivation.

Although we detected no cases of morbid viremia and just one occurrence of minimal HBV DNA during follow-up, this was not necessarily inconsistent with evidence that anti-HBs negativity increases the risk of HBV reactivation in patients with HBsAg–/anti-HBc+ serostatus. Anti-HBs may remain persistently low or negative during treatment, with HBV DNA detected periodically but without progression to morbid reactivation [5, 6, 11, 12]. Reported rates of HBV DNA manifestation during/after immunosuppressive therapy in patients with HBsAg–/anti-HBs–/anti-HBc+ serostatus are in the order of 1–10%, with symptomatic reactivation in a smaller fraction of cases [9–12]; therefore, 23 cases may have been too few to detect occasional reactivation

Table 1 Baseline characteristics of cases and controls treated with biologic DMARDs

Data show mean ± standard deviation, mean [range], or number (%)	Cases	Controls
Number	23	311
Age (years)	52.2 ± 17.9	47.5 ± 14.2
Sex		
Female	15 (65.2%)	148 (47.6%)
Male	8 (34.8%)	163 (52.4%)
Rheumatic disease		
Rheumatoid arthritis	13 (56.5%)	155 (49.8%)
Ankylosing spondylitis	5 (21.7%)	100 (32.2%)
Psoriatic arthritis/Psoriasis	4 (17.4%)	52 (16.7%)
Juvenile idiopathic arthritis	1 (4.4%)	4 (1.3%)
Detectable HBV DNA (≥10 IU/ml)	0	0
Anti-HBV core antigen positive	15 (65.2%)	189 (60.8%)
Baseline serum anti-HBs titer (mIU/ml)		
Mean [Min–Max]	22.6 [10.1–64.7]	284.5 [11.5–1000][a]
≤ 100	23 (100%)	128 (41.2%)
> 100	0	183 (58.8%)
Biologic DMARDs		
Anti-TNF (Etanercept, Adalimumab, Golimumab)	14 (60.9%)	231 (74.3%)
Not anti-TNF	9 (39.1%)	80 (25.7%)
Abatacept	1 (4.4%)	11 (3.5%)
Rituximab	1 (4.4%)	11 (3.5%)
Tocilizumab	2 (8.7%)	12 (3.9%)
Tofacitinib	3 (13.0%)	19 (6.1%)
Ustekinumab	2 (8.7%)	25 (8.0%)
Secukinumab	0	2 (0.6%)
Conventional DMARDs (accumulated dose)		
Methotrexate (mg)	536 ± 869	537 ± 734
Leflunomide (mg)	748 ± 2083	707 ± 3021
Sulfasalazine (g)	350 ± 354	242 ± 318
Hydroxychloroquine (g)	67 ± 102	54 ± 100
Cyclosporine (g)	9 ± 22	8 ± 27
Prednisolone (accumulated dose, mg)	2244 ± 2614	1422 ± 1910
Comorbidities		
Prior alanine transaminase elevation[b]	2 (8.7%)	10 (3.2%)
Hepatitis C virus antibody positive	2 (8.7%)	11 (3.5%)
Diabetes mellitus	4 (17.4%)	12 (3.9%)
Chronic liver disease	5 (21.7%)	30 (9.7%)
Chronic kidney disease	3 (13.0%)	3 (1.0%)

HBV Hepatitis B virus, *DNA* Deoxyribonucleic acid, *Anti-HBs* HBV surface antibody, *IU* International Units, *DMARD* Disease-modifying anti-rheumatic drug, *TNF* Tumor necrosis factor

[a]Maximum detectable limit

[b]More than five-fold upper reference of 40 IU/L

events. The follow-up duration (median 30 months after anti-HBs loss) may also have been insufficient. HBV DNA in such patients usually appears late, after several cycles of therapy have diminished anti-HBs to undetectable levels [6], and clinical reactivation may not occur until several years since commencing immunosuppressive

Table 2 Risk factors associated with loss of HBV surface antibody

	Univariate analysis		Multivariate analysis	
	Risk ratio (95% CI)	*p*-value	Risk ratio (95% CI)	*p*-value
Age	1.02 (0.99–1.05)	0.153		
Sex				
Female	1 (reference)	0.097		
Male	0.48 (0.20–1.14)			
Rheumatic disease				
Rheumatoid arthritis	1 (reference)	0.582		
Ankylosing spondylitis	0.60 (0.21–1.72)			
Psoriatic arthritis/Psoriasis	0.87 (0.28–2.76)			
Juvenile idiopathic arthritis	2.73 (0.29–25.57)			
Anti-HBV core antigen positive	1.23 (0.51–2.95)	0.641		
Baseline serum anti-HBs titer (mIU/ml)				
Lower vs higher (continuous)	0.93 (0.89–0.97)	0.001	0.93 (0.88–0.97)	0.002
> 100	1 (reference)		1 (reference)	
≤ 100	46.8 (10.09–∞)	< 0.001	43.98 (9.34–∞)	< 0.001
Biologic DMARDs				
Anti-TNF	1 (reference)	0.204		
Not anti-TNF	1.80 (0.73–4.49)			
Conventional DMARDs				
Methotrexate	1.00 (1.00–1.00)	0.942		
Sulfasalazine	1.00 (1.00–1.00)	0.135		
Hydroxychloroquine	1.00 (1.00–1.01)	0.515		
Cyclosporine	1.00 (0.99–1.02)	0.888		
Leflunomide	1.00 (1.00–1.00)	0.958		
Prednisolone	1.00 (1.00–1.00)	0.064		
Comorbidity				
Prior alanine transaminase elevation[a]	2.93 (0.59–14.54)	0.188		
Hepatitis C virus antibody positive	2.64 (0.54–12.92)	0.232		
Diabetes mellitus	4.76 (1.48–15.30)	0.009	0.85 (0.19–3.92)	0.838[b]
Chronic liver disease	2.62 (0.90–7.66)	0.079		
Chronic kidney disease	14.00 (2.22–88.23)	0.005	45.68 (2.39–871.5)	0.011[c]

Anti-HBs Hepatitis B virus surface antibody, *DMARD* Disease-modifying anti-rheumatic drug, *TNF* Tumor necrosis factor
[a]More than five-fold upper reference of 40 IU/L
[b]Baseline anti-HBs as continuous variable
[c]Baseline anti-HBs continuous + chronic kidney disease + diabetes mellitus

therapy [10–12]; median time from starting immunosuppressive therapy to HBV reactivation in a cohort of 1042 rheumatic disease patients with resolved HBV infections was 66 months [12]. However, 18/23 cases in our study had total follow-up of < 66 months.

This is the first indication of which we know that chronic kidney disease might be a risk factor for loss of anti-HBs in patients treated with biologic DMARDs. This is an important contemporary issue because chronic kidney disease is prevalent among patients with rheumatic diseases, consequent to older age, diabetes-related nephropathy, and widespread use of nephrotoxic medications such as non-steroidal anti-inflammatory drugs or cyclosporine. Studies have shown that patients with chronic kidney disease lose anti-HBs faster than healthy subjects do [21, 22]; anti-HBs loss in chronic kidney disease or dialysis patients has been attributed to diminished interleukin-2 secretion, impaired macrophage function, decreasing memory B cell counts, and a weak amnestic response [23–25].

Consistent with reports of increased likelihood of anti-HBs loss in patients with diabetes mellitus [26, 27], we

Table 3 Characteristics of patients with anti-HBs loss during treatment with biologic DMARDs

Baseline			Time to anti-HBs loss (months)	Medication when anti-HBs loss occurred							Comorbidities				Total follow-up (months)	HBV status and treatment after anti-HBs loss		
Disease	Serum HBV antibodies			Biologic DMARD	Conventional DMARD (accumulated dose, g)						HCV	Chronic liver disease[a]	DM	CKD		Viral load (IU/ml)[b]	HBV reactivation[c]	Antiviral therapy
	HBs (mIU/ml)	HBc			Pd	MTX	LEF	HCQ	SSZ	CsA								
RA	10.1	–	15	TOF	3.0	0.6	0	181	236	0	–	ND	–	–	32	ND	–	–
RA	13.2	+	25	ETA	3.9	0	0	280	699	34	+	Fatty liver	+	+	74	U	–	–
RA	13.4	–	11	TOF	0	0.8	0	141	0	0	–	ND	–	–	23	ND	–	–
RA	14.8	–	13	TOF	2.1	0.5	0	90	394	0	–	ND	–	–	30	U	–	–
RA	16.1	+	22	TCZ	4.4	0	9.2	0	713	0	–	PLD[d]	+	–	47	U	–	–
RA	16.5	+	17	ABT	2.6	0	0	40	588	0	–	ND	–	+	39	U	–	–
RA	17.3	+	7	ADA	1.1	0.5	0	84	294	0	–	Normal	+	–	65	10[e]	–	–
RA	17.7	+	61	GOL	7.2	3.3	0	363	714	0	–	ND	–	–	61	U	–	–
RA	18.3	+	18	ETA	2.7	1.2	0	218	1092	0	–	Normal	–	–	68	U	–	–
RA	23.4	+	60	ADA	5.8	2.6	0	74	0	0	–	Normal	–	–	76	ND	–	–
RA	41.9	+	3	ETA	0.7	0	0	45	224	4	–	Normal	–	–	80	U	–	–
RA	44.7	+	10	RTX	2.5	0.6	0	28	182	8	+	PLD	–	–	57	U	–	–
RA	56.3	–	42	TCZ	9.8	1.3	3.8	6	1295	0	–	Normal	–	+	54	ND	–	–
AS	11.5	+	22	GOL	0	0	0	0	172	0	–	Normal	–	–	33	U	–	–
AS	14.3	–	7	GOL	0	0	0	0	163	0	–	Normal	–	–	51	ND	–	–
AS	21.7	+	34	ADA	0.4	0	0	0	294	0	–	Normal	–	–	75	U	–	–
AS	26.3	–	42	ADA	0.4	0	0	0	456	0	–	Normal	–	–	60	ND	–	–
AS	64.7	–	4	ADA	0.3	0	0	0	228	0	–	Normal	–	–	36	U	–	–
PsO	10.1	+	5	GOL	0.6	0	2.8	0	0	22	–	Fatty liver	+	–	46	U	–	–
PsO	12.3	+	16	UST	0	0.5	0	0	0	90	–	Normal	–	–	62	U	–	–
PsO	17.3	+	17	UST	0	0	0	0	0	53	–	Fatty liver	–	–	47	U	–	–
PsA	27	+	28	ADA	3.8	0	1.4	0	56	0	–	ND	–	–	35	U	–	–
JIA	10.1	–	4	ETA	0.4	0.3	0	0	256	0	–	Normal	–	–	60	ND	–	–

RA Rheumatoid arthritis, *AS* Ankylosing spondylitis, *PsO* Psoriatic arthritis, *PSA* Psoriasis, *JIA* Juvenile idiopathic arthritis, *HBV* Hepatitis B virus, *HBs* HBV surface antigen, *HBc* HBV core protein, *DMARD* Disease-modifying anti-rheumatic drug, *Pd* Prednisolone, *MTX* Methotrexate, *LEF* Leflunomide, *HCQ* Hydroxychloroquine, *SSZ* Sulfasalazine, *CsA* Cyclosporine, *TOF* Tofacitinib, *ETA* Etanercept, *TCZ* Tocilizumab, *ABT* Abatacept, *ADA* Adalimumab, *GOL* Golimumab, *RTX* Rituximab, *UST* Ustekinumab, *HCV* Hepatitis C virus, *DM* Diabetes mellitus, *CKD* Chronic kidney disease, *PLD* Parenchymal liver disease, *U* Undetectable, *ND* Not done

[a]Based on ultrasound findings

[b]At any serial 6-monthly check during follow-up

[c]HBV replication > 2 log increase from baseline or a new appearance of HBV DNA to > 100 IU/ml in people with previously stable or undetectable levels

[d]In Taiwan, ultrasound findings intermediate between "normal" and "cirrhosis" based on sonographic evaluation criteria for liver surface, liver parenchyma, hepatic vessels and spleen size, are diagnosed as "parenchymal liver disease" [16]

[e]First prescribed biologic DMARD May 2013, anti-HBs loss December 2013; HBV DNA detected only once, in September 2017, with no recurrence as of August 2020

found a significant association in univariate analysis; however, statistical significance was lost in multivariate analysis, probably because only 4/23 cases had diabetes.

Previous guidelines or reviews have propounded baseline anti-HBs screening prior to using biologic DMARDs, because patients with baseline anti-HBs− serostatus have higher risk of HBV reactivation [1, 5, 7, 8]. However, current guidelines, particularly those focused on biologic DMARDs users, neither describe nor elucidate the potential risk of anti-HBs loss during biologic DMARDs therapy [2, 5, 8]. Our results imply that there is a window of opportunity to prevent morbid HBV reactivation in patients at increased risk. We contend that clinicians should closely monitor patients with low baseline anti-HBs titer (≤ 100 mIU/ml) and/or chronic kidney disease during subsequent biologic DMARDs therapy, including follow-up of anti-HBs and HBV DNA titers upon anti-HBs loss, to enable timely intervention with appropriate prophylaxis to preempt potential HBV reactivation. Expert opinion supports this approach; for example, advocating HBV follow-up and immunization to reduce the risk of reactivation during anti-TNF treatment [4].

This study had limitations, foremost the small sample size. With few cases or control group patients with chronic kidney disease, the result of multivariate analysis could reflect over-fitting, as the wide confidence interval suggests; larger-scale studies are warranted to corroborate this novel but tentative finding. We acknowledge that direct serum HBV DNA assays are the ideal way to monitor patients at risk of HBV reactivation; nevertheless, based on our findings, monitoring patients with risk factors for anti-HBs loss may be a convenient and cost-effective way of targeting hepatitis B prevention, especially in HBV-endemic regions. Admittedly, only direct monitoring can detect HBV reactivation due to immune-escape HBsAg mutations in anti-HBs+ biologic DMARDs recipients; however, this is a very rare phenomenon [28, 29] and, excepting such cases, detectable HBV DNA loads in anti-HBs+ patients otherwise occur only sporadically, and are self-limiting and clinically benign [11]. Despite considerable research into whether or not the risks of anti-HBs loss or HBV reactivation differ between biologic DMARDs, results to date have been inconclusive [30, 31]; with only 23 cases, we were unable to ascertain whether individual biologic DMARDs carried similar risks of anti-HBs loss.

Conclusions

This prospective single-center study found that lower baseline anti-HBs titer (≤ 100 mIU/ml) and chronic kidney disease strongly predicted loss of anti-HBs in patients having biologic DMARDs therapy for rheumatic diseases. These insights can be applied to identify patients at increased risk of becoming anti-HBs− and monitor them for potential HBV reactivation from the onset of biologic DMARDs therapy. More research is needed to elucidate other risk factors for loss of anti-HBs and so refine the monitoring strategy to prevent HBV reactivation in patients receiving biologic DMARDs to treat rheumatic diseases.

Abbreviations

HBV: Hepatitis B virus; HBsAg: HBV surface antigen; anti-HBc: Antibody to HBV core antigen; anti-HBs: Antibody to HBV surface antigen; DNA: Deoxyribonucleic acid; anti-TNF: Tumor necrosis factor inhibitor; DMARD: Disease-modifying anti-rheumatic drug

Acknowledgements

David Neil, of Dr. Word Ltd., Taiwan, provided professional editorial services, which were funded by Dr Ying-Ming Chiu. Ya-Chu Yang provided technical assistance with laboratory work.

Authors' contributions

MHH made substantial contributions to conceiving and designing the study, analyzing and interpreting data, and drafting the manuscript. YMC made substantial contributions to conceiving and designing the study, analyzing and interpreting data, and critical revision of the manuscript for intellectually important content. YCT was involved in revising the manuscript. All authors had full control of all primary data, read and approved the final article, and agree to be accountable for all aspects of the work described.

Authors' information

Not applicable.

Author details

[1]Division of Allergy, Immunology and Rheumatology, Department of Internal Medicine, Changhua Christian Hospital, 135 Nanxiao St., Changhua City 500-06, Taiwan. [2]Department of Allergy, Immunology, and Rheumatology, Tungs' Taichung MetroHarbor Hospital, 699, Sec. 8, Taiwan Blvd., Taichung City 43503, Taiwan.

References

1. Sarin SK, Kumar M, Lau GK, Abbas Z, Chan HL, Chen CJ, et al. Asian-Pacific clinical practice guidelines on the management of hepatitis B: a 2015 update. Hepatol Int. 2016;10:1–98.
2. Perrillo RP, Gish R, Falck-Ytter YT. American Gastroenterological Association Institute technical review on prevention and treatment of hepatitis B virus reactivation during immunosuppressive drug therapy. Gastroenterology. 2015;148:221–244.e3.
3. Di Bisceglie AM, Lok AS, Martin P, Terrault N, Perrillo RP, Hoofnagle J. Recent US Food and Drug Administration warnings on hepatitis B reactivation with immune-suppressing and anticancer drugs: just the tip of the iceberg? Hepatology. 2015;61:703–11.
4. Murdaca G, Negrini S, Pellecchio M, Greco M, Schiavi C, Giusti F, et al. Update upon the infection risk in patients receiving TNF alpha inhibitors. Expert Opin Drug Saf. 2019;18:219–29.
5. Loomba R, Liang TJ. Hepatitis B reactivation associated with immune suppressive and biological modifier therapies: current concepts, management strategies, and future directions. Gastroenterology. 2017;152: 1297–309.
6. Hoofnagle JH. Reactivation of hepatitis B. Hepatology. 2009;49(5 Suppl): S156–65.
7. European Association For The Study Of The Liver. EASL clinical practice guidelines: management of chronic hepatitis B virus infection. J Hepatol. 2012;57:167–85.
8. Koutsianas C, Thomas K, Vassilopoulos D. Hepatitis B reactivation in rheumatic diseases: screening and prevention. Rheum Dis Clin N Am. 2017; 43:133 49.

9. Su YC, Lin PC, Yu HC, Wu CC. Hepatitis B virus reactivation in patients with resolved hepatitis B virus infection receiving chemotherapy or immunosuppressive therapy. Eur J Gastroenterol Hepatol. 2018;30:925–9.
10. Kuo MH, Tseng CW, Lee CH, Tung CH, Tseng KC, Lai NS. Moderate risk of hepatitis B virus reactivation in HBsAg⁻/HBcAb⁺ carriers receiving rituximab for rheumatoid arthritis. Sci Rep. 2020;10:2456.
11. Tien YC, Yen HH, Li CF, Liu MP, Hsue YT, Hung MH, et al. Changes in hepatitis B virus surface antibody titer and risk of hepatitis B reactivation in HBsAg-negative/HBcAb-positive patients undergoing biologic therapy for rheumatic diseases: a prospective cohort study. Arthritis Res Ther. 2018;20:246.
12. Fukuda W, Hanyu T, Katayama M, Mizuki S, Okada A, Miyata M, et al. Incidence of hepatitis B virus reactivation in patients with resolved infection on immunosuppressive therapy for rheumatic disease: a multicentre, prospective, observational study in Japan. Ann Rheum Dis. 2017;76:1051–6.
13. Paul S, Dickstein A, Saxena A, Terrin N, Viveiros K, Balk EM, et al. Role of surface antibody in hepatitis B reactivation in patients with resolved infection and hematologic malignancy: a meta-analysis. Hepatology. 2017;66:379–88.
14. Pei SN, Ma MC, Wang MC, Kuo CY, Rau KM, Su CY, et al. Analysis of hepatitis B surface antibody titers in B cell lymphoma patients after rituximab therapy. Ann Hematol. 2012;91:1007–12.
15. Chen YH, Chien RN, Huang YH, Chen DY, Lan JL, Lu LY, et al. Screening and management of hepatitis B infection in rheumatic patients scheduled for biologic therapy: consensus recommendations from the Taiwan Rheumatology Association. Formos J Rheumatol. 2012;26:1–7.
16. Hung CH, Lu SN, Wang JH, Lee CM, Chen TM, Tung HD, et al. Correlation between ultrasonographic and pathologic diagnoses of hepatitis B and C virus-related cirrhosis. J Gastroenterol. 2003;38:153–7.
17. Partlett C, Hall NJ, Leaf A, Juszczak E, Linsell L. Application of the matched nested case-control design to the secondary analysis of trial data. BMC Med Res Methodol. 2020;20:117.
18. Rothman KJ. Case-control studies. In: Rothman KJ, Greenland S, Lash TL, editors. Modern epidemiology. 3rd ed. Philadelphia: Williams & Wilkins; 2008. p. 111–27.
19. Suissa S. Novel approaches to pharmacoepidemiology study design and statistical analysis. In: Strom B, editor. Pharmacoepidemiology. 4th ed. New York: Wiley; 2005. p. 811–29.
20. Dixon WG, Kezouh A, Bernatsky, Suissa S. The influence of systemic glucocorticoid therapy upon the risk of non-serious infection in older patients with rheumatoid arthritis: a nested case-control study. Ann Rheum Dis. 2011;70:956–60.
21. Buti M, Viladomiu L, Jardi R, Olmos A, Rodriguez JA, Bartolome J, et al. Long-term immunogenicity and efficacy of hepatitis B vaccine in hemodialysis patients. Am J Nephrol. 1992;12:144–7.
22. Tsouchnikas I, Dounousi E, Xanthopoulou, Papakonstantinou S, Thomoglou V, Tsakiris D. Loss of hepatitis B immunity in hemodialysis patients acquired either naturally or after vaccination. Clin Nephrol. 2007;68:228–34.
23. Sester U, Sester M, Hauk M, Kaul H, Köhler H, Girndt M. T-cell activation follows Th1 rather than Th2 pattern in haemodialysis patients. Nephrol Dial Transplant. 2000;5:1217–23.
24. Pesanti EL. Immunologic defects and vaccination in patients with chronic renal failure. Infect Dis Clin N Am. 2001;15:813–32.
25. Descamps-Latscha B, Chatenoud L. T cells and B cells in chronic renal failure. Semin Nephrol. 1996;16:183–91.
26. Leonardi S, Vitaliti G, Garozzo MT, Miraglia del Giudice M, Marseglia G, La Rosa M. Hepatitis B vaccination failure in children with diabetes mellitus? The debate continues. Hum Vaccin Immunother. 2012;8:448–52.
27. Joo EJ, Yeom JS, Kwon MJ, Chang Y, Ryu S. Insulin resistance increases loss of antibody to hepatitis B surface antigen in nondiabetic healthy adults. J Viral Hepat. 2016;23:889–96.
28. Lazarevic I, Banko A, Miljanovic D, Cupic M. Immune-escape hepatitis B virus mutations associated with viral reactivation upon immunosuppression. Viruses. 2019;11:778.
29. Westhoff TH, Jochimsen F, Schmittel A, Stoffler-Meilicke M, Schafer JH, Zidek W, et al. Fatal hepatitis B virus reactivation by an escape mutant following rituximab therapy. Blood. 2003;102:1930.
30. Tamori A, Koike T, Goto H, Wakitani S, Tada M, Morikawa H, et al. Prospective study of reactivation of hepatitis B virus in patients with rheumatoid arthritis who received immunosuppressive therapy: evaluation of both HBsAg-positive and HBsAg-negative cohorts. J Gastroenterol. 2011; 46:556–64.
31. Papalopoulos I, Fanouriakis A, Kougas N, Flouri I, Sourvinos G, Bertsias G, et al. Liver safety of non-tumour necrosis factor inhibitors in rheumatic patients with past hepatitis B virus infection: an observational, controlled, long-term study. Clin Exp Rheumatol. 2018;36:102–9.

8

Flow cytometry evaluation of CD14/CD16 monocyte subpopulations in systemic sclerosis patients

Laiana Schneider[1,2*], Natália Aydos Marcondes[3], Vanessa Hax[1], Isadora Flesch da Silva Moreira[4], Carolina Yuka Ueda[4], Rafaella Romeiro Piovesan[4], Ricardo Xavier[1,2] and Rafael Chakr[1,2]

Abstract

Background: Systemic sclerosis (SSc) is a chronic autoimmune disease characterized by vasculopathy and fibrosis, which can be subclassified into diffuse cutaneous (dSSc) and limited cutaneous (lSSc) subtypes. Previous studies suggest that an increase in monocytes can be a hallmark of various inflammatory diseases, including SSc. Our aim was to evaluate circulating blood monocyte subpopulations (classical, intermediate and non-classical) of SSc patients and their possible association with disease manifestations.

Methods: Fifty consecutive patients fulfilling the 2013 ACR/EULAR classification criteria for SSc were included in a cross-sectional study. Monocyte subpopulations were identified based on their expression of CD64, CD14 and CD16, evaluated by flow cytometry, and were correlated with the clinical characteristics of the patients; furthermore, the expression of HLA-DR, CD163, CD169 and CD206 in the monocytes was studied. Thirty-eight age- and sex-matched healthy individuals were recruited as a control group.

Results: SSc patients had an increased number of circulating peripheral blood monocytes with an activated phenotypic profile compared to healthy subjects. Absolute counts of CD16+ (intermediary and non-classical) monocyte subpopulations were higher in SSc patients. There was no association between monocyte subpopulations and the clinical manifestations evaluated.

Conclusion: We identified higher counts of all monocyte subpopulations in SSc patients compared to the control group. There was no association between monocyte subpopulations and major fibrotic manifestations. CD169 was shown to be more representative in dSSc, being a promising marker for differentiating disease subtypes.

Keywords: Systemic sclerosis, Monocytes, Monocyte subpopulations, Flow cytometry, Pathogenesis

* Correspondence: laia_schneider@hotmail.com
[1]Serviço de Reumatologia, Hospital de Clínicas de Porto Alegre, Universidade Federal do Rio Grande do Sul, 2350 Ramiro Barcelos St, Room 645, Porto Alegre, RS 90035-903, Brazil
[2]Programa de Pós Graduação em Medicina: Ciências Médicas, Universidade Federal do Rio Grande do Sul, Porto Alegre, Brazil

Background

Systemic sclerosis (SSc) is a chronic inflammatory systemic disease, mainly characterized by expansion of the secondary extracellular matrix due to an exaggerated protein production, especially collagen. Collagen is deposited as a result of the abnormal interaction between endothelial cells, mononuclear cells (lymphocytes and monocytes) and fibroblasts. Monocytes express several receptors, which monitor and detect environmental changes. Those cells present great plasticity and heterogeneity and have the ability to modify their functional phenotype in response to stimulation [1]. There seems to be a relationship between the monocytes/macrophages activation and migration [2, 3], and SSc pathogenesis [4].

Evidences from human and murine studies suggest that an increase in monocytes can be an indicator of various inflammatory diseases and that these cells could differentiate into inflammatory or anti-inflammatory subgroups [5]. For almost two decades studies have shown the presence of two subsets of cells: classical and non-classical monocytes. Classical monocytes, characterized by expression of CD14++CD16-, represent about 80% of all monocytes and have phagocytic function, with production of reactive oxygen species and secretion of pro- and anti-inflammatory cytokines in response to agonist stimulation of toll-like receptor-4 (TLR-4) [6]. Whereas non-classical monocytes, which express CD16+, have a higher activity in response to viruses and produce proinflammatory cytokines through TLR-8 and TLR-9 [7, 8].

In recent years, a third group of monocytes has been proposed, dividing the CD16+ population into non-classical and intermediate monocytes (respectively, CD14+/−CD16++ and CD14 + CD16+) [8–10]. These CD16+ monocytes appear to be related to alternative activated M2 macrophages, and their activation pathway showed that they are associated with T helper (Th) 2 response [5, 11]. The differences between these monocyte subsets have been made clear, with distinct phenotypes and different functions, such as defense against pathogens, homeostasis and tissue repair [9, 10, 12].

Evaluation of mannose receptor-1 (MRC1 or CD206) and CD163 (macrophage scavenger receptors) that are typical of M2 macrophage activation pathway, showed an association of these markers with tissue repair and fibrosis [13], and in SSc patients those markers are associated with high pulmonary artery pressure and increased mortality [14]. Other marker that may play a key role in the monocyte activation present in SSc is CD169 (sialic acid-binding Ig-like lectine I or Siglec-1), also known as sialoadhesin, which has been shown to have a higher expression in a subset of SSc patients monocytes [15]. Monocytes of SSc patients have a greater expression of these molecules, which is even higher in patients with tissue disease and pulmonary artery hypertension.

Peripheral blood monocytes heterogeneity still lacks a clear comprehension of its role in SSc pathophysiology and clinical manifestations. The aim of our study was to characterize the three monocytes subpopulations of SSc patients, analyze the expression of CD163, CD169, CD206 and HLA-DR (function and activation monocytes receptors), and their association with clinical findings.

Methods

Patients

Fifty consecutive patients fulfilling the 2013 ACR/EULAR classification criteria for SSc [16] were recruited from the Outpatient Rheumatology Clinic of the Hospital de Clínicas de Porto Alegre, Brazil. Clinical form of disease was classified as diffuse SSc (dSSc) or limited SSc (lSSc) according to the revised classification of LeROY [17, 18]. Medications under use were obtained from medical records and were confirmed during medical appointments. Patients receiving immunosuppressive drugs for SSc at the time of inclusion were carefully evaluated since those medications can influence monocytes counts and function [9]. Only patients that received cyclophosphamide treatment at least 6 months prior to the interview were included. Disease duration was defined as the time interval since the onset of Raynaud's phenomenon or skin symptoms (whichever came first). Severity of skin involvement was assessed using the modified Rodnan skin score [19]. Laboratory test results including serology, presence of autoantibodies and pulmonary function tests such as assessment of lung diffusion capacity for carbon monoxide (DLCO) and forced vital capacity (FVC) performed in the period of 3 months before or after the peripheral blood sample collection were obtained in medical records. Patients with scleroderma in overlap syndrome with other connective tissue disease and/or infectious diseases (HIV, hepatitis C or B) were excluded.

Controls

Thirty-eight subjects age- and sex-matched to the SSc patients, with no previous history of autoimmune or hematological diseases and a normal complete blood cell (CBC) count (hemoglobin > 11.0 g/dl; white blood cells > $4 \times 10^3/mm^3$ and $< 12 \times 10^3/mm^3$; and platelets $> 150 \times 10^3/mm^3$) were recruited from a local blood donation center and at a Primary Health Care Service unit. The criteria for inclusion were the same as those used in blood donation.

Study design

This was a monocentric cross-sectional study carried out from October, 2016, to May, 2017.

Flow cytometry protocol

Peripheral blood samples were collected in ethylenediaminetetraacetic acid (EDTA) coated tubes. CBC was performed in a Sysmex XE-2100™ (Sysmex, Kobe, JPN) hematological counter and the total amount of peripheral blood monocytes was determined.

Flow cytometry immunophenotyping (FCI) to identify and characterize monocyte subpopulations was performed less than 4 h after blood sampling. About 1,000, 000 cells were placed into polystyrene tubes and were subjected to surface staining by incubation with titrated amounts of fluorochrome-conjugated monoclonal antibodies (MoAbs) against CD14 APC-H7 (clone MϕP9), CD64 BV421 (clone 10.1), CD16 BV510 (clone 3G8), HLA-DR PerCP-Cy5.5 (clone G46–6), CD206 APC (clone 19.2), CD169 BB515 (clone 7–239) and CD163 PE (clone GHI/61) for 30 min at room temperature and protected from light. All MoAbs were purchased from BD Biosciences (San Diego, USA). Red blood cells were lysed by incubation with 2 ml of lysing buffer (BD Biosciences) for 10 min. Samples were washed and resuspended in phosphate buffered saline (PBS). At least 30, 000 gated monocytes were acquired in an 8-color BD FACSCanto™ II flow cytometer (BD Biosciences) using FACSDiva™ software (BD Biosciences). Flow cytometer technical parameters were automatically set with BD Cytometer Setup and Tracking Beads (BD Biosciences). Daily internal quality control (QC) was performed with IMMUNO-TROL Cells (BD Biosciences).

Phenotypic analysis of monocyte subpopulations

Figure 1 shows the gating strategy used. Initially, doublets were excluded and total nucleated cells were selected based on FSC (forward scatter) versus SSC (side scatter) distribution. Monocytes were gated based on cell size and complexity, as well as CD64+ expression [20], and were plotted in a CD14 versus CD16 graph in order to characterize all three monocyte subpopulations: classical monocytes (CD14++CD16-), intermediate monocytes (CD14++CD16+) and non-classical monocytes

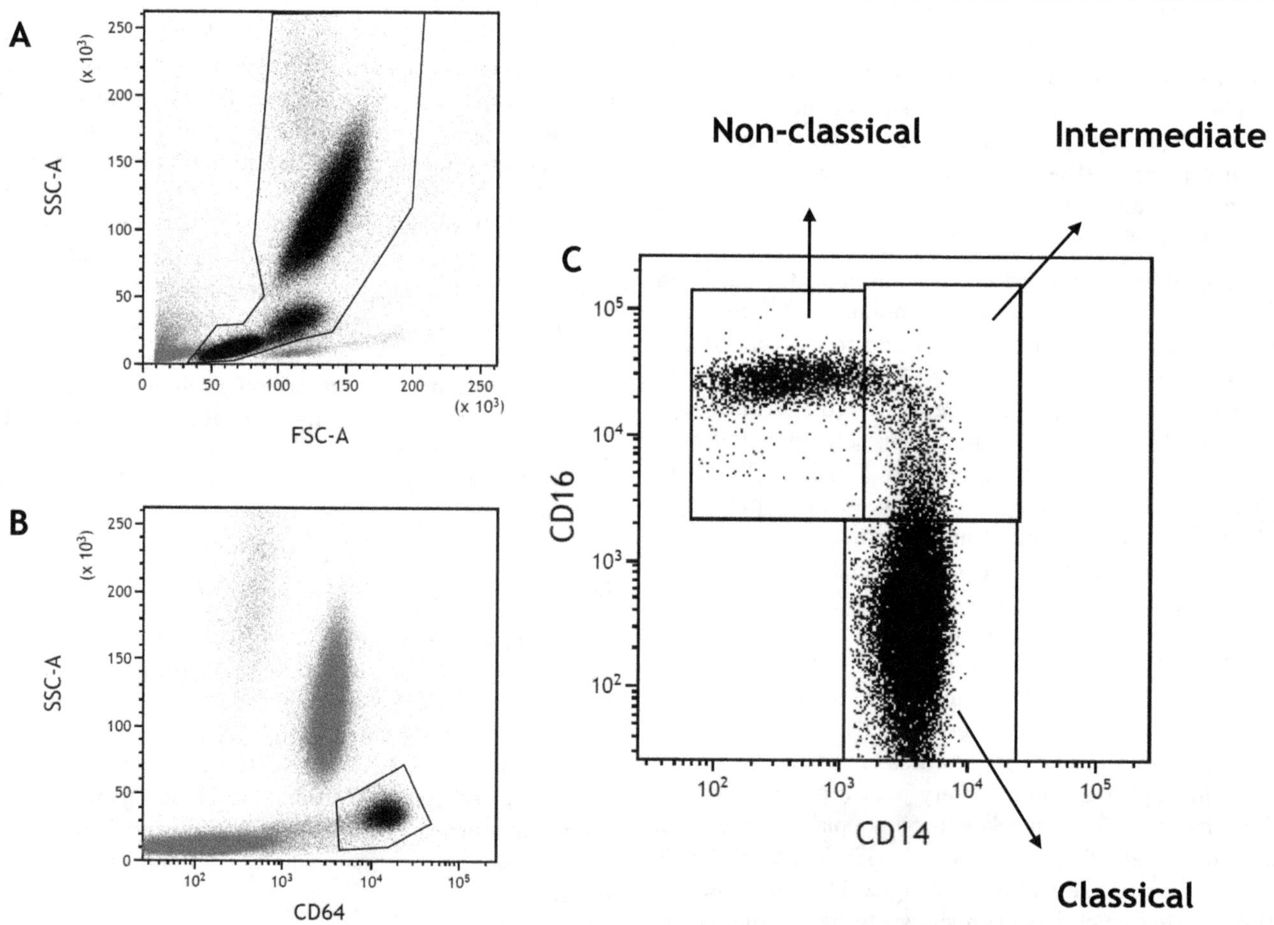

Fig. 1 Identification of monocyte subpopulations. **a** Cells were gated based on FSC (forward scatter) versus SSC (side scatter) distribution and doublets were excluded. **b** Monocytes were gated based on cell size and complexity, as well as CD64 expression. **c** Monocyte subpopulations were plotted in a CD14 versus CD16 expression in a representative healthy donor

(CD14+/−CD16++). Fluorescence-minus-one (FMO) methodology was used to differentiate autoflourescent events from events with low concentrations of cell surface markers [21]. All values obtained in this analysis were considered FMO limit and all values of fluorescence above the limit were considered as true positive. Percentage of expression and mean fluorescence intensity (MFI) of any given marker within the defined monocyte subpopulation were recorded. All FCI data were analyzed using Kaluza Analysis Software (Beckman Coulter Life Sciences, Indianapolis, USA) by two experienced operators concomitantly.

Compliance with ethical standards

This study was approved by the Research Ethics Committee of the institution (CAAE number

Table 1 Demographic, clinical, and laboratory features of systemic sclerosis patients and controls

	Systemic sclerosis patients (*n* = 50)	Healthy controls (*n* = 38)
Female gender (%)	47 (94.0) [a]	36 (94.7) [a]
Age (years)	57.2 ± 12.8 [b]	55.2 ± 11.4 [b]
European-derived (%)	40 (80)	24 (68.6)
Smoking status (%)		
Never	25 (50)	23 (65.7)
Previous	21 (42)	30 (29.7)
Current	4 (8)	2 (5.7)
Disease duration (years)	15 (7–21)	
Diffuse cutaneous involvement (%)	14 (28.0)	
Modified Rodnan skin score	6 (2.8–10.3)	
Renal crisis	4 (8.0)	
Gastrointestinal symptoms (%)		
Heartburn	25 (50.0)	
Dysphagia	26 (52.0)	
Diarrhea / constipation	21 (42.0)	
DLCO (% predicted)	70.1 ± 16.3	
Reduced DLCO (< 80% predicted)	52.9 (15.9)	
FVC (% predicted)	79.2 ± 18.9	
Reduced FVC (< 80% of predicted)	22 (44)	
PASP	31.7 ± 14.4	
Pulmonary hypertension (PASP ≥40 mmHg) (%)	5 (10)	
Autoantibodies (%)		
ANA	39/50 (78.0)	
Anti-Ro/SSA	1/45 (2.2)	
Anti-La/SSB	0/45 (0)	
Anti-Scl-70	4/44 (9.1)	
RF	35/50 (75.0)	
Medications (%)		
Prednisolone < 20 mg/day	6 (12)	
Mycophenolate mofetil	4 (8)	
Previous methotrexate administration	10 (20)	
Previous rituximab administration	2 (4)	
Previous cyclophosphamide administration	12 (24)	

Data are shown as mean (± standard deviation), median (interquartile ranges) or number (n)

ANA anti-nuclear antibodies, *Anti-dsDNA* anti-double-stranded DNA, *Anti-Scl70* antitopoisomerasel, *DLCO* diffusion capacity of carbon monoxide, *FVC* forced vital capacity, *PASP* arterial systolic pressure on Doppler echocardiography, *RF* rheumatoid factor, *SSc* systemic sclerosis

[a] Mann-Whitney test, $p = 1.000$

[b] Student's T test, $p = 0.448$

49299515.0.0000.5327) and was conducted in accordance with the Declaration of Helsinki and current laws in Brazil. Participants were included after written informed consent.

Statistical analysis

Variables distribution was analyzed by Shapiro-Wilk's test and continuous variables were compared by Student's T or Mann–Whitney's U test, whereas proportions were compared by Pearson's chi-square or Fisher's exact test. ANOVA or Kruskall-Wallis, with a Tukey or Dunn correction test was used for multiple comparisons. Pearson or Spearman correlation test was used to evaluate association between variables. The statistical significance level adopted was 5% ($p < 0.05$). Data analysis was carried out with SPSS version 21.0® (IBM, Chicago, USA) and Prisma 8 software (Graphpad Inc. San Diego, USA).

Results

Patients and controls characteristics

Demographic data and clinical characteristics of SSc and healthy control (HC) subjects are shown in Table 1. SSc patients mean age was 57.2 years and 94% were female. Limited form of disease was present in 72% of SSc patients. Median Rodnan skin score was 5 (2.0–8.0) in lSSc patients and 11 (3.8–16.8) in the dSSc patients (p = 0.007). Pulmonary function also differed among disease subgroups when comparing forced vital capacity (FVC%predicted) results: lSSc subjects had higher mean values when compared to dSSc patients (83.8 ± 17.4% versus 67.5 ± 18.2%, p = 0.005).

Circulating monocyte subpopulations

Main results of monocytes evaluation are show in Fig. 2. SSc patients had higher absolute and relative number of circulating monocytes when compared to HC (459.6 (322.9–550.3)/mm^3 versus 273.9 (179.3–352.2)/mm^3, $p < 0.001$), this difference remained significant when comparing lSSc or dSSc patients with HC independently (478.2 (342.9–555.5)/mm^3 versus 273.9 (179.3–352.2)/mm^3, $p < 0.001$; and 387.4 (310.4–551.1)/mm^3 versus 273.9 (179.3–352.2)/mm^3, $p = 0.002$, respectively) (data not shown). Among monocyte subpopulations, SSc patients had higher absolute counts of all subpopulations (classical, intermediate and non-classical) when compared to HC (classical monocytes 346.2 (260.9–450.8)/mm^3 versus 209.8 (146.1–287.1)/mm^3, $p < 0.001$; intermediate monocytes 38.2 (24.6–47.1)/mm^3 versus 25.4 (12.6–41.2)/mm^3, $p = 0.005$; non-classical monocytes 41.2 (20.8–58.3)/mm^3 versus 28.3 (11.5–46.1)/mm^3, p = 0.006) (data not shown). Regarding disease subtype, lSSc patients presented increased absolute values of all monocyte subpopulations when compared to HC (classical monocytes 363.2 (262.9–451.8)/mm^3 versus 209.8 (146.1–287.1)/mm^3, $p < 0.001$ (A); intermediate monocytes 38.5 (24.7–47.5)/mm^3 versus 25.4 (12.6–41.2)/mm^3, $p = 0.009$ (B); non-classical monocytes 42.5 (20.8–69.0)/mm^3 versus 28.3 (11.5–46.1)/mm^3, $p = 0.005$) (C). While in dSSc patients, only classical monocytes had increased absolute counts compared to HC (209.8 (146.1–287.1)/mm^3 versus 326.5 (231.2–461.9)/mm^3, $p = 0.003$) (A). There was no difference in monocytes absolute or relative values between lSSc and dSSc subgroups (p = 0.450 and p = 0.914, respectively).

Circulating CD16+ monocyte subpopulations

When analyzing intermediate and non-classical monocytes as a single group of CD16+ monocytes, we identified a higher absolute count of this subpopulation in lSSc patients compared to HC (79.9 (53.4–103.5)/mm^3 versus 55.9 (26.8–85.8)/mm^3, $p = 0.003$) (Fig. 2d).

Monocyte subpopulations and clinical manifestations

Absolute counts of monocyte subpopulations did not correlate with severity of cutaneous fibrosis assessed by the modified Rodnan skin score, pulmonary involvement assessed by DLCOc/VA, FVC and pulmonary artery systolic pressure, or disease duration when evaluated among the total of patients or in lSSc and dSSc subtypes (Fig. 3) (Additional files 1 and 2).

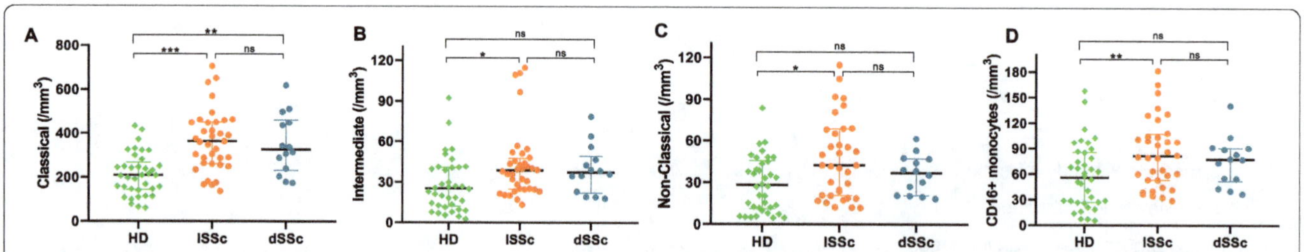

Fig. 2 Monocyte subpopulations according to their membrane expression of CD14 and CD16 in systemic sclerosis patients with limited (lSSc) (n = 36) and diffuse (dSSc) (n = 14) subtypes, and in healthy controls (HC) (n = 38). The absolute count of all monocyte subpopulations - classical **a**, intermediate **b** and non-classical **c** - is increased in lSSc compared to HC. **d** When analyzing intermediate and non-classical monocytes as a single group of CD16+ monocytes, their absolute value is increased in lSSc compared to HC. *$p < 0.05$; **$p < 0.01$; ***$p < 0.001$

Expression of surface receptors in monocyte subpopulations

Results of surface expression of HLA-DR, CD206, CD169 and CD163 receptors are shown in Fig. 4 and Additional file 3. There were different expression patterns among the evaluated monocyte subpopulations. HLA-DR, an activation marker, was consistently expressed in all monocytes from SSc and HC, and its intensity of expression was higher in all monocyte subsets from lSSc and dSSc patients when compared to control. CD206 expression varied among the monocyte subsets, the percentage of expression was higher in classical and intermediate monocytes of SSc patients when compared to HC and its MFI expression was lower in SSc as compared to HC. When analyzing SSc subgroups, percentage of CD206, the mannose receptor-1, expression was higher only in classical monocytes of lSSc patients compared to HC and in intermediate monocytes of lSSc and dSSc compared to HC; whereas MFI of CD206 expression was lower in both lSSc and dSSc classical monocytes when compared to HC. CD163, macrophage scavenger receptor, was more expressed in classical (percentage and MFI) and intermediate (percentage) monocytes of SSc patients as compared to HC. In subgroup analysis, a difference in CD163 expression was demonstrated in classical monocytes of lSSc subjects compared to the HC group. CD169 receptor had a higher percentage of expression in SSc versus HC. When evaluating SSc subtypes, classical and intermediate monocytes from dSSc patients had higher MFI and percentage of CD169 expression than lSSc and HC, whereas non-classical monocytes of dSSc patients had higher percentage of this marker expression (Fig. 4).

Further analyses were performed for comparison of the markers MFI of expression among the different monocyte subpopulations. Except for CD163 expression, the monocyte subpopulations exhibited distinct expression patterns when compared to one another,

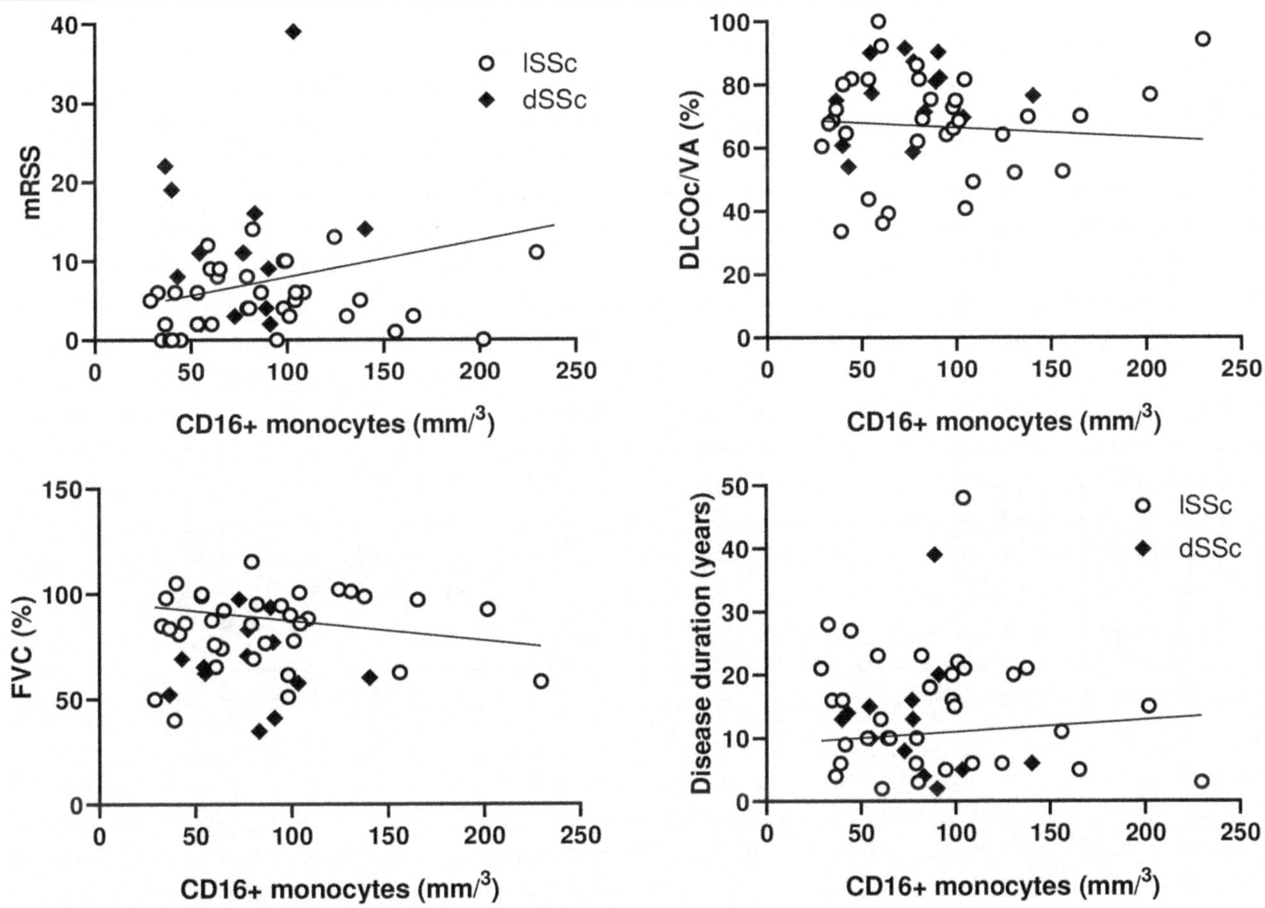

Fig. 3 Correlations regarding the CD16+ monocyte subpopulation. The CD16+ monocyte subpopulation of SSc patients ($n = 50$) and in the subgroup of patients presenting lSSc ($n = 36$) and dSSc ($n = 14$) was tested for association with cutaneous fibrosis assessed by the modified Rodnan skin score (mRSS), pulmonary involvement assessed by DLCOc/VA and FVC. Disease duration was not associated with CD16 + values. DLCO: diffusion capacity for carbon monoxide; FVC: forced vital capacity

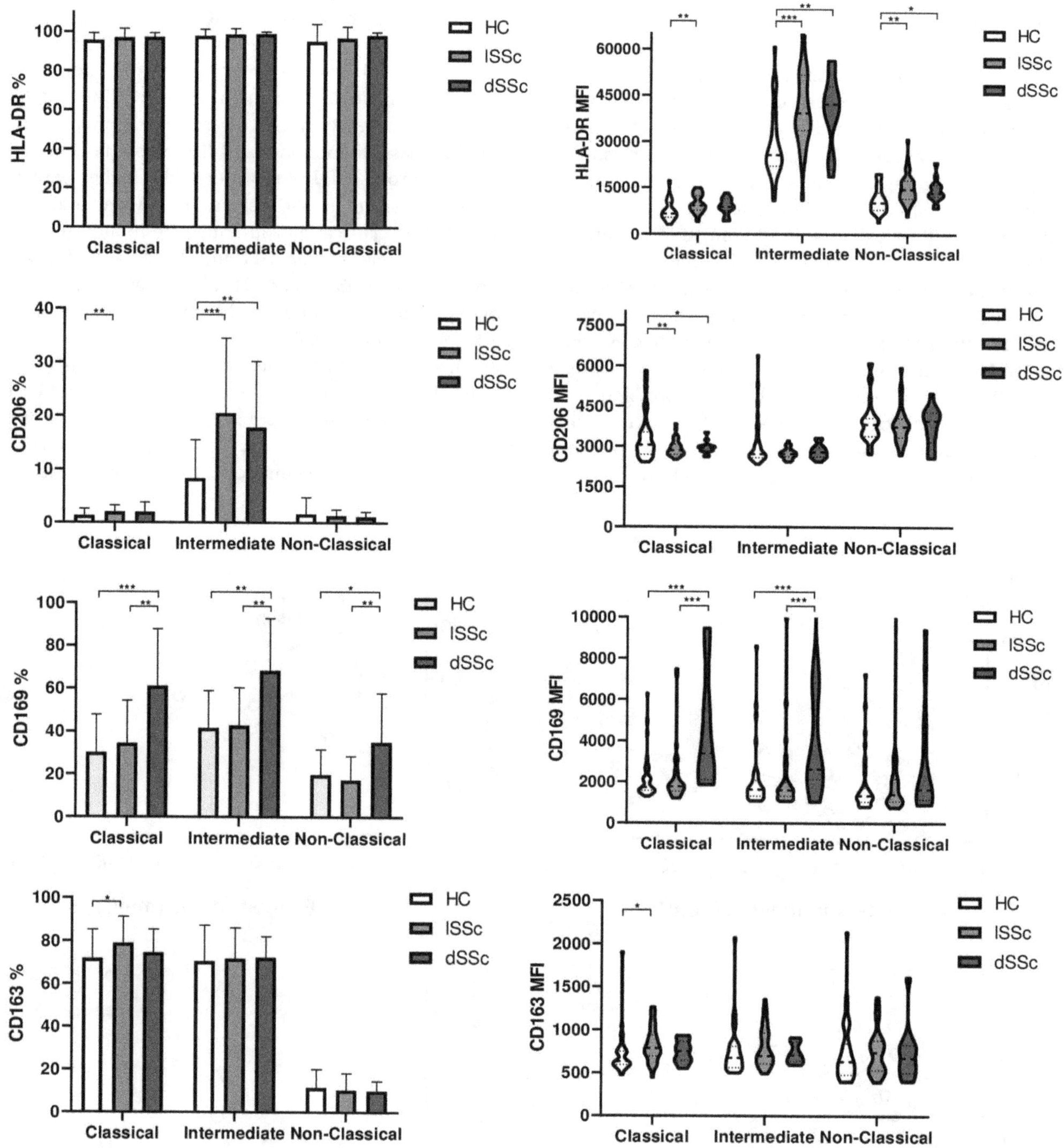

Fig. 4 Expression of surface receptors under study on monocyte subpopulations of systemic sclerosis patients divided by disease subtype in lSSc ($n = 36$) and dSSc ($n = 14$) compared with healthy controls (HC) ($n = 38$). ANOVA with Tukey correction for symmetric distribution and Kruskal-Wallis with Dunn correction for asymmetric distribution. MFI: mean fluorescence intensity. SSc: systemic sclerosis; HC: healthy controls; lSSc: limited systemic sclerosis; dSSc: diffuse systemic sclerosis. $^*p < 0.05$; $^{**}p < 0.01$; $^{***}p < 0.001$

which was similar among patients and HC subgroups (Additional file 3).

Discussion

In our study, monocytes percentage and absolute count were significantly increased in SSc patients as compared to healthy subjects, regardless of disease subtype. Monocytosis in SSc patients has been reported previously [5, 22]. Assessment of CD14 and CD16 receptors expression allowed the identification of all three monocyte subpopulations, as already described for healthy individuals and some disease states [9, 23–25]. However, our study is the first to describe these subpopulations in SSc patients, using specific markers CD14 and CD16 for such distinction according to positivity and MFI of expression.

We identified an increase in all monocyte subpopulations in SSc patients, which was even more significant in patients with lSSc. Interestingly, lSSc patients showed an increase of all three monocyte subpopulations compared to controls, whereas in dSSc patients that increase was at expense of classical monocytes, indicating that in this form of disease the CD16+ monocyte subpopulations does not increase. Recent studies in SSc patients have shown an increase in CD16+ monocytes in the peripheral blood of these patients, however, these studies did not distinguish between intermediate and non-classical subpopulations [5, 22].

Previous studies have shown a significant correlation of the absolute CD16+ monocyte subpopulation count and severity of skin fibrosis and pulmonary fibrosis [5 26]. In our study, we did not find correlations between monocyte subpopulations and the clinical manifestations evaluated. This difference may be related with intermediate and non-classical monocyte subpopulations grouped into CD16+ monocytes. Although differences among intermediate and non-classical monocyte subsets have been stablished [9, 10, 12], there is a strong proximity between them [9], suggesting a direct developmental relationship, where gain of CD16 expression and decrease in CD14 expression may be indicative of maturation [27] and inflammatory activation for these cells to be recruited to the periphery, where they begin to act in localized inflammatory processes [5]. In addition, there are resident tissue macrophages originated from the yolk sac or from fetal liver progenitors [28], that have long tissue life and self-renewing ability by in situ proliferation, even in the absence of recruitment from circulating monocytes [29–31]. The role of these macrophages in tissues during inflammation is still unclear and further research is needed on the role of circulating monocytes for their activation and proliferation, especially in inflammation models.

Our data corroborate the results obtained by Lescoat et al. (2017) and Trombetta et al. (2018) concerning the increased amount of circulating monocytes with CD16+ monocytes as the main representative monocyte subset in SSc patients [5, 32]. Nevertheless, our results differ regarding correlations with clinical manifestations. The fact that we did not find a correlation of monocyte subsets with clinical manifestations reinforces the hypothesis of cellular modulation and activation in loco, since the different tissues are able to direct the inflammatory response in order to exacerbate inflammation with pro-inflammatory mediators or into resolution and repair [33]. Hence, findings of monocyte/macrophage activation in the bloodstream may not be observed at the tissue level, specifically, in internal organs affected by SSc.

HLA-DR is a cell activation marker, so it is consistent to find a greater expression intensity of this marker in patients with autoimmune diseases when compared to normal subjects. We found an increase in MFI expression of HLA-DR in all monocyte subpopulations of SSc patients compared to HC. MFI of HLA-DR expression in CD16+ monocyte subpopulations (intermediate and non-classical) was significantly higher than that of CD16- classical monocytes, indicating a greater activation of CD16+ antigen-presenting cells, which is expected in an autoimmune state.

Other molecules, such as capture receptor CD163 and CD206 were also associated with M2 macrophages and could be involved into further differentiation processes. A previous study comparing the expression of monocyte and macrophage markers in peripheral blood and skin biopsy specimens showed higher percentages of circulating cells expressing CD204, CD163 and CD14, furthermore these findings were correlated with skin involvement [22].

Additionally, circulating CD14+ monocytes/macrophages with CD206 coexpression have been shown to be associated with pulmonary artery hypertension [13]. It has also been shown that macrophages derived from circulating monocytes have coexpression of CD206, CD163 and CD169, and that the expression of these markers is significantly higher in patients with pulmonary interstitial disease [3]. In our study, a higher percentage of classical and intermediate monocytes with CD206 expression were identified in SSc patients compared to HC, which demonstrates a greater amount of M2-like cells in those monocyte subgroups of SSc patients.

Using a flow cytometry approach for assessing surface markers from circulating monocytes/macrophages, Soldano et al. (2018) demonstrated that SSc patients have higher expression of the M2 related markers CD14, CD206, CD163 and CD204; or that there is a coexpression of M1 and M2 surface markers in those cells [34]; providing evidence of plasticity in the expression of this markers in circulating monocyte/macrophage and that monocytes can evolve to exhibit features that are shared by more than one macrophage population.

Previous studies have suggested that CD169 may be a phagocyte activity marker in inflammatory disorders. CD169 has been identified as a marker of highly pathogenic phagocytes in multiple sclerosis patients. Also, an increased expression of Siglec-1 on peripheral blood monocytes as well as its role in cell reactivity to autoantigen has been shown in rheumatoid arthritis [35, 36]. CD169 expression in renal macrophages has been correlated with proteinuria and tissue damage in glomerulonephritis [37], however its expression in peripheral blood cells was not assessed. CD169 expression has also been associated with involvement in the immune system regulation [38]. Biological functions of CD169 in macrophages and monocytes have yet to be elucidated. In our study, there was an increased expression of CD169 in classical monocytes from SSc patients compared to controls, and CD169 expression was higher in all monocyte subpopulations of dSSc patients compared to lSSc and controls. This finding could represent a greater disease activity in this subgroup of patients.

As to the use of medications, no association of these with subpopulations of monocytes was found. There were no differences between patients monocyte subpopulations regarding corticosteroids use ($n = 6$). Patients included in the study used low doses (less than 20 mg per day), similar to previous reports [5].

Our study has some limitations. First of all, the patient population appears to be relatively small. However, there were many restrictions for patient inclusion in order to minimize treatment interference and disease overlap. Evaluation of exclusively circulating cells is also a limitation. There is a need for simultaneous assessment of circulating cells and tissue biopsies to better understand the participation of macrophages derived from circulating monocytes in tissue fibrosis. We have evidence that monocytes and macrophages actually participate in SSc pathogenesis and that there are slight differences between tissues [1, 39], nevertheless, we need better strategies to analyze these cells and studies assessing different tissues and peripheral blood to determine whether these macrophages are derived from circulating monocytes or other cells. In addition, our findings should be interpreted in light of our sample characteristics. Considering the pathophysiological and clinical changes observed in SSc over time, different monocyte subpopulations could be observed in early phases of the disease. Also, monocytes activation may be influenced by different levels of immunosuppression and distinct mechanisms of action of immunosuppressive drug treatment.

Conclusions

In conclusion, our results showed that SSc patients have increased absolute counts of all three monocyte subpopulations and that there is no difference among monocyte subpopulations between lSSc and dSSc disease subtypes. Monocytes from SSc patients presented a more activated phenotypic profile which was suggestive of M2 cells, with higher expression of CD206. Opposing to previous reports, we did not find an association between monocyte subpopulations and major fibrotic manifestations. The intermediate and non-classical monocyte subpopulations of SSc patients have increase expression of HLA-DR. CD169 appears to be more representative marker for dSSc subtype, however, more studies are necessary to confirm that this is a good marker for differentiation of disease subtype.

Abbreviations

CBC: Complete blood cell; DLCO: Lung diffusion capacity for carbon monoxide; dSSc: Diffuse cutaneous systemic sclerosis; EDTA: Ethylenediaminetetraacetic acid; FCI: Flow cytometry immunophenotyping; FMO: Fluorescence-minus-one; FSC: Forward scatter; FVC: Forced vital capacity; HC: Healthy control; lSSc: Limited cutaneous systemic sclerosis; MFI: Mean fluorescence intensity; MoAbs: Monoclonal antibodies; MRC1: Mannose receptor-1; PBS: Phosphate buffered saline; QC: Quality control; Siglec-1: Sialic acid-binding Ig-like lectine I; SSc: Systemic sclerosis; SSC: Side scatter; Th: T helper; TLR: Toll-like receptor

Supplementary Information

Additional file 1: Table S1. Spearman correlation coefficient values between monocyte subpopulations and clinical data.

Additional file 2: Table S2. Analysis of the absolute of CD16 + in relation to the time of disease separated by tercil.

Additional file 3: Table S3. Comparison of the markers MFI of expression among the different monocyte subpopulations.

Acknowledgements

We would like to thank Fabiane Spagnol Pedrazzani, at the Department of Specialized Diagnostics of the Hospital de Clínicas de Porto Alegre, for her assistance in the design of the technical parameters for the flow cytometry protocol.

Authors' contributions

LS, VH, RX and RC designed the project. LS, NAM, VH, IFSM, CYU and RRP collected the data and were responsible for data analysis. LS standardized and performed the flow cytometry experiments. LS and NAM wrote the manuscript. VH, RX and RC reviewed the manuscript. All authors read and approved the final manuscript.

Author details

[1]Serviço de Reumatologia, Hospital de Clínicas de Porto Alegre, Universidade Federal do Rio Grande do Sul, 2350 Ramiro Barcelos St, Room 645, Porto Alegre, RS 90035-903, Brazil. [2]Programa de Pós Graduação em Medicina: Ciências Médicas, Universidade Federal do Rio Grande do Sul, Porto Alegre, Brazil. [3]Laboratório Zanol, Porto Alegre, Brazil. [4]Faculdade de Medicina, Universidade Federal do Rio Grande do Sul, Porto Alegre, Brazil.

References

1. Taroni JN, Greene CS, Martyanov V, Wood TA, Christmann RB, Farber HW, et al. A novel multi-network approach reveals tissue-specific cellular

modulators of fibrosis in systemic sclerosis. Genome Med. 2017;9(1):27.
2. Bossini-Castillo L, Simeon CP, Beretta L, Vonk MC, Callejas-Rubio JL, Espinosa G, et al. Confirmation of association of the macrophage migration inhibitory factor gene with systemic sclerosis in a large European population. Rheumatology (Oxford). 2011;50(11):1976–81. https://doi.org/10.1093/rheumatology/ker259.
3. Lescoat A, Ballerie A, Augagneur Y, Morzadec C, Vernhet L, Fardel O, et al. Distinct properties of human M-CSF and GM-CSF monocyte-derived macrophages to simulate pathological lung conditions in vitro: application to systemic and inflammatory disorders with pulmonary involvement. Int J Mol Sci. 2018;19(3):894.
4. Becker H, Willeke P, Schotte H, Domschke W, Gaubitz M. Macrophage migration inhibitory factor may contribute to vasculopathy in systemic sclerosis. Clin Rheumatol. 2008;27(10):1307–11. https://doi.org/10.1007/s10067-008-0960-7.
5. Lescoat A, Lecureur V, Roussel M, Sunnaram BL, Ballerie A, Coiffier G, et al. CD16-positive circulating monocytes and fibrotic manifestations of systemic sclerosis. Clin Rheumatol. 2017;36(7):1649–54. https://doi.org/10.1007/s10067-017-3597-6.
6. Ziegler-Heitbrock HW, Ströbel M, Kieper D, Fingerle G, Schlunck T, Petersmann I, et al. Differential expression of cytokines in human blood monocyte subpopulations. Blood. 1992;79(2):503–11. https://doi.org/10.1182/blood.V79.2.503.503.
7. Cros J, Cagnard N, Woollard K, Patey N, Zhang SY, Senechal B, et al. Human CD14dim monocytes patrol and sense nucleic acids and viruses via TLR7 and TLR8 receptors. Immunity. 2010;33(3):375–86. https://doi.org/10.1016/j.immuni.2010.08.012.
8. Auffray C, Sieweke MH, Geissmann F. Blood monocytes: development, heterogeneity, and relationship with dendritic cells. Annu Rev Immunol. 2009;27(1):669–92. https://doi.org/10.1146/annurev.immunol.021908.132557
9. Wong KL, Yeap WH, Tai JJ, Ong SM, Dang TM, Wong SC. The three human monocyte subsets: implications for health and disease. Immunol Res. 2012; 53(1–3):41–57. https://doi.org/10.1007/s12026-012-8297-3.
10. Passlick B, Flieger D, Ziegler-Heitbrock HW. Identification and characterization of a novel monocyte subpopulation in human peripheral blood. Blood. 1989;74(7):2527–34. https://doi.org/10.1182/blood.V74.7.2527.2527.
11. González-Domínguez É, Domínguez-Soto Á, Nieto C, Flores-Sevilla JL, Pacheco-Blanco M, Campos-Peña V, et al. Atypical activin a and IL-10 production impairs human CD16+ monocyte differentiation into anti-inflammatory macrophages. J Immunol. 2016;196(3):1327–37. https://doi.org/10.4049/jimmunol.1501177.
12. van Furth R. Origin and turnover of monocytes and macrophages. Curr Top Pathol. 1989;79:125–50. https://doi.org/10.1007/978-3-642-73855-5_6.
13. Christmann RB, Hayes E, Pendergrass S, Padilla C, Farina G, Affandi AJ, et al. Interferon and alternative activation of monocyte/macrophages in systemic sclerosis-associated pulmonary arterial hypertension. Arthritis Rheum. 2011; 63(6):1718–28. https://doi.org/10.1002/art.30318.
14. Gundra UM, Girgis NM, Ruckerl D, Jenkins S, Ward LN, Kurtz ZD, et al. Alternatively activated macrophages derived from monocytes and tissue macrophages are phenotypically and functionally distinct. Blood. 2014; 123(20):e110–22. https://doi.org/10.1182/blood-2013-08-520619.
15. York MR, Nagai T, Mangini AJ, Lemaire R, van Seventer JM, Lafyatis R. A macrophage marker, Siglec-1, is increased on circulating monocytes in patients with systemic sclerosis and induced by type I interferons and toll-like receptor agonists. Arthritis Rheum. 2007;56(3):1010–20. https://doi.org/10.1002/art.22382.
16. van den Hoogen F, Khanna D, Fransen J, Johnson SR, Baron M, Tyndall A, et al. 2013 classification criteria for systemic sclerosis: an American College of Rheumatology/European league against rheumatism collaborative initiative. Arthritis Rheum. 2013;65(11):2737–47. https://doi.org/10.1002/art.38098.
17. Johnson SR, Feldman BM, Hawker GA. Classification criteria for systemic sclerosis subsets. J Rheumatol. 2007;34(9):1855–63.
18. LeRoy EC, Medsger TA. Criteria for the classification of early systemic sclerosis. J Rheumatol. 2001;28(7):1573–6.
19. Clements P, Lachenbruch P, Siebold J, White B, Weiner S, Martin R, et al. Inter and intraobserver variability of total skin thickness score (modified Rodnan TSS) in systemic sclerosis. J Rheumatol. 1995;22(7):1281–5.
20. Wong KL, Tai JJ, Wong WC, Han H, Sem X, Yeap WH, et al. Gene expression profiling reveals the defining features of the classical, intermediate, and nonclassical human monocyte subsets. Blood. 2011;118(5):e16–31. https://doi.org/10.1182/blood-2010-12-326355.
21. Roederer M. Compensation in flow cytometry. Curr Protoc Cytom. 2002; Chapter 1:Unit 1.14.
22. Higashi-Kuwata N, Jinnin M, Makino T, Fukushima S, Inoue Y, Muchemwa FC, et al. Characterization of monocyte/macrophage subsets in the skin and peripheral blood derived from patients with systemic sclerosis. Arthritis Res Ther. 2010;12(4):R128. https://doi.org/10.1186/ar3066.
23. Rossol M, Kraus S, Pierer M, Baerwald C, Wagner U. The CD14(bright) CD16+ monocyte subset is expanded in rheumatoid arthritis and promotes expansion of the Th17 cell population. Arthritis Rheum. 2012;64(3):671–7. https://doi.org/10.1002/art.33418.
24. Cavaliere FM, Prezzo A, Bilotta C, Iacobini M, Quinti I. The lack of BTK does not impair monocytes and polymorphonuclear cells functions in X-linked agammaglobulinemia under treatment with intravenous immunoglobulin replacement. PLoS One. 2017;12(4):e0175961. https://doi.org/10.1371/journal.pone.0175961.
25. Burbano C, Vasquez G, Rojas M. Modulatory effects of CD14+CD16++ monocytes on CD14++CD16- monocytes: a possible explanation of monocyte alterations in systemic lupus erythematosus. Arthritis Rheum. 2014;66(12):3371–81. https://doi.org/10.1002/art.38860.
26. Mahoney JM, Taroni J, Martyanov V, Wood TA, Greene CS, Pioli PA, et al. Systems level analysis of systemic sclerosis shows a network of immune and profibrotic pathways connected with genetic polymorphisms. PLoS Comput Biol. 2015;11(1):e1004005. https://doi.org/10.1371/journal.pcbi.1004005.
27. Lambert C, Preijers FWMB, Yanikkaya Demirel G, Sack U. Monocytes and macrophages in flow: an ESCCA initiative on advanced analyses of monocyte lineage using flow cytometry. Cytometry B Clin Cytom. 2017; 92(3):180–8.
28. Yona S, Kim KW, Wolf Y, Mildner A, Varol D, Breker M, et al. Fate mapping reveals origins and dynamics of monocytes and tissue macrophages under homeostasis. Immunity. 2013;38(1):79–91. https://doi.org/10.1016/j.immuni.2012.12.001.
29. Davies LC, Rosas M, Jenkins SJ, Liao CT, Scurr MJ, Brombacher F, et al. Distinct bone marrow-derived and tissue-resident macrophage lineages proliferate at key stages during inflammation. Nat Commun. 2013;4(1):1886. https://doi.org/10.1038/ncomms2877.
30. Hashimoto D, Chow A, Noizat C, Teo P, Beasley MB, Leboeuf M, et al. Tissue-resident macrophages self-maintain locally throughout adult life with minimal contribution from circulating monocytes. Immunity. 2013;38(4): 792–804. https://doi.org/10.1016/j.immuni.2013.04.004.
31. Jenkins SJ, Ruckerl D, Cook PC, Jones LH, Finkelman FD, van Rooijen N, et al. Local macrophage proliferation, rather than recruitment from the blood, is a signature of TH2 inflammation. Science. 2011;332(6035):1284–8. https://doi.org/10.1126/science.1204351.
32. Trombetta AC, Soldano S, Contini P, Tomatis V, Ruaro B, Paolino S, et al. A circulating cell population showing both M1 and M2 monocyte/macrophage surface markers characterizes systemic sclerosis patients with lung involvement. Respir Res. 2018;19(1):186. https://doi.org/10.1186/s12931-018-0891-z.
33. Matzinger P, Kamala T. Tissue-based class control: the other side of tolerance. Nat Rev Immunol. 2011;11(3):221–30.
34. Soldano S, Trombetta AC, Contini P, Tomatis V, Ruaro B, Brizzolara R, et al. Increase in circulating cells coexpressing M1 and M2 macrophage surface markers in patients with systemic sclerosis. Ann Rheum Dis. 2018;77(12): 1842–5. https://doi.org/10.1136/annrheumdis-2018-213648.
35. Bogie JF, Boelen E, Louagie E, Delputte P, Elewaut D, van Horssen J, et al. CD169 is a marker for highly pathogenic phagocytes in multiple sclerosis. Mult Scler. 2018;24(3):290–300. https://doi.org/10.1177/1352458517698759.
36. Xiong YS, Cheng Y, Lin QS, Wu AL, Yu J, Li C, et al. Increased expression of Siglec-1 on peripheral blood monocytes and its role in mononuclear cell reactivity to autoantigen in rheumatoid arthritis. Rheumatology (Oxford). 2014;53(2):250–9. https://doi.org/10.1093/rheumatology/ket342.
37. Ikezumi Y, Suzuki T, Hayafuji S, Okubo S, Nikolic-Paterson DJ, Kawachi H, et al. The sialoadhesin (CD169) expressing a macrophage subset in human proliferative glomerulonephritis. Nephrol Dial Transplant. 2005;20(12):2704–13. https://doi.org/10.1093/ndt/gfi105.
38. Oetke C, Vinson MC, Jones C, Crocker PR. Sialoadhesin-deficient mice exhibit subtle changes in B- and T-cell populations and reduced immunoglobulin M levels. Mol Cell Biol. 2006;26(4):1549–57. https://doi.org/10.1128/MCB.26.4.1549-1557.2006.
39. Stifano G, Christmann RB. Macrophage involvement in systemic sclerosis: do we need more evidence? Curr Rheumatol Rep. 2016;18(1):2. https://doi.org/10.1007/s11926-015-0554-8.

9

Unstimulated whole salivary flow in Sjögren's Syndrome

María Alejandra Martínez-Ceballos[1*], Natalia Aguilera[1], Kenny Carolina Garzón-González[2], Jairo Cajamarca-Baron[3], Juan Pablo Alzate-Granados[1] and Adriana Rojas-Villarraga[4]

Abstract

Background: Sjögren's Syndrome compromises the exocrine function, producing xerostomia and xerophthalmia. It can appear as an isolated condition or associated with other autoimmune diseases (polyautoimmunity). The Unstimulated Salivary Flow rate (UWSF) is used to quantify saliva production. There is no objective evidence to differentiate the values in patients with Sjögren's versus healthy people or patients with non-Sjögren's sicca. The objective of the present review was to evaluate the UWSF in patients with Sjögren's syndrome in comparison to controls (healthy and non-Sjögren's sicca patients).

Methods: A systematic literature review was carried out (PRISMA guidelines). Analytical observational studies of cases and controls, cross-sectional studies, cohort studies and randomized clinical trials (including healthy controls) were considered. The Medline/OVID, Lilacs, Embase, and Cochrane/OVID databases were consulted. MeSH, DeCS, keywords, and Boolean operators were used. The meta-analysis (RevMan 5.2) was done through the random-effects model [mean difference (MD)]. Level and quality of evidence were evaluated by the Oxford Center Levels of Evidence and Joanna Brigs list respectively.

Results: Thirty-two articles were included (20 were case-control studies, 6 were cross-sectional, 2 prospective cohort, 2 retrospective cohort, and 2 studies were abstracts) and 28 were meta-analyzed. The unstimulated whole salivary flow rate in the Sjögren's group was lower than in controls (healthy and patients with non-Sjögren Sicca syndrome) (MD-0.18 ml/min; 95% CI, − 0.24 to − 0.13; chi^2-P-value < 0.00001). Heterogeneity was 97% and there was publication bias (funnel plot). The level of evidence was mostly 3 or 4. The quality of evidence was met (97% of items valued).

Conclusion: For the first time, the unstimulated whole salivary flow rate is found to be lower in patients with Sjögren's syndrome compared to controls (healthy and non-SS sicca) through a meta-analysis.

Trial registration: PROSPERO CRD42020211325.

Keywords: Sjögren's syndrome, Salivary glands, Xerostomia, Autoimmune diseases, Autoimmunity

* Correspondence: mariamace9@gmail.com

[1] Research Division Fundación Universitaria de Ciencias de la Salud (FUCS), Bogotá, Colombia

Introduction

Sjögren's Syndrome (SS) is a chronic autoimmune disease that compromises the function of the exocrine glands in the skin and mucosa of the eyes, mouth, etc. and it results in predominantly xerophthalmia and xerostomia [1]. SS could appear as an isolated disease (Primary Sjögren Syndrome (pSS)), or associated with another autoimmune pathology (Secondary Sjögren Syndrome (sSS)) such as autoimmune thyroid disease (15–30%), rheumatoid arthritis (4–31%), systemic lupus erythematosus (9–19%), and systemic sclerosis (14%). Recently this association was named polyautoimmunity [2].

SS is among the most frequent systemic autoimmune rheumatic diseases. The prevalence is around 0.3 to 1 case per 1000 persons [3], and it has an annual incidence of 6.92 cases per 100,000 people [4]. It is a frequent condition in women with a 9:1 female/male ratio and a high frequency of diagnosis at the age of 50 [3].

The physio-pathological mechanisms of SS are unknown. However, the epithelial destruction of the exocrine gland by an abnormal T (especially Th1 and Th17) and B cell response to specific auto-antigens such as Ro/SSA and La/SSB (autoimmune epithelitis) is described. The etiology for the development of this disease is multifactorial and includes genetic, epigenetic, hormonal, and environmental factors [5].

SS is classified according to American College of Rheumatology/European League against Rheumatism (ACR/EULAR) criteria. It includes the presence of ocular (objective tests) or oral gland hypofunction (by means of sialometry), specific autoantibodies, and focal lymphocytic infiltrates in the minor salivary gland. The ACR/EULAR criteria have to be applied to patients with suspected SS due to dry eye and dry mouth symptoms (at least one positive response from five established dryness questions), salivary gland enlargement, or extraglandular compromise (at least one item from ESSDAI (EULAR Sjögren's syndrome disease activity index)) [6].

Up to 80% of patients suffer dry eye and dry mouth symptoms, the key manifestations of SS. The clinical picture is also associated with systemic (e.g. asthenia and articular pain) or extraglandular manifestations in 40% [3].

There are procedures that objectively measure saliva production. The sample can be taken from an isolated salivary gland or several that are combined during rest [Unstimulated Whole Salivary Flow (UWSF)] or with stimulation [Stimulated Whole Salivary Flow (SWSF)] [7]. The measurement of UWSF is a quick, easy, and non-invasive test, and it is an item in the classification criteria for SS. Recently, the EULAR developed recommendations for the management of Sjögren's syndrome with topical and systemic therapies [8]. They emphasized that the therapeutic approach to oral dryness should be driven by the baseline measurement of salivary glandular function (UWSF), and not by the patient's subjective feelings since environmental and personal stress factors may influence the subjective feeling of dryness.

The main concern here is the production of saliva measured by the UWSF. Several studies, including systematic literature reviews and meta-analyses have evaluated saliva production in patients with xerostomia in different non-SS autoimmune diseases such as systemic lupus erythematosus, type I diabetes mellitus [9], autoimmune thyroid diseases, oral lichen planus [10, 11], systemic sclerosis [12], juvenile idiopathic arthritis [13]. All of these have shown a lower rate of saliva production compared to healthy controls. Nevertheless, we were unable to find saliva production results for patients with SS as a primary disease in our search.

In the context of SS, a value of ≤0.1 ml/min is included in the ACR/EULAR SS criteria [14]. Nevertheless, this cut-off point went through a transition over a period of years, and it is included in or excluded from the different proposed international criteria [6, 14–20]. However, the justification for these changes is not clear in the literature even though it is a diagnostic criterion with the same weight as eye tests (Schirmer and ocular staining score) for an SS diagnosis. The established values in these criteria differentiated salivary gland hypofunction only in patients with sicca symptoms versus healthy controls, but not in patients with SS.

Therefore, in this systematic literature review and meta-analysis, the intention is to evaluate the saliva production through the UWSF in SS patients compared to non-SS patients with sicca symptoms and healthy controls in order to show objective differences between the diverse study groups.

Materials and methods

Search strategy

A systematic literature review was done to identify the articles that report UWSF values in patients with SS versus healthy subjects or patients with non-SS sicca symptoms. PRISMA guidelines [21] were followed for reporting systematic reviews and meta-analysis. Medline/OVID, Lilacs, Embase, and Cochrane/OVID were searched up to July 20th, 2020. Medical Subject Heading terms (MesH): "Adult," "Sjogren's Syndrome," "Sjogrens, " "Sjögren," "Sjögren's," "Sjogren," "Gougerot," "Gougerot-Sjogren," "Gougerot-Sjögren," "Primitive Gougerot-Sjögren," "Gougerot-Sjögren," "Gougerot-Houwers-Sjögren," "Unstimulated salivary flow," "USF," "Unstimulated whole salivary flow," "Whole unstimulated salivary flow," "Unstimulated saliva," "Basal salivary flow," "Sialometry," "Whole unstimulated salivation" were used. MeSH terms were crossed with keywords using boolean operators (OR, AND, NOT) and wild cards (Table 1). The search was not restricted by year,

Table 1 Search Strategy

Population:

Adult [Mesh]

Exposition:

"Sjogren's Syndrome"[Mesh]
Sjögren's syndrome
Sjogren syndrome
Sjögren syndrome
Sjogren disease
Sjögren disease
Sjogren's disease
Sjögren's disease
Sjögren
Sjögren's
Sjogren
Sjogren's
Gougerot
Gougerot Sjogren
Gougerot Sjögren
Gougerot-Sjogren
Gougerot-Sjögren
Gougerot Sjogren syndrome
Gougerot Sjögren syndrome
Gougerot-Sjogren syndrome
Gougerot-Sjögren syndrome
Gougerot Sjogren disease
Gougerot Sjögren disease
Gougerot-Sjogren disease
Gougerot-Sjögren disease
Gougerot Sjogren
Gougerot Sjögren
Gougerot-Sjogren
Gougerot-Sjögren
Gougerot Sjogren syndrome
Gougerot Sjögren syndrome
Gougerot-Sjogren syndrome
Gougerot-Sjögren syndrome
Gougerot Sjogren disease
Gougerot Sjögren disease
Gougerot-Sjogren disease
Gougerot-Sjögren disease
Primitive Gougerot-Sjögren syndrome
Gougerot-Houwers-Sjögren syndrome
Gougerot-Houwers-Sjögren disease

Outcome:

Unstimulated salivary flow
USF

Table 1 Search Strategy *(Continued)*

Unstimulated salivary flow rate
Unstimulated whole salivary flow
Whole unstimulated salivary flow
Whole USF
Unstimulated saliva
Decreased unstimulated saliva
Unstimulated saliva measurement
Basal salivary flow
Basal sialometry
Unstimulated sialometry
Unstimulated whole sialometry
Whole unstimulated sialometry
Whole unstimulated salivation
"Salivary elimination"[Mesh]

Search Strategy:

1. Adult/exp
2. Adult.tw
3. Adults.tw
4. Sjogren's Syndrome/exp
5. (Sjogren's Syndrome).tw
6. Sjogrens.tw
7. Sjögren.tw
8. Sjögren's.tw
9. Sjogren.tw
10. Sjogren's.tw
11. Gougerot.tw
12. Gougerot-Sjogren.tw
13. Gougerot-Sjögren.tw
14. (Primitive Gougerot-Sjögren).tw
15. (Primitive adj3 Gougerot-Sjögren).tw
16. Gougerot-Houwers-Sjögren.tw
17. (Unstimulated salivary flow).tw
18. (Unstimulated adj3 salivary adj3 flow).tw
19. USF.tw
20. (Unstimulated whole salivary flow).tw
21. (Unstimulated adj3 whole adj3 salivary adj3 flow).tw
22. (Whole unstimulated salivary flow).tw
23. (Whole adj3 unstimulated adj3 salivary adj3 flow).tw
24. (Unstimulated saliva).tw
25. (Unstimulated adj3 saliva).tw
16. (Basal salivary flow).tw
27. (Basal adj3 salivary adj3 flow).tw
28. sialometry.tw
29. (Whole unstimulated salivation).tw
30. (Whole adj3 unstimulated adj3 salivation).tw

language, or country of origin, but filters for species (humans) and ages (Adult) were applied. This review was registered in the international prospective registry of systematic reviews (PROSPERO) with registration number CRD42020211325.

Inclusion criteria

Study design

Analytical observational studies of cases and controls, cross-sectional studies, cohort studies and randomized clinical trials (including healthy controls).

Population

Patients 18 years of age or older, with sicca symptoms and SS diagnosis based on established criteria: ACR/EULAR, AECG (American-European Consensus Group), and Fox et al. [14, 18, 22].

Intervention

UWSF measurement by any method of collection.

Control group

Patients with non-SS sicca symptoms and/or healthy subjects.

Exclusion criteria

Studies that compare with other autoimmune diseases.
Pregnant women.

Data extraction and quality assessment

Two reviewers (NA and CG) independently screened titles and abstracts to determine the initial eligibility. After the screening phase, the same two reviewers evaluated the selected abstracts and full text independently (software Mendeley Desktop v1.19.2) to evaluate their inclusion based on the established criteria. Another two reviewers (ARV and MAM) resolved disagreements by discussing them until they reached a final consensus.

The level of evidence and methodological quality assessment was done by two independent reviewers (NA and ARV) using the Oxford Centre for Evidence-Based Medicine 2011 Levels of Evidence Question (OCEBM) [23] and Joanna Briggs Checklists [24].

Two independent reviewers (MAM and JPA) extracted the data using a Microsoft Excel® (v. 2013) database. The UWSF measures were unified to ml/min, and the values reported in the subgroups were averaged. The central tendencies and dispersion measures (mean and standard deviation) were imputed. The expert reviewer (ARV) independently verified the abovementioned values. Two authors (JPA and MAM) registered the extracted data in the Review Manager Software 5.2® and the two authors inconsistencies were corrected.

The following data were taken out: First author name, study year, study design, objective of the study, country, number of cases with SS (primary SS and SS with polyautoimmunity), number of controls (non-SS sicca symptoms and/or healthy subjects), number of women, age, disease duration, UWSF, stimulated salivary flow rate (SSF), comorbidities, and pharmacological therapy in cases and controls.

Data analysis

Statistical analysis was done with Review Manager Software® (RevMan 5.2). After that, data from the articles chosen were merged using the random-effects model (DerSimonian and Laird) due to the studies' high heterogeneity (sample size, saliva collection technique, and classification criteria for SS) to establish a global summary measure (overall effect).

The meta-analysis measurement considered the possible effects of the exposure as an average of ranges. The final effect size was presented as a mean difference with a confidence interval and the respective *P*-value. The forest plot was used to show the weight of each study.

Heterogeneity was assessed using the Chi^2 statistic, and the I^2 (Higgins). I^2 values of 25, 50, and 75% corresponding to low, medium, and high levels of heterogeneity respectively were considered. In addition, substantial heterogeneity was established if the value of the Chi^2 test was less than one. To evaluate the robustness of results and to identify the potential sources of heterogeneity, a sensitivity analysis and a subgroup analysis were done. Publication bias was graphically assessed by visual inspection of the funnel plot and confirmed using the Egger's regression test.

Results

Search results

The first search identified 569 articles. Two reviewers evaluated the studies by title and abstract and chose 133 without duplicates. The second round was done based on full text and 32 articles were selected. There was a total of 28 studies included in the quantitative synthesis. Figure 1 shows the PRISMA flow-diagram. Causes of exclusion are detailed in Table 2.

Of the articles included by full text, 20 were case-control studies, 6 were cross-sectional, 2 prospective cohort, 2 retrospective cohort, and 2 studies were abstracts and there was not enough information to establish the type of study and quality of evidence. The level and quality of evidence are shown in Table 3. The level of evidence for most of the articles was 3 or 4 using OCEBM guidelines and the quality of evidence was around 97% for all articles.

The 32 articles included correspond to approximately 3262 patients. Of these, 46.8% (1528) were cases, and

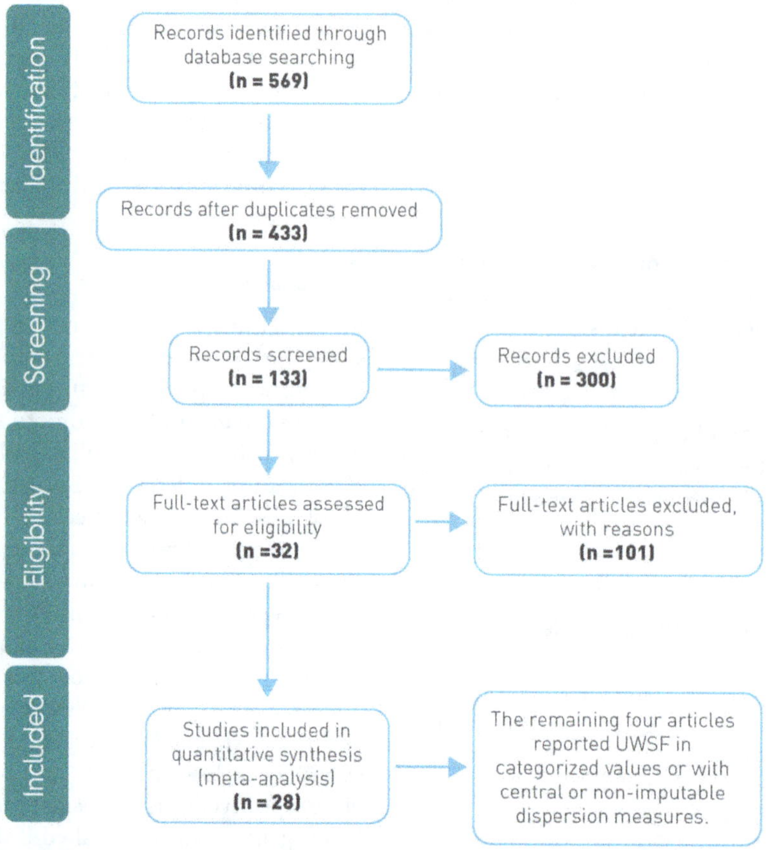

Fig. 1 PRISMA Flow-Diagram of article selection

53.2% (1734) were controls. The age range of cases was 39 to 63 years old while the age range was 24 to 69 for controls. The female sex was the most frequent in both groups. With respect to patients with SS, 66% (1010) had pSS, around 25.3% (386) had SS, and 8.6% (132) suffered from polyautoimmunity. Furthermore, patients with non-SS sicca came to 54.5% (946), and healthy people were 45.5% (788) of the group of controls. In total, 28 articles were meta-analyzed to evaluate the differences in UWSF between patients with SS and controls (healthy subjects and patients with non-SS sicca). The UWSF in the remaining four articles could not be analyzed because the authors did not report absolute values. The total number of people in these 28 articles was 2759 patients and of these, 49.1% (1356) were cases. Of these, 63.8% (866) had pSS, 26.5% (359) had SS, and 9.7% (131) had polyautoimmunity. Around 93% (725) were female. Of the total, 50.9% (1403) were controls, and of the controls, 43.8% (615) had non-SS sicca symptoms and 56.2% (788) were healthy subjects. Female sex was also predominant and accounted for about 83.74% (567).

Of the studies included in the meta-analysis, 13 were based on standardized methods of which the most widely used is that of Navazesh et al. [25], followed by Vitali et al. [26], and Sreebny et al. [27]. The method used by Navazesh et al. [25], requires fasting, no smoking, no chewing gum, nor having any oral cavity procedures done for at least 1 h before the exam. It also requires 5 min of rest prior to the test during which orofacial movements must be minimized. Then, residual saliva must be swallowed before starting the procedure, and saliva must be expelled every minute for a period of 15 min during it.

Meta-analysis results

The pooled analysis demonstrated a lower UWSF in patients with SS [Mean difference (MD) -0.18 ml/min; 95% CI, − 0.24 to − 0.13; chi^2-P-value < 0.00001] compared to controls (healthy subjects and patients with non-SS sicca) under a random-effects model. The I^2 statistic, which estimates the total variability in the effect size, was calculated to be 97% (Fig. 2) and could be attributed to heterogeneity among the true effects.

A subgroup analysis (heterogeneity of 98%) of patients with pSS reported that they had a lower UWSF compared to controls (healthy subjects and patients with non-SS sicca) (MD − 0.24 ml/min; 95% CI, − 0.32 to − 0.16; chi^2-P-Value < 0.00001). The comparison of pSS versus non-SS

Table 2 Reasons for excluding the discarded articles

Authors	Reason
T. A Alfaya et al.	A case report
S. Furness et al.	A narrative review
S. Nusair, et al.	A literature Review
D. Guellec et al.	A systematic review
L. J Dawson et al.	All patients had SS
K. Haldorsen et al.	
A. K Johansson et al.	
D. Zoukhri et al.	
N. L Rhodus et al.	
Atkinson JC, et al.	
Lundström IM, et al	
Haga, HJ, et al.	
Fei YY, et al.	
A. M. Al-Hamad et al.	
K. Marton et al.	All the patients had sicca symptoms, but no confirmed diagnosis of SS
J. M Meijer et al.	Clinical trial with rituximab in patients with pSS
T. E Daniels et al.	Controls not included
Kojima, I et al.	
Koh, JH et al.	
Liu, X et al.	
J. Y Kang et al.	Correlations between scintigraphic parameters and whole salivary flow rate mentioned
T. Mandl et al.	Data difficult to obtain. UWSF values are categorized
A. Ardita et al.	Included only patients with SS and another autoimmune disease. UWSF VNM
I.Castro et al.	Inclusion criteria not fulfilled
M. R Hillen et al.	It is a letter to the editor. UWSF VNM
C. Manterola Delgado et al.	It is a study about esophageal motility. UWSF VNM
C. Vitali et al.	It is hard to obtain the data
K. Ayar et al.	It is not clear which patients with celiac disease had SS
M. T Brennan et al.	Measure of saliva production only reported by submandibular and parotid gland
H. J. Haga et al.	No healthy controls or patients with non-SS sicca
H. F Oliveira et al.	
J. P Aitken-Saavedra et al.	
S. Gotoh et al.	Only measure of saliva production by labial gland reported
Y. J Lee et al.	Other autoimmune non-SS diseases included
H. Asashima et al.	Patients with primary and polyautoimmunity compared
H. Ben-Aryeh et al.	Patients with sicca symptoms compared, but the SS group of patients not reported
H. Flink et al.	Patients with SS not included
Hernández C, et al.	Saliva is measured in mm with a filter paper.
E. M Hay et al.	The patients did not have SS diagnosis
A.M Lindvall et al.	They did not state how they diagnosed SS
E. Benedek -spät et al.	They report only a measurement of saliva production by parotid gland
K. Márton et al.	UWSF in patients with dental prostheses reported. No SS subjects mentioned
N. L. Rhodus et al.	UWSF of patients with SS vs sicca symptoms not distinguished. Values of entire population with xerostomia mentioned
A. Bookman et al.	UWSF values are categorized
C. N Carvalho et al.	
S. Retamozo et al.	

Table 2 Reasons for excluding the discarded articles *(Continued)*

Authors	Reason
J. W Kim et al.	
T. Mandl et al.	UWSF values in controls not mentioned
S. Dugonjić et al.	
Y. Fleissig et al.	
S. S De Rossi et al.	
S. Dugonjić et al.	
A. K. Rosztóczy et al.	
D. Martini et al.	
S. Gotoh et al.	
B. M Liquidato et al.	UWSF values not mentioned, and data is duplicated from previous article
Y. Zhao et al.	UWSF values not reported and control group included patients with other autoimmune diseases
L. P Longman et al.	UWSF values per group not mentioned
Y. T Konttinen et al.	UWSF VNM
S. K Mandal et al.	
M. Schiodt et al.	
A. Alunno et al.	
L. T. H Jacobss et al.on	
L. P. Longman et al.	
C. Aguilera et al.	
J. Rostron et al.	
J. Booker et al.	
M. Koseki et al.	
B.M Liquidato et al.	
M. H Munshed, et al.	
K. Yamamoto et al.	
Nikolov N, et al.	
S. Osailan et al.	
G. Proctor et al.	
T. Fujibayashi et al.	
W. P. G. Holbrook et al.	
S. Yamachika et al.	
H.J Haga et al.	
C. Baldini et al.	
T. Jarai et al.	
N. Luciano et al.	
A. Rasmussen et al.	
L. Gueiros et al.	
K. M Leehan et al.	
J.Jayakanthan et al.	
P. Wei et al.	
E. Mossel et al.	
A. Vissink et al.	
D. Cornec et al.	
J. A Ice et al.	
E. J Nam et al.	
D. S Hammenfors et al.	
E. Mossel et al.	
J. Riega-Torres et al.	
C. H Shiboski et al.	
B. Tashbayev et al.	
S. K Mandal et al.	
B. M Liquidato et al.	
W. W. I Kalk et al.	Values of saliva production by submandibular and parotid gland reported

UWSF Unstimulated Whole Salivary Flow, *pSS* Primary Sjögren's Syndrome, *SS* Sjögren's Syndrome, *VNM* Values not mentioned

sicca disclosed a difference in the UWSF (MD-0.10 ml/min; 95% CI, − 0.13 to − 0.06; chi^2-*P*-value< 0.00001 with a heterogeneity of 82%). As for the subgroup analysis (heterogeneity of 99%) of patients with pSS versus healthy people, a difference in UWSF was observed (MD-0.43 ml/min; 95% CI − 0.49 to − 0.27; chi^2-*P*-value < 0.00001). In a subgroup analysis (heterogeneity of 97%) by type of study design, the results were different but consistent with the pooled results from all subgroups with the exception of the cross-sectional study group in which there were no significant differences (Fig. 3).

No statistically significant difference was found (MD-0.06 ml/min; 95% CI − 0.14 a 0.01; I^2 93%, chi2-*s*-value

Table 3 Main results of the studies included in the meta-analysis

	Study	Year	Cases	Controls	Age (Years) in cases (Mean ± SD)	Age (Years) in controls	UWSF (ml/min) in cases (Mean SD)	UWSF (ml/min) in controls (Mean SD)	Quality of evidence[a]
1	A.M Nahir et al.	1987	9	20	NA	NA	0,06±0,02	0,25±0,1	10/10
2	F.N. Skopouli	1989	81	188	NA	NA	0,094±0,1	0,406±0,272	Not Enough Information
3	T. Filho	1993	41	193	NA	NA	1,18±0,99	2,47±0,99	Not Enough Information
4	U. Hakansson et al.	1994	17	42	63 (53–72)[b]	69 (57–72)[b]	0,025± 0,042	0,14±0,16	10/10
5	N. Rhodus et al.	1997	18	9	54,5 (37–74)[c]	56,1 (38–74)[c]	0,0216±0,004	0,431 SE 0,092	9/10
6	N.L Rhodus et al.	1998	10	10	57,2 (37–74)[b]	57,4 (41–80)[b]	0,0094±0,004	0,096 SE 0,16	10/10
7	S.L Wang et al.	1998	30	23	39 (28–62)[b]	42 (29–69)[b]	0,070±0,089	0,330±0,188	10/10
8	A.M Pedersen et al.	1999	16	27	61,5 (40–82)[c]	50 (39–70)[c]	0,05 (0–0,1)	0.31 (0,14-0,90)	10/10
9	A. Vissink et al.	2003	57	36	53±14	48±12	0,05±0.08	0.23±0.15	10/10
10	A. Negoro et al.	2004	31	47	55,2±13,1	32,3±5,9	0,07±0,07	0,282±0,22	10/10
11	K. Márton et al.	2006	49	43	55±11	NA	0,12±0,13	0,37±0,24	9/10
12	I Van Den Berg et al	2009	62	114	NA	NA	0,08±0,13	0,22±0,18	11/11
13	A. Bookman et al.	2010	265	70	NA	NA	0,046±0,086	0,093±0,093	8/8
14	T. Kitagawa et al.	2011	45	54	60,9±9,9	67,1±11,3	0,015±0,026	0,071±0.058	8/8
15	E. H. Kang et al.	2011	30	55	49,9±9	51,5±10	0,06±0,05	0,15±0,12	10/10
16	C. Baldini et al.	2011	55	10	52,4±10,5	56±10,7	1,05±0,77	1,02±0,78	10/10
17	B. Busamia et al.	2012	32	41	53	NA	0,22±0,03	0,36±0,05	8/8
18	M. A. D. Anjos Corvo et al	2012	19	12	60	44	0,127±0,106	0,402±0,16	9/10
19	G. Mumcu et al.	2013	14	10	51,3±5,03	43,4±9,5	0,04±0,01	1,73±1,3	9/10
20	N. Berman et al.	2014	104	121	53,8±13,7	51,9±13,2	0,46±0,24	0,85±0,3	9/10
21	M.A.D Anjos Corvo et al	2014	12	11	56,25±8,6	56,1±12,7	0,16±0,162	0,26±0,144	10/10
22	K. Ohyama et al.	2015	90	36	61,9±9,8	42,4±15,1	0,5±0,1	0,25±0,15	10/10
23	C. Baldini et al.	2015	50	57	47±13	53±12	0,153±0,173	0,32±0,226	8/8
24	N.M.A Chaudhury et al.	2015	24	30	55,25 SE 3,29	56,53 SE 3,43	0,14±0,03	0,42±0,05	10/10
25	E.C Barbosa et al.	2016	10	7	NA	NA	0,18	0,67	10/10
26	S. Rusthen et al.	2017	31	33	52±12,4	50,1±12,7	0,08±0,07	0,29±0,17	9/10
27	Fernández-Martínez et al.	2018	60	60	55,5±14,3	55,7±8,1	0,016±0,004	0,12±0,7	10/10
28	K-A Lee et al.	2018	94	44	55,6±12,2	59,2±11,8	0,146±0,15	0,226±0,23	10/11

Most of values are expressed on mean and standard deviation or median and interquartile rank. All the values were converted to ml/min units. To the articles which report UWSF in subgroups, a mean was calculated

UWSF Unstimulated Whole Salivary Flow, *NA* Not available, *SE* Standard Error

[a]Joanna Briggs Checklist., [b] Mean (Range), [c] Median (Interquartile range)

< 0.11 with a heterogeneity of 93%) when UWSF in patients with pSS was compared to those with polyautoimmunity.

As for publication bias, visual inspection of the funnel plot shows asymmetry (Fig. 4), and that was confirmed by an Egger's regression test (*P*=0.0001).

Discussion

Here, for the first time (to our knowledge), a meta-analysis shows that the unstimulated whole salivary flow rate is lower in patients with Sjögren's syndrome compared to controls (healthy and non-SS sicca patients). A mean difference value of – 0.18 ml/min (95% CI,-0.24 to-0.13, *P*-value < 0.00001) is disclosed.

The above result is important given the role that saliva plays in oral health. For example, saliva provides the teeth with protection and lubrication and fosters their remineralization. It also cooperates with the transportation of digestive enzymes. It has antimicrobial properties and plays a part in chewing and swallowing. It is estimated that the saliva production rate is 0.5 to 1.5Lt/day in healthy adults [7, 28]. The glands responsible for

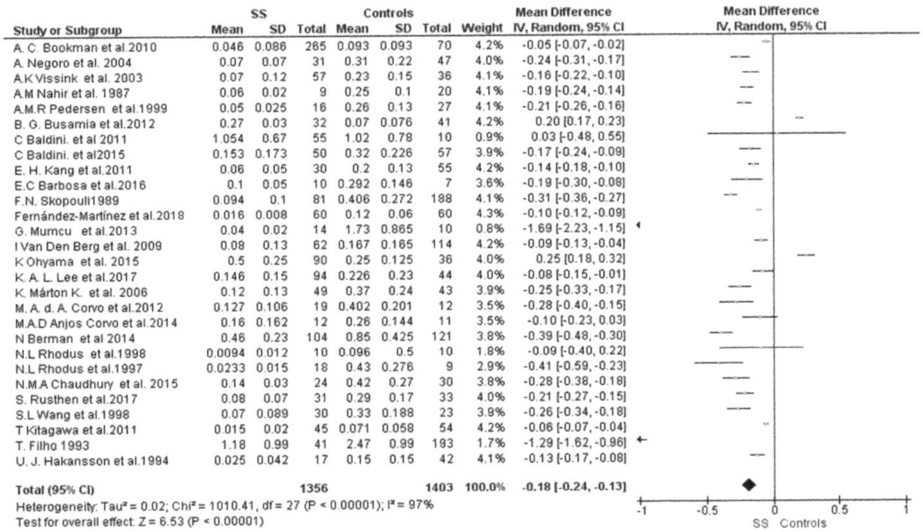

Fig. 2 Forest plot (random-effects model Mean Differences) of the unstimulated whole salivary flow rate in patients with Sjögren's Syndrome compared to controls (healthy subjects and patients with sicca non-SS). This forest plot summarizes the results of studies evaluating the unstimulated whole salivary flow rate in patients with Sicca symptoms (SS vs controls). The numbers on the x-axis measure mean difference. The small green boxes represent the point estimate of the effect size and sample size of each study. The black lines on either side of the box represent a 95% confidence interval. The solid vertical line represents a mean difference of 0 or no effect. The overall pooled mean difference and 95% CI is indicated by a diamond at the bottom. Names of the first author's studies are shown on the left. CI: Confidence Interval; df: degree freedom; Chi2: chi-squared test; I2: Higgins heterogeneity test; SD: Standard deviation; SS: Sjögren's Syndrome

saliva production are the major salivary glands (parotid, sublingual, and submandibular) and account for 90% of it. The remaining 10% of saliva production is attributed to the minor salivary glands that are diffusely distributed in the oral mucosa [7, 29].

Diminished production of the salivary flow rate implies the hypo-function of salivary glands. Therefore, it is essential to find out what the main causes of the compromised flow rate are. The adverse effects of medication, therapeutic irradiation, and SS are common causes of decreased salivary flow. The ACR/EULAR criteria are used for the SS diagnosis. They include the UWSF rate, and if the salivary production is ≤ 0.1 ml/min or ≤ 1.5 ml in 15 min, the criteria assign one point to the final calculation. Unfortunately, in the majority of the cases, this test is only applied when the patient does not have dry eye by objective measures (Schirmer test or ocular staining score) [30]. In general terms, there is a consensus in the literature on the UWSF cut-off point that demonstrates glandular hypofunction when its value is ≤ 0.1 ml / min. However, it has been suggested that values between 0.1 to 0.2 ml/min could be the lower threshold, and that values > 0.2 ml/min are found in healthy people [31].

The value of ≤0.1 ml/min includes all the people with dry eye/mouth symptoms resulting from causes that cannot be differentiated from SS. Traditionally, this cut-off point of UWSF is used for the SS diagnosis. However, the origin of this value is not clear in the literature review (Table 4). In 1975, Daniels et al. said that there were no established specific criteria for determining the presence of the oral component of SS, but since then, the abovementioned cut-off point has been used in different sets of criteria for patients with suspected SS with no solid scientific support [15]. Thus, this Systematic Literature Review (SLR) and meta-analysis were developed to evaluate the difference using an objective measure. In the present study, the difference in the value of the UWSF for controls and the one for SS was found to be − 0.18 ml/min. Note that out of the 1403 controls included, a considerable group were healthy subjects (n= 788). That is why, when a subgroup analysis is done to evaluate the difference in UWSF between pSS and healthy people, it shows a higher than expected difference, − 0.43 ml/min.

Furthermore, the controls with non-SS sicca in the present results include subjects with sialosis, fibromyalgia, radiotherapy, burn mouth syndrome, diabetes, arterial hypertension, sodium retention syndrome, dyslipidemia, positive serology for hepatitis C, hyperthyroidism, hypothyroidism, osteoarthritis, and neoplasia. A minor difference in the saliva production (− 0.10 ml/min) was found in the subgroup analysis of patients with pSS and non-SS sicca as was expected. In a 2016 systematic literature review that evaluated the level of xerostomia, hypo-salivation, and salivary flow rate in patients with diabetes, the UWSF rate was found to be 0.16 to 0.55 ml/min in the group of patients and 0.26 to 0.75

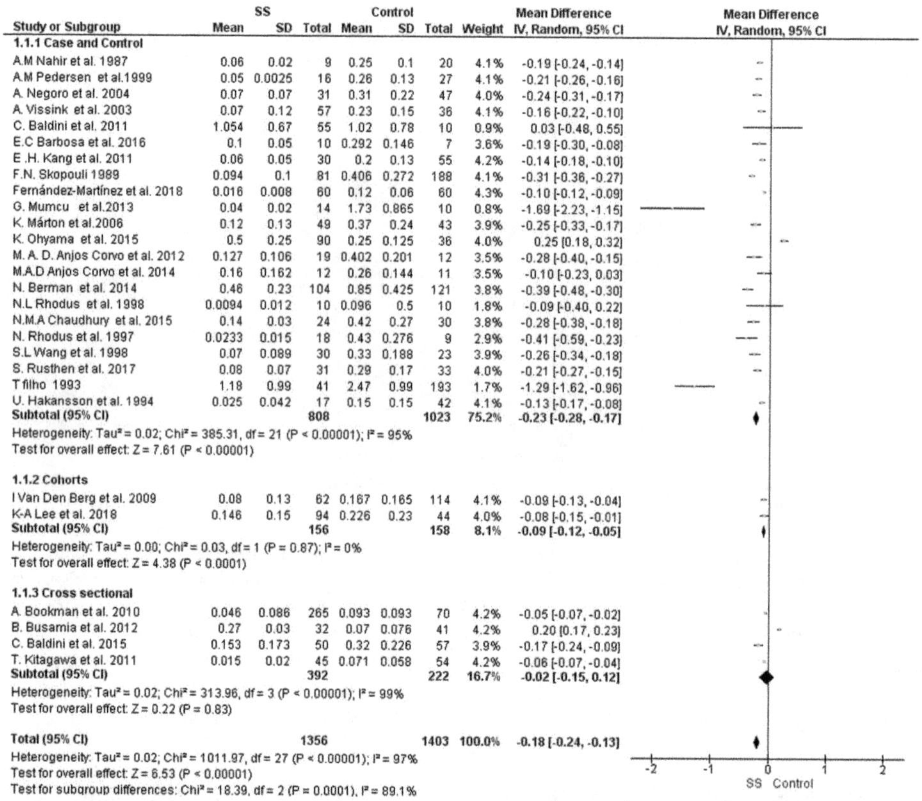

Fig. 3 Forest plot (random-effects model Mean Differences) of the unstimulated whole salivary flow rate in patients with Sjögren's Syndrome compared to controls (healthy subjects and patients with sicca non-SS) by study design type. Names of the first author's studies are shown on the left. CI: Confidence Interval; df: degree freedom; Chi2: chi-squared test; I2: Higgins heterogeneity test; SD: Standard deviation; SS: Sjögren's Syndrome

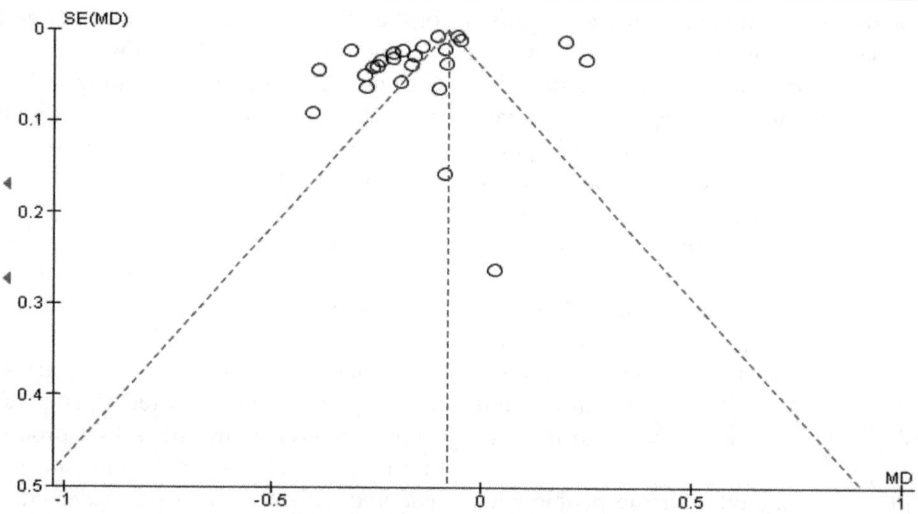

Fig. 4 Funnel plot of published studies evaluating the unstimulated whole salivary flow rate in patients with Sjögren's Syndrome compared to controls (healthy subjects and patients with non-SS sicca). It shows an important publication bias with an asymmetric article distribution. A funnel plot of standard error versus the unstimulated whole salivary flow difference in means is shown. Visual inspection of the funnel plot (scatter diagram) shows asymmetric article distribution confirmed by an Egger's regression test (*P*=0.0001). MD: mean difference; SE: Standard error

Table 4 Historical criteria background for saliva production in Sjögren's syndrome diagnosis

Author	Year	Objective dry mouth evaluation included for diagnosis.	Value
Daniels et al.	1975	There are no established objective criteria for determining the presence of the oral component of SS.	NA
Manthorpe et al.	1975–1976	No	NA
Skopoul et al.	1986	No, they mention subjective xerostomia and stimulated modified whole sialometry	NA
Fox et al.	1986	No	Just mention decreased basal and stimulated salivary flow rate
Vitali et al.	1993	Objective evidence of salivary gland involvement determined based on a positive result from at least 1 of the following 3 tests: Salivary scintigraphy, parotid sialography, USF.	USF ≤1,5 ml/15 min
Fujibayashi et al.	1999	Optional in an item, gum or Saxon test	NA
Vitali et al.	2002	Yes	UWSF ≤1,5 ml/15 min
Fujibayashi et al.	2004	Yes	Flow rate ≤10 ml/10 min
Shiboski et al.	2012	No	NA
Shiboski et al.	2016	Yes	UWSF ≤0,1 ml/min

NA Not available, *USF* Unstimulated Salivary Flow, *UWSF* Unstimulated Whole Salivary Flow

ml/min in the control group. This is similar to the present results even though this population corresponds to non-autoimmune diabetes (Type 2) [32].

Another meta-analysis from 2018 involved subjects with autoimmune thyroid diseases and oral lichen planus. SS was eliminated from the study, and it included 130 patients in the end. The authors analyzed UWSF values and found a diminished production of UWSF in the group of patients compared to controls (– 1.09; – 1. 49, – 0.7; *P*-value < 0.001) [10]. It reveals the lack of studies that include patients with other autoimmune diseases. However, it shows evidence of a greater difference in the mean value of UWSF in cases versus controls in comparison to our meta-analysis of values of UWSF of patients with SS versus controls.

The clinical usefulness and practical implications of the present results show that cases have – 0.18 ml/min of unstimulated salivary flow compared to controls. This implies that in 1 h, patients present a saliva production of 11 ml less than controls, directly impacting previously mentioned basic physiological functions. The present meta-analysis results could be involved in future studies to define new UWSF cut-off points that better discriminate between patients with SS vs. sicca non-SS by analyzing sensitivity, specificity, and through ROC curves.

In addition, this could guide new research focused on modifying the pre-stablished cut-off point for making treatment decisions. In fact, the recent EULAR recommendations for the management of Sjögren's syndrome [8] suggested a first evaluation considering the UWSF measurement, and if the value is < 0.1 ml/min, they proposed to classifying the patients according to SWSF values (> 0.7 ml/min: normal/mild, 0.7–0.1 ml/min: moderate and < 0.1 ml/min: severe dysfunction). If SWSF values showed severe dysfunction, saliva substitution should be considered the preferred therapeutic approach to alleviate symptoms. This would be needed given that in patients with no residual glandular function (severe glandular dysfunction), salivary glands cannot be stimulated, either by pharmacological or non-pharmacological interventions. The present meta-analysis results might guide new discussions regarding practical implications with respect to not only the diagnostic process, but also, treatment decisions given the limitations on developing the SWSF measurement. This is a complicated test in daily practice and not always available in all clinical settings as was mentioned by the EULAR panel in their recommendations. It might be feasible to discuss avoiding the SWSF test and using the UWSF instead given the objective saliva production measurement based on the present results.

The limitations of the present study include its heterogeneity through the I^2 test and the publication bias as evinced in the funnel plot due to the fact that it had a preponderance of studies with a small sample size (95% smaller than a n=100). Additionally, there are variations in the saliva collection technique and the sampling time in the different articles. Therefore, the results have to be taken with caution. Nonetheless, this exercise supports the need to unify criteria for clinical evaluation, monitor patients with sicca symptoms, and set up epidemiological studies with larger sample sizes and greater homogeneity in their comorbidities.

Moreover, the study design included articles that were mostly cross-sectional and cohort studies with a three or four level of evidence. There were fewer articles that compared SS patients with diagnoses of other autoimmune diseases (polyautoimmunity) to pSS patients and, as a result, no difference was found. Therefore, this could be an important step for future research.

Unfortunately, the articles did not provide enough information to do a meta-regression. Furthermore, some of them were not clear with respect to whether or not the cases and controls were receiving pharmacological treatments or had comorbidities or other diseases that could have an influence on the values of the UWSF.

Conclusion

For the first time, the difference in the values of the UWSF rate in patients with SS compared to controls (non-SS sicca subjects and healthy people) was objectively demonstrated through a meta-analysis. The purpose behind this study is to challenge the different specialists in oral health and rheumatology regarding the importance of the use of UWSF, which has the same weight within the classification criteria [14] for SS as the Schirmer test or the ocular staining score test. This takes into account the fact that eye tests are done more frequently than the UWSF in real-life conditions in the context of SS diagnosis. The results of our research will make it possible to understand the objective assessment of cut-off points for UWSF in SS and in other causes of xerostomia.

Acknowledgments

We would like to recognize Cecile Dunn for her technical support concerning the English language and the Internal call for the improvement of English scientific manuscripts from the Fundación Universitaria de Ciencias de la Salud -FUCS.

Authors' contributions

Dr. Adriana Rojas had full access to all the data in the study and takes responsibility for the integrity of the data and the accuracy of the data analysis. Concept and design: M. A Martínez-Ceballos, N Aguilera, JP Alzate-Granados, K. C Garzón-González, J. Cajamarca, A. Rojas-Villarraga. Acquisition, analysis or interpretation of data: M. A Martínez-Ceballos, N Aguilera, JP Alzate- Granados, K. C Garzón-González, J. Cajamarca, A. Rojas-Villarraga. Drafting of the manuscript: M. A Martínez-Ceballos, N Aguilera, JP Alzate-Granados, K. C Garzón-González, J. Cajamarca, A. Rojas-Villarraga. Critical revisión of the manuscript for important intellectual content: M. A Martínez-Ceballos, N Aguilera, JP Alzate- Granados, K. C Garzón-González, J. Cajamarca, A. Rojas-Villarraga. Statistical analysis: A Rojas-Villarraga, JP Alzate- Granados, M. Martínez-Ceballos. Administrative, technical, or material support: M. A Martínez-Ceballos, N Aguilera, JP Alzate- Granados, K. C Garzón-González, J. Cajamarca, A. Rojas-Villarraga. Supervision: A Rojas-Villarraga, JP Alzate-Granados. The author(s) read and approved the final manuscript.

Author details

[1] Research Division Fundación Universitaria de Ciencias de la Salud (FUCS), Bogotá, Colombia. [2]Internal Medicine Department, Fundación Universitaria de Ciencias de la Salud (FUCS). Hospital San José, Bogotá, Colombia. [3]Rheumatology Department, Fundación Universitaria de Ciencias de la Salud (FUCS), Bogotá, Colombia. [4]Research Institute, Fundación Universitaria de Ciencias de la Salud (FUCS), Bogotá, Colombia.

References

1. Rostron J, Rogers S, Longman L, Kaney S, Field EA. Health-related quality of life in patients with primary Sjögren's syndrome and xerostomia: a comparative study. Gerodontology. 2002;19(1):53–9.
2. Anaya JM, Rojas-Villarraga A, Mantilla RD, Arcos-Burgos M, Sarmiento-Monroy JC. Polyautoimmunity in Sjögren Syndrome. Rheum Dis Clin North Am. 2016;42:457–72 W.B. Saunders.
3. Mariette X, Criswell LA. Primary Sjögren's syndrome. N Engl J Med. 2018; 378(10):931–9.
4. Qin B, Wang J, Yang Z, Yang M, Ma N, Huang F, et al. Epidemiology of primary Sjögren's syndrome: a systematic review and meta-analysis. Ann Rheum Dis. 2015 Nov;74(11):1983–9.
5. Brito-Zerón P, Baldini C, Bootsma H, Bowman SJ, Jonsson R, Mariette X, et al. Sjögren Syndrome. Nat Rev. 2016;2:1–20.
6. Shiboski SC, Shiboski CH, Criswell LA, Baer AN, Challacombe S, Lanfranchi H, et al. American College of Rheumatology Classification Criteria for Sjögren's Syndrome: a data-driven, expert consensus approach in the SICCA cohort. Arthritis Care Res (Hoboken). 2012;64(4):475–87.
7. Navazesh M, Kumar SK. Measuring salivary flow Challenges and opportunities. J Am Dent Assoc. 2008;139:5S–40S.
8. Ramos-Casals M, Brito-Zerón P, Bombardieri S, Bootsma H, De Vita S, Dörner T, et al. EULAR recommendations for the management of Sjögren's syndrome with topical and systemic therapies. Ann Rheum Dis. 2020;79(1): 3–18.
9. Hoseini A, Mirzapour A, Bijani A, Shirzad A. Salivary flow rate and xerostomia in patients with type I and II diabetes mellitus. Electron Physician. 2017;9(9): 5244–9.
10. Moosavi M-S, Barati H. Salivary gland performance in autoimmune diseases: review and meta-analysi. Acta Clin Belg. 2020;75(1):19–25. https://doi.org/10.1080/17843286.2018.1540164. Epub 2018 Oct 30.
11. Naik M, Vaishnavee V. Qualitative and quantitative salivary changes and subjective oral dryness among patients with thyroid dysfunction. Indian J Dent Res. 2018;29(1):16.
12. Knaś M, Zalewska A, Waszkiewicz N, Szulimowska J, Dziezcioł J, Sierakowski S, et al. Salivary: flow and proteins of the innate and adaptive immunity in the limited and diffused systemic sclerosis. J Oral Pathol Med. 2014;43(7): 521–9.
13. Kobus A, Kierklo A, Zalewska A, Kuźmiuk A, Szajda SD, Ławicki S, et al. Unstimulated salivary flow, pH, proteins and oral health in patients with juvenile idiopathic arthritis. BMC Oral Health. 2017;17(1):94.
14. Shiboski CH, Shiboski SC, Seror R, Criswell LA, Labetoulle M, Lietman TM, et al. 2016 American College of Rheumatology/European league against rheumatism classification criteria for primary Sjögren's syndrome a consensus and data-driven methodology involving three international patient cohorts. Ann Rheum Dis. 2017;76:9–16.
15. Daniels TE, Silverman S, Michalski J, Greenspan J, Path M, Sylvester R, et al. The oral component of Sjögren's syndrome. Oral Surgery, Oral Med Oral Pathol. 1975;39(6):875–88.
16. Manthorpe R, Oxholm P, Prause JU, Schiødt M. The Copenhagen Criteria for Sjögren's syndrome. Scand J Rheumatol. 1986;61:19–21.
17. Skopouli FN, Drosos AA, Papaioannou T, Moutsopoulos HM. Preliminary diagnostic criteria for Sjögren's syndrome. Scand J Rheumatol. 1986; 15(Suppl. 61):22–5.
18. Fox RI, Robinson CA, Curd JG, Kozin F, Howell F. Sjögren syndrome proposed criteria for classification. Arthritis Rheum. 1986;29(5):577–85.
19. Balestrieri G, Bencivelli W, Bernstein RM, Bjerrum KB, Braga S, Coll J, et al. Preliminary criteria for the classification of Sjogren' S Syndrome results of a prospective concerted action supported by the European Community. Arthritis Rheum. 1993;36(3):340–7.
20. Fujibayashi T, Sugai S, Miyasaka N, Hayashi Y, Tsubota K. Revised Japanese criteria for Sjögren's syndrome (1999): availability and validity. Mod Rheumatol. 2004;14(6):425–34.
21. Liberati A, Altman DG, Tetzlaff J, Mulrow C, Gøtzsche PC, Ioannidis JPA. The PRISMA statement for reporting systematic reviews and meta-analyses of studies that evaluate health care interventions: explanation and elaboration. J Clin Epidemiol. 2009;62:e1 34.

22. Vitali C, Bombardieri S, Jonsson R, Moutsopoulos HM, Alexander EL, Carsons SE, et al. Classification criteria for Sjögren's syndrome: a revised version of the European criteria proposed by the American-European Consensus Group. Ann Rheum Dis. 2002;61(6):554–8 Available from: http://www.pubmedcentral.nih.gov/articlerender.fcgi?artid=1754137&tool=pmcentrez&rendertype=abstract. [cited 2011 Oct 11].
23. OCEBM Levels of evidence working group, et al. "The Oxford 2011 Levels of Evidence". Oxford Centre for Evidence-Based Medicine. 2011. http://www.cebm.net/index.aspx?o=5653.
24. The Joanna Briggs Institute. Critical appraisal tools. 2018.
25. Navazesh M. Methods for collecting saliva. Ann N Y Acad Sci. 1993;694(1):72–7.
26. Vitali C, Bombardieri S, Moutsopoulos HM, Balestrieri G, Bencivelli W, Bernstein RM, et al. Preliminary criteria for the classification of Sjögren's syndrome. Results of a prospective concerted action supported by the European community. Arthritis Rheum. 1993;36(3):340–7.
27. Herrera JL, Lyons MF, Johnson LF. Saliva: its role in health and disease. J Clin Gastroenterol. 1988;10(5):569–78.
28. Han P, Suarez-Durall P, Mulligan R. Dry mouth: a critical topic for older adult patients. J Prosthodont Res. 2015;59:6–19.
29. Furness S, Bryan G, Mcmillan R, Hv W. Interventions for the management of dry mouth: non- pharmacological interventions (Review). Cochrane Database Syst Rev. 2013;8.(Art.No.: CD009603:1–38.
30. Shiboski CH, Shiboski SC, Seror R, Criswell LA, Labetoulle M, Lietman TM, et al. 2016 American College of Rheumatology/European league against rheumatism classification criteria for primary Sjögren's syndrome: a consensus and data-driven methodology involving three international patient cohorts. Arthritis Rheumatol. 2017;69(1):35–45.
31. Flink H, Tegelberg Å, Lagerlöf F. Influence of the time of measurement of unstimulated human whole saliva on the diagnosis of hyposalivation. Arch Oral Biol. 2005;50(6):553–9.
32. López-pintor RM, Casañas E, González-serrano J, Serrano J, Ramírez L, De Arriba L, et al. Xerostomia, Hyposalivation, and salivary flow in diabetes patients. J Diabetes Res. 2016;2016:1–16.

10

Increased modifiable cardiovascular risk factors in patients with Takayasu arteritis

Alexandre Moura dos Santos[1], Rafael Giovani Misse[1], Isabela Bruna Pires Borges[1], Bruno Gualano[1], Alexandre Wagner Silva de Souza[2], Liliam Takayama[1], Rosa Maria R. Pereira[1] and Samuel Katsuyuki Shinjo[1*]

Abstract

Background: Modifiable cardiovascular risk factors (MCRFs), such as those related to aerobic capacity, muscle strength, physical activity, and body composition, have been poorly studied in Takayasu arteritis (TAK). Therefore, the aim of the study was to investigate MCRFs and their relationships with disease status and comorbidities among patients with TAK.

Methods: A multicenter cross-sectional study was conducted between 2019 and 2020, in which 20 adult women with TAK were compared with 16 healthy controls matched by gender, age, and body mass index. The following parameters were analyzed: aerobic capacity by cardiopulmonary test; muscle function by timed-stands test, timed up-and-go test, and handgrip test; muscle strength by one-repetition maximum test and handgrip test; body composition by densitometry; physical activity and metabolic equivalent by IPAQ, quality of life by HAQ and SF-36; disease activity by ITAS2010 and NIH score; and presence of comorbidities.

Results: Patients with TAK had a mean age of 41.5 (38.0–46.3) years, disease duration of 16.0 (9.5–20.0) years, and a mean BMI of 27.7±4.5 kg/m^2. Three out of the 20 patients with TAK had active disease. Regarding comorbidities, 16 patients had systemic arterial hypertension, 11 had dyslipidemia, and two had type 2 diabetes mellitus, while the control group had no comorbidities. TAK had a significant reduction in aerobic capacity (absolute and relative VO_2 peak), muscle strength in the lower limbs, increased visceral adipose tissue, waist-to-hip ratio, reduced walking capacity, decreased weekly metabolic equivalent, and quality of life ($P< 0.05$) as compared to controls. However, there were no correlations between these MCRFs parameters and disease activity.

Conclusions: TAK show impairment in MCRFs; therefore, strategies able to improve MCRF should be considered in this disease.

Keywords: Aerobic capacity, Cardiovascular diseases, Muscle strength, Vasculitis

Introduction

Takayasu arteritis (TAK) is a primary systemic vasculitis characterized mainly by large-diameter vessels involvement, such as the aorta and major branches. Epidemiological studies have shown that the disease mainly affects women under the age of 40 years of age [1, 2].

Patients with TAK have a high prevalence of cardiovascular disease (CVD) and its risk factors. Additionally, 60–70% of patients present dyslipidemia [3, 4]. During follow-up, approximately 85% of patients developed systemic arterial hypertension [5, 6], and an increased prevalence of metabolic syndrome in TAK [6]; altogether, these factors may lead to increased morbidity and mortality in TAK.

CVD risk factors, morbidity, and mortality rate can be divided into modifiable and non-modifiable. Modifiable cardiovascular risk factors (MCRFs) include impairment

* Correspondence: samuel.shinjo@usp.br
[1]Division of Rheumatology, Faculdade de Medicina FMUSP, Universidade de Sao Paulo, Sao Paulo, Brazil

in aerobic capacity [7, 8], muscle strength [9, 10], physical activity levels [11, 12], and body composition [13], among others. MCRFs may be relevant for predicting traditional CVD risk factors in healthy individuals and those patients with rheumatic diseases.

Furthermore, MCRFs are closely interconnected, and the alteration of one of the factors may worsen one or more other factors. Moreover, they seem to have additive responses in morbidity and mortality [14, 15]. However, few studies have currently analyzed MCRF parameters in patients with TAK [16, 17].

For example, reduced aerobic capacity has been described in several systemic autoimmune diseases [18–20]. This reduction is accompanied by a decline in physical capacity, muscle strength, and physical activity, which can worse body composition, increase fatigue, and predispose to a higher prevalence of CVD and its risk factors in rheumatic diseases [19, 21].

Oliveira et al. [17] showed that patients with TAK had reduced aerobic capacity. However, the authors did not evaluate other MCRFs, such as visceral adipose tissue and the waist and hip index, which are relevant CVD risk factors [3–6]. In addition, limitations may exist in the analysis of its findings regarding aerobic capacity, strength, and muscle function, due to the size of your sample.

Therefore, the aim of this study was to evaluate MCRFs and their relations with the disease status and comorbidities in patients with TAK.

Patients and methods

This is a multicenter cross-sectional study, conducted between 2019 and 2020, in which adult women with TAK. Patients had an age between 18 and 50 years and fulfilled at least three of the six items of classification criteria for TAK [22]. The study was approved by the local ethics committee and registered with ClinicalTrials (#NCT03750929).

The following exclusion criteria were adopted: patients with severe or decompensated diseases (e.g., endocrinopathies) that could interfere with the results interpretation and the physical testing safety; presence or history of critical/symptomatic aortic stenosis, congestive heart failure, arrhythmias or electrocardiographic changes in the ST segment, coronary artery disease; presence or history of peripheral atherosclerosis disease; sciatica or neurogenic claudication; with impaired walking (osteoarticular disorders in limbs), precluding exercise testing; pregnancy or lactation; and smoking in the previous 6 months of the study.

Interviews were conducted with eligible TAK patients, and medical records were systematically reviewed. In the control group, the volunteers were matched for age, gender, and body mass index (BMI) to patients with TAK. The following data were collected:

- Demographic data: age and ethnicity;
- Quality of life: Health Assessment Questionnaire (HAQ) [23], Short Form Health Survey (SF-36) [24]
- Clinical data: age at disease diagnosis, duration of disease, the Edinburgh Claudication Questionnaire (ECQ) [25], Walking Impairment Questionnaire (WIQ) [26], Indian Takayasu's Arteritis Activity Score (ITAS2010) [27];
- Laboratory data: serum levels of C-reactive protein (CRP) and an erythrocyte sedimentation rate (ESR), total cholesterol, high-density lipoprotein (HDL), low-density lipoprotein (LDL), triglycerides;
- Pharmacological therapy: previous and current (glucocorticoids, immunosuppressive, immunomodulator and/or immunobiologicals drugs);
- Disease activity: ITAS 2010 [27], and National Institute of Health (NIH) score [28] (only in TAK);
- Comorbidities and their risk factors for CVD: type 2 diabetes mellitus was defined when the fasting glycemic test ≥ 126 mg/dL and/or the result of the oral glucose tolerance test ≥ 200 mg/dL [29]; systemic arterial hypertension was considered when blood pressure had systolic values ≥ 130 mmHg and/or diastolic values ≥ 85 mmHg [30]; dyslipidemia was defined when total plasma cholesterol ≥ 200 mg/dL, HDL-cholesterol ≤ 50 mg/dL, LDL-cholesterol ≥ 130 mg/dL and/or triglycerides ≥ 150 mg/dL [31]; or previously medical diagnosis and drug treatment for these comorbidities.
- Vascular images taken routinely and recently in the outpatient clinic (< 6 months after the inclusion of patients in the present study): data referring to vascular lesions in the aorta and the major branches (magnetic resonance-angiography and/or computed tomography-angiography) (only in TAK).

Physical activity level and weekly caloric expenditure

These parameters were obtained from the International Physical Activity Questionnaire (IPAQ, short version eight), translated into Portuguese and validated for the Brazilian population [32].

Anthropometry and body composition

The following parameters were collected: body mass (using a digital scale), height (using stadiometer), hip, waist and abdominal circumference, BMI, and waist-to-hip ratio. Dual X-ray absorptiometry was used to assess body composition, including lean mass, fat mass, and visceral adipose tissue, through iDXA equipment (GE Lunar Medical Systems, Madison, WI).

Aerobic capacity

A treadmill cardiopulmonary test was conducted. The test was carried out according to the previous description [33].

Muscle strength

Maximum repetition test (1RM) was performed to determine muscle strength. The 1RM test was performed using the bench press and the 45° leg press. A familiarization trial was carried out, and it was followed by a 48 h-interval, followed by two tests performed on non-consecutive days, in which reproducibility was accepted as soon as the coefficient of variation was < 0.5%. The warm-up consisted of eight repetitions at 50% of 1RM with an interval of 2 min of rest. After that, three repetitions were performed at 70% of 1RM between 3-min intervals. To determine the 1RM, five attempts were made, and the highest recorded value was regarded as the maximum load. The interval between each attempt was 3 min [34].

Muscle function

Timed-Stands test (TST) [35], and Timed Up-and-Go (TUG) test [36] were applied beyond the handgrip test [37]. We performed a familiarization that was preceded by at least 48 h of interval before the tests. The coefficient of variation for all tests was < 0.5%.

As a control group (CTR), healthy volunteers were matched for age, gender, and BMI to patients with TAK. In addition, individuals in the CTR group had no systemic autoimmune diseases and were not smokers in the previous 6 months of the study.

Statistical analysis

Data distribution was evaluated using the Shapiro-Wilk test. Data with normal distribution were expressed as mean ± standard deviation, while data with asymmetric distribution were expressed as the median and the interquartile range (25–75%). The existence of differences between quantitative variables and normal distribution was analyzed using the Student's *t*-test. For the quantitative variables with asymmetric distribution, the Mann-Whitney U test was used. The categorical data were expressed as a percentage (%), and the differences were analyzed using Fisher's exact test. The correlation between variables with symmetric distribution was analyzed using the Pearson correlation coefficient, while that with asymmetric distribution was analyzed using the Spearman coefficient ρ [38]. Furthermore, the correlations were classified as poor (< 0.3), fair (0.3–0.5), moderately strong (0.6–0.8), and very strong (> 0.8) [39]. The differences were considered statistically significant when values of $P < 0.05$. The analyzes were performed with the GraphPad Prism® software, version 6.01 for Windows (San Diego, California, USA).

Results

One hundred eight patients with TAK were interviewed. Of these patients, 56 did not meet the inclusion criteria, and 32 refused to participate for various personal reasons (e.g., lack of time, a long distance from home, and lack of interest); therefore, 20 patients were included in the study (Fig. 1).

TAK and 16 CTR were comparable regarding age, ethnicity distribution, and BMI parameters (Table 1). There no evidence of any chronic disease and comorbidities in the CTR group (Table 2).

Half of the patients with TAK had a type V angiographic classification by Hata et al. [40], followed by four type III patients, three type IV patients, two type IIb patients, and one type I patient (Table 1).

Regarding the drug treatment, only two patients were treated with prednisone at the time of data collection (doses were 10 mg/day and 5 mg/day over the past 3 months). Eleven (55.0%) patients used one or more immunosuppressive and/or immunobiological drugs: six used methotrexate, two azathioprine, and one leflunomide. Moreover, two patients were treated with infliximab, and one was treated with tocilizumab. Moreover, according to the ITAS2010 and NIH questionnaires, three (15.0%) patients were classified as presenting active disease (Table 1).

Systemic arterial hypertension and claudication of lower limbs were respectively present in 80.0 and 65.0% of patients with TAK, and two patients had type 2 diabetes mellitus. In addition, 11 (55.0%) of the patients had dyslipidemia under treatment, with two (10.0%) patients having diabetes mellitus. No individuals from the CTR group had systemic arterial hypertension, dyslipidemia, limb claudication or type 2 diabetes mellitus, and none of them used any type of medication other than contraceptives. No smokers were reported in the TAK and control groups (Table 2).

In the treadmill cardiopulmonary test, there were no differences between the TAK and CTR groups with respect to estimated maximum heart rate, anaerobic threshold, respiratory compensation point, and time-to-exhaustion (Table 3).

However, in comparison with the CTR group, patients achieved a lower maximum heart rate during the test, as well as a significant decrease in the absolute and relative VO_2 peak (Table 3).

Five out of 20 patients with TAK were excluded due to possible cardiopulmonary diseases; therefore, 15 patients participated in muscle strength and function tests (Table 3).

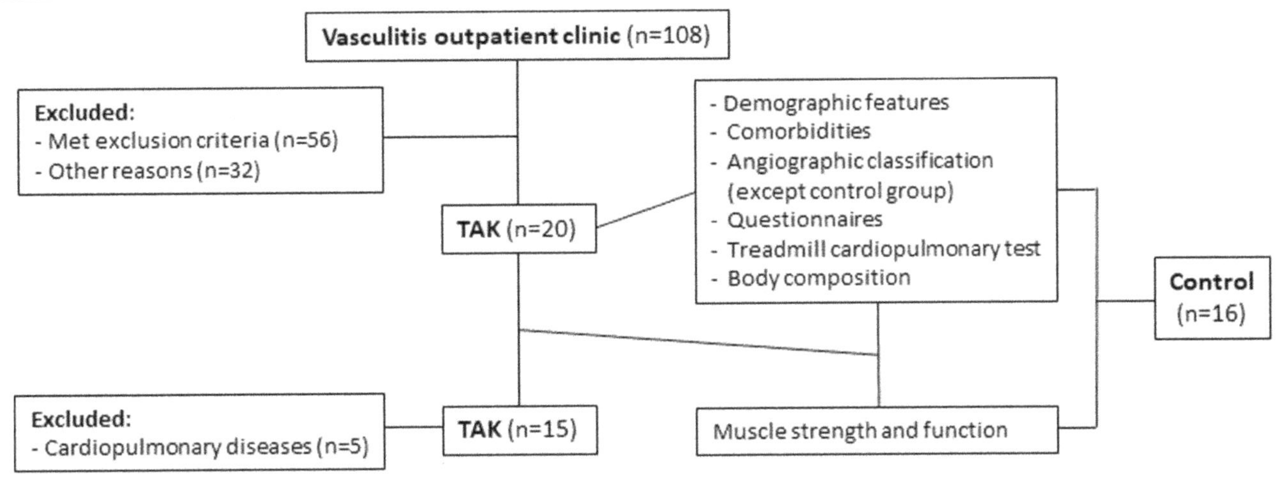

Fig. 1 Study flowchart. Legends: Control group; TAK: Takayasu arteritis

Regarding muscle strength, the TAK group did not show significant reductions in the muscle strength of the upper limbs, assessed via the bench press. However, compared to the CTR group, a significant decrease in the strength of the lower limbs, assessed via leg press, was found in the TAK group (Table 3).

The TST, TUG, and handgrip strength in both hands were similar between the TAK and CTR groups (Table 3). Concerning the CTR group, patients with TAK presented a significant reduction in the ability to perform activities of daily living, assessed using the HAQ questionnaire (Table 4).

In the domains of the SF-36 questionnaire, in comparison with the CTR, the TAK group showed more significant impairment, in terms of functional capacity, physical function, pain, general health, and mental health. In the walking impairment questionnaire (WIQ), compared to CTR, patients showed a reduction in all the variables evaluated ($P < 0.05$) (Table 4).

Regarding the level of physical activity assessed through the IPAQ, 14 (60%) patients in the TAK group had lower levels of physical activity than CTR. In the TAK group, six (30%) patients had moderate physical activity levels, with no difference compared to CTR, and none of the patients was classified as having a high level of physical activity. Additionally, in comparison with CTR, the weekly caloric expenditure values of the TAK group were lower (Table 4).

In comparison with the CTR group, the body composition and anthropometric measurements were similar between the TAK and CTR groups (Table 5), except for the higher volume and mass of visceral adipose tissue, and the waist-hip ratio in patients with TAK.

Based on reduced responses in both lower limb strength and aerobic capacity, we investigated possible correlations between these two variables and variables related to functional capacity. However, no correlations were found between any of the evaluated variables (Table 6).

Table 1 General features of patients with Takayasu arteritis

	N=20
Age (years)	41.5 (38.0–46.3)
Caucasian ethnicity	11 (55.0)
Disease duration (years)	16.0 (9.5–20.0)
Angiographic classification	
Hata I	1 (5.0)
Hata IIa	0
Hata IIb	2 (10.0)
Hata III	4 (20.0)
Hata IV	3 (15.0)
Hata V	10 (50.0)
Disease activity - NIH	3 (15.0)
Disease activity - ITAS2010	3 (15.0)
Erythrocyte sedimentation rate (mm/1st hour)	12.0 (9.5–21.5)
C-reactive protein (mg/L)	3.4 (0.9–6.8)

Data are presented in median (25–75%) or percentage (%)
ITAS2010 Indian Takayasu Activity Index, *NIH* National Institute of Health score

Discussion

The present study showed patients with TAK present worse MCRF than controls. Moreover, the patients showed impaired walking capacity and increased visceral adipose tissue and waist-to-hip ratio. However, no correlations were observed between MCRF parameters or disease activity.

Despite being a rare disease, this study evaluated a sample of patients with well-characterized TAK, which were compared with well-matched healthy individuals.

Table 2 Comorbidities and traditional risk factors for cardiovascular diseases

	TAK (*n*=20)	CTR (*n*=16)	*P* value
SAH or drug treatment	16 (80)	—	—
Dyslipidemia or drug treatment	11 (55)	—	—
Type 2 diabetes mellitus or drug treatment	2 (10)	—	—
Smoker	—	—	—
Total cholesterol (mg/dL)	167.0 (143.5–188.5)	177.0 (148.0–208.0)	0.335
HDL-cholesterol (mg/dL)	60.0 (48.5–74.0)	50.0 (48.0–81.0)	0.899
LDL-cholesterol (mg/dL)	93.0 (78.5–107.0)	109.0 (109.0–120.0)	0.089
Triglycerides (mg/dL)	100.0 (74.5–114.5)	83.0 (53.0–87.0)	0.279
Fasting glucose test (mg/dL)	83.5 (80.25–92.0)	85.0 (81.0–89.0)	0.832

Data are presented as median (25–75%) or percentage (%)
CTR Control group, *SAH* Systemic arterial hypertension, *TAK* Takayasu arteritis

Furthermore, the demographic, clinical, and laboratory data, as well as imaging conditions, pharmacological treatment, comorbidities, and disease status of patients with TAK were comprehensively described.

In the present study, only women were selected due to the higher prevalence of this gender in TAK [1, 2]. Individuals over 50 years of age were excluded to minimize the inclusion of individuals with comorbidities inherent in older age groups, as well as patients with atherosclerosis and peripheral arterial disease [41], or other vasculitis such as giant cell arteritis [42]. The inclusion of such group of patients would have undermined the accuracy of the diagnosis and symptoms.

Even with rigorous selection criteria, it was necessary to exclude five out of 20 TAK patients who had already been recruited to the study. The exclusion of these patients was due to arrhythmias, severe systemic arterial hypertension, or decompensated increase in heart rate observed during maximum stress in the cardiopulmonary test. Hence, we were unable to proceed with a cardiopulmonary test protocol. Therefore, these patients were excluded from muscle strength and function tests because they may pose a risk to personal safety and health.

A large gap exists in the literature regarding the assessment of MCRFs in TAK, specifically in the assessment of VO_2 peak. However, our study obtained

Table 3 Parameters of aerobic capacity, strength and functional capacity of patients with Takayasu arteritis and the control group

	TAK (*n*=20)	CTR (*n*=16)	*P* value
Aerobic capacity			
Estimated maximum heart rate (bpm)	180.5±7.2	180.2±6.1	0.907
Maximum heart rate in test (bpm)	149.3±15.7	172.9±18.2	0.002
Anaerobic threshold (min)	4.5±1.6	3.8±0.6	0.111
Respiratory compensation point (min)	7.7±1,9	7.9±1,7	0.730
Time-to-exhaustion (min)	10.7±2.6	10.5±2.3	0.847
VO_2 peak relative (mL/kg/min)	17.4±4.6	26.3±8.0	0.004
VO_2 peak absolute (L/min)	1.2±0.3	1.6±0.4	0.007
Muscle strength and function			
Bench press 1RM (kg)	25.3±4.3	28.0±5.4	0.311
Leg press 1RM 45° (kg)	122.7±35.9	174.2±37.3	0.018
Handgrip test			
Right (kg)	28.4±5.4	30.0±5.4	0.543
Left (kg)	26.1±5.7	28.5±5.2	0.378
Timed-Stands test (reps)	15.5±2.4	18.8±3.4	0.068
Timed Up and Go test (s)	6.7±0.6	6.3±0.5	0.199

Data are presented as mean ± standard deviation
CTR Control group, *RM* Repetition maximum, *TAK* Takayasu arteritis, VO_2 Volume of oxygen uptake

Table 4 Ability to perform activities of daily living, quality of life and level of physical activity of patients with Takayasu arteritis and the control group

	TAK (*n*=20)	CTR (*n*=16)	*P* value
HAQ (0.00–3.00)	0.56 (0.12–0.87)	0.00 (0.00–0.00)	< 0.001
SF-36 (0–100)			
Functional Capacity	62.5 (46.2–88.7)	100.0 (95.0–100.0)	< 0.001
Physical function	50.0 (0.0–100.0)	100.0 (100.0–100.0)	0.008
Pain	41.0 (34.2–63.5)	84.0 (69.2–100.0)	< 0.001
General health	61.0 (43.2–80.7)	92.0 (79.5–97.7)	< 0.001
Vitality	55.0 (35.0–72.5)	77.5 (55.0–85.0)	0.066
Social aspects	88.0 (66.0–100.0)	100.0 (84.7–100.0)	0.194
Emotional aspects	100.0 (33.0–100.0)	100.0 (67.0–100.0)	0.195
Mental health	60.0 (53.0–84.0)	82.0 (75.0–97.0)	0.034
WIQ (0–100)			
Walking distance	68.0 (37.3–100.0)	100.0 (100.0–100.0)	< 0.001
Walking speed	64.1 (38.6–79.9)	100.0 (97.3–100.0)	< 0.001
Ability to climb stairs	58.3 (42.7–85.4)	100.0 (96.7–100.0)	< 0.001
Overall score	64.4 (42.4–86.9)	100.0 (88.9–100.0)	< 0.001
IPAQ-SF (%)			
Low	14 (60.0)	3 (18.7)	0.013
Moderate	6 (30.0)	9 (56.2)	0.080
High	0	2 (12.5)	–
METs per week	453.0 (240.0–751.7)	1693 (1089.0–2206.0)	< 0.001

Data are presented as median (25–75%) or percentage (%)
CTR Control group, *HAQ* Health Assessment Questionnaire, *IPAQ-SF* International Physical Activity Questionnaire Short Version, *METs* Metabolic equivalent, *SF-36* Short Form Health Survey, *TAK* Takayasu arteritis, *WIQ* Walking Impairment Questionnaire

Table 5 Body composition of patients with Takayasu arteritis and the control group

	TAK (*n*=20)	CTR (*n*=16)	*P* value
Body mass (kg)	69.8±13.7	67.1±13.3	0.564
Height (cm)	158.3±6.1	159.7±6.7	0.508
Body mass index (kg/m2)	27.7±4.5	26.2±3.8	0.264
Fat body mass (kg)	29.4±9.4	26.0±11.5	0.347
Lean body mass (kg)	38.0±5.3	40.5±7.1	0.255
Bone mineral content (kg)	2.3±0.3	2.3±0.4	0.580
Visceral adipose tissue (cm^3)	804.0±432.5	506.4±307.8	0.022
Visceral adipose tissue (g)	760,1±408,7	477,8±290,3	0.021
Abdominal circumference (cm)	91.6±10.7	85.5±7.7	0.172
Waist circumference (cm)	83.5±9.7	77.4±5.8	0.100
Hip circumference (cm)	104.3±11.0	104.8±8.0	0.919
Waist-hip ratio	0.8±0.1	0.7±0.0	0.016

Data are presented as mean ± standard deviation
CTR Control group, *TAK* Takayasu arteritis

Table 6 Correlation between functional variables, lower limb strength and peak relative VO_2 of patients with Takayasu arteritis

	TAK (*n*=15)	
	rho/r	*P* value
Lower limb strength (leg press)		
HAQ	−0.291	0.293
WIQ - Overall score	0.069	0.806
SF36 - Functional capacity	0.171	0.543
SF36 - Physical aspect	−0.057	0.838
IPAQ-SF - METs	0.295	0.285
VO_2 peak relative (mL/kg/min)	0.024	0.933
VO2 peak relative (mL/kg/min)		
HAQ	0.158	0.517
WIQ - Overall score	−0.193	0.427
SF36 - Functional capacity	−0.122	0.619
SF36 - Physical aspect	−0.114	0.641
IPAQ-SF - METs	−0.051	0.835
Lower limb strength (leg press)	0.024	0.933

HAQ Health Assessment Questionnaire, *IPAQ-SF* International Physical Activity Questionnaire Short Version, *METs* Metabolic equivalent, *SF-36* Short Form Health Survey, *TAK* Takayasu arteritis, VO_2 Volume of oxygen

results similar to cardiopulmonary treadmill test by Oliveira et al. [17] Lanzi et al. [16] evaluated (even though indirectly) the 6-min walk test, finding low values. However, they did not use a control group and employed one "gold standard" test, making comparisons difficult.

Furthermore, as seen in ANCA-associated vasculitis [43] and other rheumatic diseases [20, 21], our patients showed a significant reduction in maximum oxygen consumption; that is, a reduction in the capacity to absorb, transport, and use oxygen [44]. This reduction and poor test performance can be attributed to two main purported mechanisms:

a) Impairment of the cardiopulmonary system is expected for this population with major cardiovascular impairments, such as stenosis or occlusion of the branches of the aorta, valve problems, etc.
b) The presence of vascular claudication may impair physical performance, imposing the same daily living limitation as a peripheral arterial disease [45]. Difficulty in walking produces even more impaired aerobic capacity, creating a vicious circle of reduced VO_2 peak and inactivity, as seen in peripheral arterial disease [45].

Although the disease pathogenesis is distinct, the walking capacity of TAK patients is hindered, which occurs similarly to patients with peripheral arterial disease [45].

Moreover, patients with TAK also had a reduction in functional capacity, physical strength, pain, and general and mental health, demonstrating this disease leads to impairments in multiple aspects of quality of life.

Similarly, the patients had impairments in daily living, as pointed out in the HAQ questionnaire. These findings corroborate other studies that assessed quality of life using the SF-36 and HAQ questionnaires, where a worsening was found in all domains that demonstrated a worsening of quality of life in general when compared to healthy controls [46, 47].

Another important aspect is the association between remission and improved quality of life. In our study, only 15% of patients had disease activity demonstrating regardless of activity the disease seems to deteriorate patients' quality of life [47].

As found in our patients, muscle strength is reduced due to other chronic diseases [48, 49], resulting in a significant decrease in functional capacity and quality of life. Our data are similar to outocmes found in ANCA-associated vasculitis, demonstrating a possible association between reduced strength and worsened quality of life in vasculitis patients [50].

Importantly, muscle weakness is a strong and independent risk factor for all-cause morbidity and mortality in some populations [9, 10, 48, 49].

A critical factor in our results is the reduction in the total level of weekly caloric expenditure and physical activity. As seen in other rheumatic diseases, the reduction may be associated with a worsening of quality of life [51].

Similar to Margiotta et al.'s [52] study of paitents with systemic lupus erythematosus, our TAK patients presented low levels and intensities of physical activity that did not meet the recommendations of the World Health Organization (i.e., at least 150 min per week of moderate-intensity physical activity or 75 min of vigorous-intensity activity) [53].

Similar to outcomes in the healthy population, physical inactivity may worsen the health of patients with rheumatic diseases, which may lead to higher risk of CVD and comorbidities and increase the number and length of hospital stays [54].

Far from our findings, Akar et al. [49] demonstrated no differences in body composition in patients with rheumatoid arthritis, with the exception of bone mass density. Ours results found TAK patients showed a significant increase in waist-to-hip ratio and visceral adipose tissue compared to controls, signaling an impairment of body composition in this population.

However, patients with rheumatic diseases who present worse body composition, specifically adipose tissue, show an association with greater inflammation, disease activity, glucocorticoid use, and disease severity, but mainly increased cardiovascular risk, as seen in systemic lupus erythematosus [55].

Adipose tissue has long been related to morbidity and mortality. In addition to this traditional relationship, another important link is adipose tissue's pro-inflammatory nature, where adipokines are linked to immune response through their link with cytokines that lead to the inflammatory process in rheumatic diseases, such as interleukin-6 and tumor necrosis factor-alpha [56]. The result is the hypothetical maintenance of vicious circle of inflammation in rheumatic diseases, which can favor the process of atherosclerosis, cardiovascular risk, and mortality in this population [57].

In addition, BMI should not be the sole parameter to assess by which to assess boody composition in TAK. In our study, the BIM parameter was shown to be inaccurate, as it was in other populations, for evaluating adipose tissue and obesity [58].

Traditionally, patients with TAK have a higher risk of developing CVD and a greater presence of its risk factors. A series of studies corroborate our findings, as they observed the increase in systemic arterial hypertension and dyslipidemia in TAK [4, 6].

Markers such as LDL, total cholesterol, triglycerides were close to or within the normal range compared to healthy subjects, as shown in our study. These findings make it difficult to assess possible long-term risks, probably due to previous treatment of lipoproteins in patients with TAK.

The focus of this study is to assess the MCRFs, which corroborate the higher risk of morbidity and mortality [7–15, 59]. In our study, we found that most of the factors studied were deteriorating in TAK patients, such as reduced aerobic capacity, decreased muscle strength, reduced physical activity, low intensity of physical activity, and increased visceral adipose tissue.

As demonstrated by Crump et al. [14, 15], even though the analysis of these factors was conducted in studies including most men, the sum of these MCRFs seem to represent an aggravated risk, with a 2.5-fold increase in CVD.

Additionally, the MCRFs did not show significant correlations in our study, which may be, however, probably due to the sample size. In addition, drug treatment can also make it challenging to detect existing correlations between these factors. Therefore, our findings need to be analyzed with caution.

Many of the factors are modifiable with changes in habits, increased physical activity level, reduced sedentary lifestyle, and physical exercise, to ultimately improve the quality of life. However, a longitudinal study is eminently necessary to assess these changes.

Conclusions

Our patients in the TAK group have significant impairment of several MCRFs. These patients require strategies that will help change the MCFR, in order to reduce morbi-mortality and improve the quality of life.

Abbreviations

BMI: Body mass index; CRP: C-reactive protein; CTR: Control group; CVD: Cardiovascular disease; ECQ: Edinburgh Claudication Questionnaire; ESR: Erythrocyte sedimentation rate; HAQ: Health Assessment Questionnaire; HDL: High-density lipoprotein; IPAQ: International Physical Activity Questionnaire; ITAS: Indian Takayasu's Arteritis Activity Score; LDL: Low-density lipoprotein; MCRFs: Modifiable cardiovascular risk factors; NIH: National Institute of Health; RM: Maximum repetition test; SF: Short Form; TAK: Takayasu arteritis; TST: Timed-Stands test; TUG: Timed Up-and-Go; WIQ: Walking Impairment Questionnaire

Acknowledgments

Not applicable.

Authors' contributions

All authors contributed equally to write and review the manuscript. The author(s) read and approved the final manuscript.

Author details

[1]Division of Rheumatology, Faculdade de Medicina FMUSP, Universidade de Sao Paulo, Sao Paulo, Brazil. [2]Division of Rheumatology, Universidade Federal de São Paulo (UNIFESP), Sao Paulo, Brazil.

References

1. Lupi-Herrera E, Sanchez-Torres G, Marcushamer J, et al. Takayasu's arteritis. Clinical study of 107 cases. Am Heart J. 1977;93:94–103.
2. Belem JMFM, Pereira RMR, Perez MO, et al. Epidemiologic features of systemic vasculitides in the southeast region of Brazil: hospital-based survey. J Clin Rheumatol. 2019;2:106–10.
3. de Carvalho JF, Pereira RM, Viana VS, et al. Lack of antilipoprotein lipase antibodies in Takayasu's arteritis. Clin Develop Immunol. 2009;2009:803409.
4. de Carvalho JF, Bonfá E, Bezerra MC, et al. High frequency of lipoprotein risk levels for cardiovascular disease in Takayasu arteritis. Clin Rheumatol. 2009; 28:801–5.
5. Sato EI, Sassaki RH Jr, Leão CS, et al. Clinical and angiographic features of Takayasu's arteritis. Rev Bras Reumatol. 1998;38:9–14.
6. da Silva TF, Levy-Neto M, Bonfa E, et al. High prevalence of metabolic syndrome in Takayasu arteritis: increased cardiovascular risk and lower adiponectin serum levels. J Rheumatol. 2013;40:1897–904.
7. Mandsager K, Harb S, Cremer P, et al. Association of cardiorespiratory fitness with long-term mortality among adults undergoing exercise treadmill testing. JAMA Netw Open. 2018;1:1–12.
8. Kodama S, Saito K, Tanaka S, et al. Cardiorespiratory fitness as a quantitative predictor of all-cause mortality and cardiovascular events in healthy men and women: a meta-analysis. JAMA. 2009;301:2024–35.
9. Artero EG, Lee DC, Lavie CJ, et al. Effects of muscular strength on cardiovascular risk factors and prognosis. J Cardiopulm Rehabil Prev. 2012; 32:351–8.
10. Katzmarzyk PT, Craig CL. Musculoskeletal fitness and risk of mortality. Med Sci Sports Exerc. 2002;34:740–4.
11. Kubota Y, Evenson KR, MacLehose RF, et al. Physical activity and lifetime risk of cardiovascular disease and cancer. Med Sci Sports Exerc. 2017;49:1599–605.
12. Arem H, Moore SC, Patel A, et al. Leisure time physical activity and mortality: a detailed pooled analysis of the dose-response relationship. JAMA Int Med. 2015;175:959–67.
13. Britton KA, Massaro JM, Murabito JM, et al. Body fat distribution, incident cardiovascular disease, cancer, and all-cause mortality. J Am Coll Cardiol. 2013;62:921–5.
14. Crump C, Sundquist J, Winkleby MA, et al. Aerobic fitness, muscular strength and obesity in relation to risk of heart failure. Heart. 2017;103:1780–7.
15. Crump C, Sundquist J, Winkleby MA, et al. Interactive effects of aerobic fitness, strength, and obesity on mortality in men. Am J Prev Med. 2017;52: 353–61.
16. Lanzi S, Calanca L, Borgeat Kaeser A, et al. Walking performances and muscle oxygen desaturation are increased after supervised exercise training in Takayasu arteritis: a case report and a review of the literature. Eur Heart J Case Rep. 2018;2:1–6.
17. Oliveira DS, Shinjo SK, Silva MG, et al. Exercise in Takayasu arteritis: effects on inflammatory and angiogenic factors and disease-related symptoms. Arthritis Care Res (Hoboken). 2017;69:892–902.
18. Hörnberg K, Sundström B, Innala L, et al. Aerobic capacity over 16 years in patients with rheumatoid arthritis: relationship to disease activity and risk factors for cardiovascular disease. PLoS One. 2017;12:1–16.
19. Stavropoulos-Kalinoglou A, Metsios GS, Veldhuijzen van Zanten JJ, et al. Individualised aerobic and resistance exercise training improves cardiorespiratory fitness and reduces cardiovascular risk in patients with rheumatoid arthritis. Ann Rheum Dis. 2013;72:1819–25.
20. Pinto AJ, Miyake CN, Benatti FB, et al. Reduced aerobic capacity and quality of life in physically inactive patients with systemic lupus erythematosus with mild or inactive disease. Arthritis Care Res (Hoboken). 2016;68:1780–6.
21. Dassouki T, Benatti FB, Pinto AJ, et al. Objectively measured physical activity and its influence on physical capacity and clinical parameters in patients with primary Sjogren's syndrome. Lupus. 2017;26:690–7.
22. Arend WP, Michel BA, Bloch DA, et al. The American College of Rheumatology 1990 criteria for the classification of Takayasu arteritis. Arthritis Rheum. 1990;33:1129–34.
23. Ekdahl C, Eberhardt K, Andersson SI, et al. Assessing disability in patients with rheumatoid arthritis. Use of a Swedish version of the Stanford Health Assessment Questionnaire. Scand J Rheumatol. 1988;17:263–71.
24. da Mota Falcão D, Ciconelli RM, Ferraz MB. Translation and cultural adaptation of quality of life questionnaires: an evaluation of methodology. J Rheumatol. 2003;30:379–85.
25. Makdisse M, Nascimento Neto R, Chagas AC, et al. Cross-cultural adaptation

and validation of the Brazilian Portuguese version of the Edinburgh Claudication Questionnaire. Arq Bras Cardiol. 2003;88:501–6.
26. Ritti-Dias RM, Gobbo LA, Cucato GG, et al. Translation and validation of the Walking Impairment Questionnaire in Brazilian subjects with intermittent claudication. Arq Bras Cardiol. 2009;92:136–49.
27. Fritsch S, Copes RM, Savioli B, et al. Translation and validation of the Indian Takayasu clinical activity score (ITAS2010) for the Brazilian Portuguese language. Adv Rheumatol. 2019;59:43.
28. Kerr GS, Hallahan CW, Giordano J, et al. Takayasu arteritis. Ann Intern Med. 1994;120:919–29.
29. Davies MJ, D'Alessio DA, Fradkin J, et al. Management of hyperglycemia in type 2 diabetes, 2018. A consensus report by the American Diabetes Association (ADA) and the European Association for the Study of Diabetes (EASD). Diabetes Care. 2018;41:2669–701.
30. Whelton PK, Carey RM, Aronow WS, et al. 2017 ACC/AHA/AAPA/ABC/ACPM/AGS/APhA/ASH/ASPC/NMA/PCNA guideline for the prevention, detection, evaluation, and management of high blood pressure in adults: executive summary: a report of the American College of Cardiology/American Heart Association Task Force on clinical practice guidelines. Hypertension. 2018;71:1269–324.
31. De Backer G, Ambrosioni E, Borch-Johnsen K, et al. European guidelines on cardiovascular disease prevention in clinical practice: third joint task force of European and other societies on cardiovascular disease prevention in clinical practice (constituted by representatives of eight societies and by invited experts). Eur J Cardiovasc Prev Rehabil. 2003;10:S1–S10.
32. Matsudo S, Araújo T, Matsudo V, et al. Questionário internacional de atividade física (IPAQ): estudo de validade e reprodutibilidade no Brasil. Rev Bras Ativ Fis Saúde. 2001;6:5–18.
33. Dos Santos AM, Missé RG, Borges IBP, et al. The aerobic capacity in patients with antisynthetase syndrome and dermatomyositis. Adv Rheumatol. 2019;60:3.
34. Brown LE, Weir JP. Asep procedures recommendation I: accurate assessment of muscular strength and power. J Exerc Physiol Online. 2001;4:1–21.
35. Newcomer KL, Krug HE, Mahowald ML. Validity and reliability of the timed-stands test for patients with rheumatoid arthritis and other chronic diseases. J Rheumatol. 1993;20:21–7.
36. Podsiadlo D, Richardson S. The timed "up & go": a test of basic functional mobility for frail elderly persons. J Am Geriatr Soc. 1991;39:142–8.
37. Innes EV. Handgrip strength testing: a review of the literature. Australian Occup Ther J. 1999;46:120–40.
38. Moye L. Statistical methods for cardiovascular researchers. Circ Res. 2016;118:439–53.
39. Chan YH. Biostatistics 104: correlational analysis. Singap Med J. 2003;44:614–9.
40. Hata A, Noda M, Moriwaki R, et al. Angiographic findings of Takayasu arteritis: new classification. Int J Cardiol. 1996;54:155–63.
41. Aboyans V, Kamineni A, Allison MA, et al. The epidemiology of subclavian stenosis and its association with markers of subclinical atherosclerosis: the multi-ethnic study of atherosclerosis (MESA). Atherosclerosis. 2010;211:266–70.
42. Machado EB, Michet CJ, Ballard DJ, et al. Trends in incidence and clinical presentation of temporal arteritis in Olmsted county, Minnesota, 1950-1985. Arthritis Rheum. 1998;31:745–9.
43. Newall C, Schinke S, Savage CO, et al. Impairment of lung function, health status and functional capacity in patients with ANCA-associated vasculitis. Rheumatology (Oxford). 2005;44:623–8.
44. Wasserman K, Whipp BJ, Koyl SN, et al. Anaerobic threshold and respiratory gas exchange during exercise. J Appl Physiol. 1973;35:236–43.
45. Parmenter BJ, Dieberg G, Smart NA. Exercise training for management of peripheral arterial disease: a systematic review and meta-analysis. Sports Med. 2015;45:231–44.
46. Yilmaz N, Can M, Oner FA, et al. Impaired quality of life, disability and mental health in Takayasu's arteritis. Rheumatology (Oxford). 2013;52:1898–904.
47. Akar S, Can G, Binicier O, et al. Quality of life in patients with Takayasu's arteritis is impaired and comparable with rheumatoid arthritis and ankylosing spondylitis patients. Clin Rheumatol. 2008;27:859–65.
48. Kilgour RD, Vigano A, Trutschnigg B, et al. Handgrip strength predicts survival and is associated with markers of clinical and functional outcomes in advanced cancer patients. Support Care Cancer. 2013;21:3261–70.
49. Swallow EB, Reyes D, Hopkinson NS, et al. Quadriceps strength predicts mortality in patients with moderate to severe chronic obstructive pulmonary disease. Thorax. 2007;62:115–20.
50. Hessels AC, van der Hoeven JH, Sanders JSF, et al. Leg muscle strength is reduced and is associated with physical quality of life in antineutrophil cytoplasmic antibody-associated vasculitis. PLoS One. 2019;14:e0211895.
51. Margiotta DPE, Basta F, Dolcini G, et al. Physical activity and sedentary behavior in patients with systemic lupus erythematosus. PLoS One. 2018;13:e0193728.
52. Akar S, Sarı İ, Çömlekci A, et al. Body composition in patients with rheumatoid arthritis is not different than healthy subjects. Eur J Rheumatol. 2014;1:106–10.
53. Bull FC, Al-Ansari Salih S, Biddle S, et al. World Health Organization 2020 guidelines on physical activity and sedentary behaviour. Br J Sports Med. 2020;54:1451–62.
54. Turesson C, Matteson EL. Cardiovascular risk factors, fitness and physical activity in rheumatic diseases. Curr Opin Rheumatol. 2007;19:190–6.
55. Li Z, Shang J, Zeng S, et al. Altered body composition and increased visceral adipose tissue in premenopausal and late postmenopausal patients with SLE. Clin Rheumatol. 2019;38:3117–27.
56. Nikiphorou E, Fragoulis GE. Inflammation, obesity and rheumatic disease: common mechanistic links. A narrative review. Ther Adv Musculoskelet Dis. 2018;10:157–67.
57. Scotece M, Conde J, Gómez R, et al. Role of adipokines in atherosclerosis: interferences with cardiovascular complications in rheumatic diseases. Mediat Inflamm. 2012;2012:125458.
58. Shah NR, Braverman ER. Measuring adiposity in patients: the utility of body mass index (BMI), percent body fat, and leptin. PLoS One. 2012;7:e33308.
59. Fox CS, Massaro JM, Hoffmann U, et al. Abdominal visceral and subcutaneous adipose tissue compartments: association with metabolic risk factors in the Framingham heart study. Circulation. 2007;116:39–48.

11

The genetic influence of the brain-derived neurotrophic factor Val66Met polymorphism in chronic low back pain

Angela Shiratsu Yamada[1*], Flavia Tasmim Techera Antunes[1], Camila Ferraz[2], Alessandra Hubner de Souza[3] and Daniel Simon[1,2]

Abstract

Background: The Val66Met polymorphism of the brain-derived neurotrophic factor (BDNF) gene is a potential biomarker of vulnerability to pain. Thus, the present study aimed to investigate the association of this polymorphism with clinical and biopsychosocial factors in patients with chronic low back pain (CLBP).

Methods: A total of 107 individuals with CLBP answered questionnaires that were validated and adapted for the Brazilian population, including the Brief Inventory of Pain, the Central Sensitization Inventory, the Roland Morris Disability Questionnaire, the Tampa Scale for Kinesiophobia, the Pain Catastrophizing Scale, the Survey of Pain Attitude-Brief, and the Hospital Anxiety and Depression Scale. All of the subjects were genotyped for the BDNF Val66Met polymorphism.

Results: The sample showed moderate scores of disability, central sensitization, and kinesiophobia, in addition to mild anxiety, hopelessness, and ruminant thoughts. No significant association was observed between the Val66Met polymorphism and the variables analyzed. Besides, there was no relationship between the BDNF Val66Met polymorphism with CSI, catastrophization, or disabilities that were generated by CLBP.

Conclusion: The results showed that the Val66Met polymorphism of the BDNF gene was not associated with clinical and biopsychosocial characteristics of CLBP in the sample studied.

Keywords: Central sensitization, Catastrophizing, BDNF, Polymorphism, Single nucleotide polymorphism, Val66Met

Background

In the populations suffering from chronic pain, low back pain is one of the most prevalent musculoskeletal disorders, affecting 70 to 85% of adults at some point in their life [1]. Regardless of the primary or secondary pathology, the consequences of persistent pain include the fear of movement, pain catastrophizing, anxiety, and central sensitization. These outcomes appear to be the major contributors of pain and disability under these conditions [2, 3].

It is well known that the experience of pain is influenced by biological, psychological, and behavioral factors. Among the biological factors, there is a growing interest in the genetic aspects, in an attempt to explain some of the differences in the pain responses between individuals [4]. Studies have considered that the genetic factors represent more than a 50% susceptibility to chronic low back pain (CLBP) [5], whereas the variation in the genes that are involved in pain perception and its modulation, transduction, transmission, and conduction by the nervous system can result in variabilities in the experience of pain [6].

The brain-derived neurotrophic factor (BDNF) is a neurotrophin that is involved in neurogenesis and synaptic plasticity in the central nervous system. The

* Correspondence: angelasyamada@gmail.com
[1]Molecular and Cellular Biology Applied to Health, Lutheran University of Brazil (ULBRA), Canoas, Brazil

Val66Met polymorphism (c.196G > A, dbSNP: rs6265) of the BDNF gene represents the replacement of valine (Val) with a methionine (Met) at codon 66. This substitution in the BDNF pro-region changes the intracellular trafficking and packaging of the pro-BDNF, its availability in the synaptic cleft, and the deterioration of synaptic plasticity, thus decreasing the BDNF secretion [7]. The Val66Met polymorphism has been considered as a marker of vulnerability to pain. Individuals with the Met allele were more likely to have chronic pain when associated with the presence and severity of chronic musculoskeletal pain in multiple sites, in studies that investigated individuals with childhood or recent life stress [8], and with an increased risk of chronic postoperative pain [9]. However, the studies on the role of BDNF, both in relation to the genotypes, their expression, and the serum protein levels in chronic pain, still show inconclusive results.

Most treatment strategies for CLBP are still based on the biomedical model, that is, structural-anatomical-mechanical [10]. However, the biopsychosocial model is based on a dynamic relationship between the biological changes, psychological status, and social context, emphasizing that these factors have different roles in chronic pain, disability, and emotional maladjustment [11]. Therefore, the present study aimed to investigate the association of the single nucleotide polymorphism (SNP) Val66Met of the BDNF gene with clinical and biopsychosocial factors in patients with CLBP.

Methods

All of the procedures complied with the requirements of Resolution 466/12 of the National Health Council. The data collection occurred after the approval by the Research Ethics Committee from the Lutheran University of Brazil (ULBRA), under protocol number 2.254.800. All of the patients gave written informed consent before their participation.

Subjects

The study was carried out in Palmas (Tocantins, Brazil), at the Lutheran University Center of Palmas (CEULP/ULBRA), in the community service center, the Clinical School of Physiotherapy (CSP). The eligibility criteria were individuals over 18 years of age of both genders, who had CLBP for over 3 months.

Procedure

The individuals with CLBP answered questionnaires that were validated and adapted for the Brazilian population, such as the Brief Inventory of Pain (BIP) [12]; the Central Sensitization Inventory (CSI) [13]; the Roland Morris Disability Questionnaire (RMDQ) [14]; the Tampa Scale for Kinesiophobia [15]; the Pain Catastrophizing Scale (PCS) [16]; and the Hospital Anxiety and Depression Scale (HADS) [17]. Afterward, 5 ml of peripheral blood was collected using sodium ethylenediaminetetraacetic acid (EDTA) as an anticoagulant, and it was then frozen.

Genetic analyses

The total DNA was purified from the blood samples and the Val66Met SNP (rs6265) was genotyped through the real-time polymerase chain reaction (PCR) when using TaqMan® SNP Genotyping assays (Thermo Fisher Scientific; catalog 4,351,379, assay ID: C__11592758_10). All of the assays were run on a StepOnePlus™ system (Biosystems Inc., Foster City, USA).

Statistical analyses

The data was analyzed using descriptive statistics, and by employing mean, standard deviations, and percentages through the SAS version 9.4 program. A bivariate analysis was performed to compare the variables under study in relation to the genotypes of Val66Met. For the qualitative variables, the Chi-square test was applied, and for the quantitative variables, the Mann-Whitney non-parametric test was applied. The allele frequencies were determined by direct counting of the alleles. The departures from the Hardy-Weinberg equilibrium were evaluated by the Chi-square test. $p < 0.05$ was considered statistically significant.

Results

The sample was composed of 107 patients (56.5% women) with CLBP. The clinical and demographic characteristics of the sample are shown in Table 1. Briefly, the mean age was 46.2 ± 14.3 years, the BMI was 26.8 ± 5.1 kg/m^2 (26.7% with obesity), with a score of 49.6 ± 14.4 in the CSI assessment, presuming central sensitization, and a score of 15.7 ± 5.3 in the RMDQ, presuming disabilities. The analysis of the BIP showed that the patients had pain in at least roughly nine body regions, summing the low back. The Tampa scores were considered moderate (45.6 ± 7.8). The PCS scores evidenced rumination thoughts. In addition, mild anxiety was observed according to the HADS scores.

In the present study, it was observed that 26 (24.3%) patients were carriers of the Met allele of SNP Val66Met in the BDNF gene. There were no significant associations between the Val66Met genotypes and either the quantitative (Table 2) or the qualitative variables studied (Table 3).

Discussion

The present study found no associations between the BDNF Val66Met genotypes and the biopsychosocial phenotypes in patients with CLBP. The Val66Met

Table 1 Characteristics of the sample studied

Variable	Mean	SD
Age	46.24	14.27
Subjective assessment of stress	5.84	2.39
BMI	26.82	5.14
Total CSI score	49.6	14.39
Total RMDQ score	15.7	5.3
BIP pain intensity		
Worst	6.49	2.59
Least	3.16	2.45
Average	5.37	2.26
Now	4.56	3.02
BIP interference		
General activity	5.83	3.34
Mood	5.5	3.52
Walking	5.41	3.32
Normal work	5.97	3.7
Relations	3.58	3.34
Sleep	5.44	3.46
Enjoyment of life	4.48	3.63
Σ pain-body regions	8.95	6.04
Total Tampa score	45.61	7.82
Total PCS score	2.17	1.2
PCS rumination	2.68	1.33
PCS helplessness	1.53	1.31
HADS-anxiety	9.04	3.47
HADS-depression	6.91	3.98

BMI body mass index, *BPI* the brief inventory of pain, *CSI* central sensitization inventory, *HADS* hospital anxiety and depression scale, *PCS* pain catastrophizing scale, *RMDQ* Rolland-Morris disability questionnaire, *SD* standard deviation

polymorphism is the most studied in the BNDF gene and it has been investigated in several pathological conditions in humans [18–20]. The Val66Met polymorphism has also been associated with the methylation patterns, and it is being related to the epigenetic regulation of the BDNF gene [21]. From a biological perspective, it is known that the responses of an organism's experience to the external environment can be reflected in the epigenetic changes. Thus, the gene expression could also be regulated by the epigenetic modifications to the chromatin structure and the patterns of DNA methylation. These adaptations can modify, among others, neuronal morphology and the activity to produce changes in behavior [22, 23]. Alterations in the chromatin structure represent mechanisms by which pain can be converted gradually and progressively into the pathological processes of neuroinflammation, central sensitization, and ultimately, chronic pain syndromes [24].

The averages of the disabilities of the patients in the present study due to CLBP were classified as moderate from the RMDQ. It is recommended to consider an assessment of the multidimensional nature of CLBP in the management of pain [25]. This could be physical (for example, disability and body composition), psychological (for example, kinesiophobia, fear-avoidance, pain catastrophizing, pain self-efficacy, depression, anxiety, and sleep quality), and/or social (social functioning and work absenteeism) factors.

Most of the evaluated patients presented overweight/obesity conditions. Adiposity may modulate pain through peripheral sensitization from increased systemic inflammation [26]. In addition, it was observed that the increased fat infiltration of the paraspinal musculature could be associated with a compromised function of the muscles that control and support the low back [27, 28]. The findings from the BIP data also showed that the worst pain affected the normal work of the patients, restricting the performance of the activities of daily living.

The individuals in the present study reported being physically inactive. The relationship between a cluster of unhealthy lifestyle behaviors (smoking, alcohol drinking, physical activity, weight control, breakfast, snacking, and sleep) and low back pain (LBP) was investigated in a cross-sectional study of over 400,000 Japanese adults showing an association of this cluster with an increased risk of LBP, regardless of age and BMI [29]. Moreover, chronic pain is at least partly attributed to a sedentary and inactive lifestyle and it could be recognized as a lifestyle-related disease. Physical activity/inactivity may also determine the genetic/epigenetic and neural factors encoded in the brain [30]. A single session of exercise and regular physical activity induce changes in the genes that regulate the nociceptive processes, the learning of fear, and the stress responses, as well as those that are involved in the pathophysiology of chronic diseases [31].

In the current study, the mean of the total scores in Tampa was moderate. Fear can be learned through associative learning. Previous study reported that conditioning to fear was able of inducing a rapid increase in methylation of the BDNF gene in the hippocampus, and it occurred during the consolidation of fear [32]. It is well known that the fear and the avoidance of particular movements could add to a disability, but the assessment and removal of these barriers to movement might, therefore, reduce the disability [33]. A psychological factor that distinctly predicts changeability in the perception of pain and the development of moderate kinesiophobia is pain catastrophizing [34]. In the present study, the CLBP patients presented scores that suggested rumination and helplessness thoughts, besides mild anxiety and central sensitization. Anxiety and stress predict chronic pain in

Table 2 Comparison of the quantitative variables according to the BDNF Val66Met genotypes

Variable	Val/ Val (*n* = 81)	Val/Met (*n* = 26)	*P*-value
Age	46.2 ± 14.3	46.5 ± 14.6	0.73
Subjective assessment of stress	5.9 ± 2.5	5.8 ± 2.1	0.62
BMI	27.1 ± 5.2	26.4 ± 4.9	0.47
Total CSI score	50.3 ± 14.6	48.0 ± 13.9	0.50
Total RMDQ score	15.6 ± 5.5	15.8 ± 4.8	0.99
BIP pain intensity			
Worst	6.5 ± 2.5	6.4 ± 2.9	0.97
Least	3.2 ± 2.4	2.8 ± 2.4	0.42
Average	5.4 ± 2.1	5.2 ± 2.8	0.52
Now	4.6 ± 3.0	4.2 ± 3.0	0.45
BIP interference			
General activity	5.9 ± 3.4	5.4 ± 3.2	0.44
Mood	5.7 ± 3.5	4.9 ± 3.7	0.36
Walking	5.4 ± 3.2	5.3 ± 3.5	0.96
Normal work	6.1 ± 3.8	5.3 ± 3.4	0.16
Relation	3.6 ± 3.4	3.5 ± 3.2	0.92
Sleep	5.4 ± 3.6	5.3 ± 3.2	0.76
Enjoyment of life	4.3 ± 3.7	5.1 ± 3.5	0.34
Summation of pain body regions	9.0 ± 5.0	8.7 ± 8.8	0.07
Total Tampa score	45.6 ± 8.1	45.9 ± 7.2	0.87
Total PCS score	2.2 ± 1.2	1.9 ± 1.1	0.32
PCS rumination	2.8 ± 1.4	2.3 ± 1.1	0.18
PCS helplessness	1.5 ± 1.3	1.4 ± 1.4	0.51
HADS anxiety	9.3 ± 3.5	8.4 ± 3.5	0.52
HADS depression	7.1 ± 3.8	6.6 ± 4.4	0.35

Values are shown as mean ± standard deviation
BMI body mass index, *BPI* the brief inventory of pain, *CSI* central sensitization inventory, *HADS* hospital anxiety and depression scale, *PCS* pain catastrophizing scale, *RMDQ* Rolland-Morris disability questionnaire
P-value for the Mann-Whitney test

the long term and they might mediate the vulnerability to pain [35]. Thus, there is plausibility that the extent of central sensitization symptoms in people with non-specific LBP might be associated with the pre-morbid trait anxiety sub-types and the abnormal trait sensory processing profiles [36, 37]. Moreover, depression and anxiety are barriers to treatment adherence in various chronic pain conditions, such as low back pain [38].

Although 74% of the patients in the present study reported themselves to be active/employed, they described the pain during a month at an intense level and with chronicity for up to 13 months. This is important since CLBP is also considered responsible for absenteeism at work, and with high rates of disability, generating high costs for the health system, social security, and society in general [39]. Moreover, non-opioids were the main medication used, and most of the patients reported a modest relief of the pain with the medication.

The importance of behavioral approaches to back pain management does not preclude the continuing need to investigate mechanisms and the potential biological determinants of non-specific low back pain [40]. The relative importance of the genetic factors in human musculoskeletal pain conditions, such as CLBP, painful temporomandibular joint disorders, fibromyalgia, and chronic widespread pain, is becoming clearer. Several polymorphisms in the genes are contributing to serotonergic and adrenergic pathways that are associated with musculoskeletal pain [41]. Despite studies demonstrating evidence that the BDNF Val66Met polymorphism influences the cortical processing of experimental electrical pain stimuli in an indirect manner [4], or in pain catastrophizing [42], the findings in the present study did not show the influence of this polymorphism in chronic pain complaints.

Certain limitations must be considered in the interpretation of the current study's findings. First, the

Table 3 Comparison of the qualitative variables according to the BDNF Val66Met genotypes

	Genotype		*P*-value
	Val/ Val N (%)	Val/Met N (%)	
Gender			
Female	45 (55.6)	16 (61.5)	0.59
Male	36 (44.4)	10 (38.6)	
Civil status			
Living alone	42 (51.8)	11 (42.3)	0.40
Living with partner	39 (48.2)	15 (57.7)	
Ethnicity			
White	14 (18.2)	8 (34.8)	
Brown	46 (59.7)	13 (56.5)	0.14
Black	17 (22.1)	2 (8.7)	
Schooling			
Until high school	63 (77.8)	16 (64.0)	0.17
Complete high school	18 (22.2)	9 (36.0)	
Have children			
No	19 (23.5)	6 (23.1)	0.97
Yes	62 (76.5)	20 (76.9)	
Healthy			
Good, very good, or great	35 (44.3)	12 (46.1)	0.87
Regular, bad, or lousy	44 (55.7)	14 (53.9)	
Chronicity pain			
3–12 months	21 (25.9)	5 (19.2)	
13–60 months	27 (33.3)	13 (50.0)	0.31
> 60 months	33 (40.8)	8 (30.8)	
Pain intensity			
Least	8 (9.9)	4 (15.4)	
Moderate	14 (17.3)	3 (11.5)	0.62
Intense	59 (72.8)	19 (73.1)	
Pain duration in the month			
Intermittent	37 (46.2)	15 (65.2)	0.11
Constant	43 (53.8)	8 (34.8)	
Comorbidities			
No	46 (56.8)	16 (61.5)	0.67
Yes	35 (43.2)	10 (38.5)	
Physical activity			
Inactive	55 (67.9)	18 (69.2)	
Insufficiently active	8 (9.9)	4 (15.4)	0.80
Moderately active	13 (16.0)	3 (11.5)	
Vigorously active	5 (6.2)	1 (3.9)	
Smoking			
No	68 (91.9)	21 (91.3)	0.93
Yes	6 (8.1)	2 (8.7)	
Alcoholism			
No	66 (89.2)	22 (95.7)	0.35
Yes	8 (10.8)	1 (4.3)	

Table 3 Comparison of the qualitative variables according to the BDNF Val66Met genotypes *(Continued)*

	Genotype		
	Val/ Val N (%)	Val/Met N (%)	*P*-value
Satisfaction			
Unsatisfied or a little satisfied	33 (51.6)	9 (40.9)	0.39
Satisfied or much satisfied	31 (48.4)	13 (59.1)	
Occupational situation			
Active/employed	62 (76.5)	18 (69.2)	0.45
Unemployed	19 (23.5)	8 (30.8)	
Low back pain in family history			
No	36 (44.4)	12 (46.2)	0.88
Yes	45 (55.6)	14 (53.8)	
Overweight/obesity			
No	32 (41.0)	11 (42.3)	0.91
Yes	46 (59.0)	15 (57.7)	
CSI			
No	14 (17.3)	4 (15.4)	0.82
Yes	67 (82.7)	22 (84.6)	
RMDQ			
No	28 (34.6)	9 (34.6)	0.97
Yes	53 (65.4)	17 (65.4)	
Medication			
Non opioid	33 (62.3)	12 (80.0)	0.20
Weak opioid	20 (37.7)	3 (20.0)	
Medication frequency			
Every 6 h	35 (66.0)	7 (50.0)	0.27
If there is pain	18 (34.0)	7 (50.0)	
Start of medication			
12 months ago	32 (68.1)	8 (80.0)	
13–60 months	7 (14.9)	1 (10.0)	0.75
More than 60 months	8 (17.0)	1 (10.0)	
Relief of pain with medication			
50% relief	32 (62.8)	5 (45.5)	0.29
More than 50% relief	19 (37.2)	6 (54.5)	
Tampa score			
Light	7 (8.6)	2 (7.7)	
Moderate	47 (58.1)	14 (53.8)	0.89
Critical	27 (33.3)	10 (38.5)	
HADS-anxiety			
No	34 (42.0)	11 (42.3)	0.98
Yes	47 (58.0)	15 (57.7)	
HADS-depression			
No	53 (65.4)	20 (76.9)	0.27
Yes	28 (34.6)	6 (23.1)	

CSI central sensitization inventory, *HADS* hospital anxiety and depression scale, *RMDQ* Rolland-Morris disability questionnaire
P-value for the Chi-square test

statistical power of the sample size that was analyzed was limited. Second, this was a cross-sectional study, which might limit the causality identification of the demographic and clinical variables that were investigated. Third, to have a better understanding of the role of BDNF in CLBP, it would be important to investigate the correlation between the genotypes and the serum levels.

Conclusion

The present study showed no association between the Val66Met BDNF polymorphism with the clinical and biopsychosocial characteristics in patients with CLBP. However, further studies are still needed to elucidate if the BDNF Val66Met polymorphism could influence other distinct subjective pain experience outcomes in different samples with CLBP.

Abbreviations

BDNF: Brain-derived neurotrophic factor; BIP: Brief inventory of pain; BMI: Body mass index; CLBP: Chronic low back pain; CSI: Central Sensitization Inventory; CEULP/ULBRA: Lutheran University Center of Palmas; HADS: Hospital anxiety and depression scale; LBP: Low back pain; Met: Methionine; NAC: Community service center; PCR: Polymerase chain reaction; PCS: Pain catastrophizing scale; RMDQ: Roland Morris disability questionnaire; SD: Standard deviation; SNP: Single nucleotide polymorphism; ULBRA: Lutheran University of Brazil; Val: Valine

Acknowledgements

The authors would like to thank the patients who participated in the study.

Authors' contributions

A.S. Yamada, A.H. de Souza, and D. Simon designed the study. A.S. Yamada and C. Ferraz collected the data. A.S. Yamada and D. Simon performed the statistical analyses. A.S. Yamada, A.H. de Souza, and D. Simon interpreted and discussed the results. A.S. Yamada and D. Simon wrote the paper. A.S. Yamada, F.T.T. Antunes, C. Ferraz, A.H. de Souza, and D. Simon contributed to the final version of the manuscript. All of the authors have reviewed and approved the final version of the article, including the authorship list.

Author details

[1]Molecular and Cellular Biology Applied to Health, Lutheran University of Brazil (ULBRA), Canoas, Brazil. [2]Human Molecular Genetics Laboratory, Lutheran University of Brazil (ULBRA), Canoas, Brazil. [3]Biochemical and Molecular Pharmacology from the Federal University of Minas Gerais, Belo Horizonte, Brazil.

References

1. Becker A, Held H, Redaelli M, Strauch K, Chenot JF, Leonhardt C, et al. Low back pain in primary care: costs of care and prediction of future health care utilization. Spine. 2010;35(18):1714–20. https://doi.org/10.1097/brs.0b013e3181cd656f.
2. Gatchel RJ, Peng YB, Peters ML, Fuchs PN, Turk DC. The biopsychosocial approach to chronic pain: scientific advances and future directions. Psychol Bull. 2007;133(4):581–624. https://doi.org/10.1037/0033-2909.133.4.581.
3. Siddall PJ, Cousins MJ. Persistent pain as a disease entity: implications for clinical management. Anesth Analg. 2004;99(2):510–20. https://doi.org/10.1213/01.ANE.0000133383.17666.3A
4. Vossen H, Kenis G, Rutten B, van Os J, Hermens H, Lousberg R. The genetic influence on the cortical processing of experimental pain and the moderating effect of pain status. PLoS One. 2010;5(10):e13641. https://doi.org/10.1371/journal.pone.0013641.
5. MacGregor AJ, Andrew T, Sambrook PN, Spector TD. Structural, psychological, and genetic influences on low back and neck pain: a study of adult female twins. Arthritis Rheum. 2004;51(2):160–7. https://doi.org/10.1002/art.20236.
6. Omair A, Mannion AF, Holden M, Fairbank J, Lie BA, Hägg O, et al. Catechol-O-methyltransferase (COMT) gene polymorphisms are associated with baseline disability but not long-term treatment outcome in patients with chronic low back pain. Eur Spine J. 2015;24(11):2425–31. https://doi.org/10.1007/s00586-015-3866-5.
7. Harrisberger F, Smieskova R, Schmidt A, Lenz C, Walter A, Wittfeld K, et al. BDNF Val66Met polymorphism and hippocampal volume in neuropsychiatric disorders: a systematic review and meta-analysis. Neurosci Behav Rev. 2015;55:107–1. https://doi.org/10.1016/j.neubiorev.2015.04.017.
8. Generaal E, Milaneschi Y, Jansen R, Elzinga BM, Dekker J, Penninx BW. The brain-derived neurotrophic factor pathway, life stress, and chronic multi-site musculoskeletal pain. Mol Pain. 2016;12:1744806916646783.https://doi.org/10.1177/1744806916646783.
9. Tian Y, Liu X, Jia M, Yu H, Lichtner P, Shi Y, et al. Targeted genotyping identifies susceptibility locus in brain-derived Neurotrophic factor gene for chronic postsurgical pain. Anesthesiology. 2018;128(3):587–97. https://doi.org/10.1097/ALN.0000000000001977.
10. Desconsi MB, Bartz PT, Fiegenbaum TR, Candotti CT, Vieira A. Treatment of patients of nonspecific chronic low back pain by physical therapists: a cross-sectional study. Fisioter Pesqui. 2019;26(1):15–21. https://doi.org/10.1590/1809-2950/17003626012019.
11. Dionísio GH, Salermo VY, Padilha A. Central sensitization and beliefs among patients with chronic pain in a primary health care unit. BrJP. 2020;3(1):42–7. https://doi.org/10.5935/2595-0118.20200010.
12. Ferreira KA, Teixeira MJ, Mendonza TR, Cleeland CS. Validation of brief pain inventory to Brazilian patients with pain. Support Care Cancer. 2011;19(4):505–11. https://doi.org/10.1007/s00520-010-0844-7.
13. Caumo W, Antunes LC, Elkfury JL, et al. The central sensitization inventory validated and adapted for a Brazilian population: psychometric properties and its relationship with brain-derived neurotrophic factor. J Pain Res. 2017;10:2109–22. https://doi.org/10.2147/JPR.S131479.
14. Nusbaum L, Natour J, Ferraz MB, Goldenberg J. Translation, adaptation and validation of the Roland-Morris questionnaire - Brazil Roland-Morris. Braz J Med Biol Res. 2001;34(2):203–10. https://doi.org/10.1590/S0100-879X2001000200007.
15. Siqueira FB, Teixeira-Salmela LF, Magalhães LC. Analysis of the psychometric properties of the brazilian version of the Tampa scale for kinesiophobia. Acta Ortop Br. 2007;15(1):19–24. https://doi.org/10.1590/S1413-78522007000100004.
16. Junior JS, Nicholas MK, Pereira IA, Pimenta CAM, Asghari A, Cruz RM. Validation of the pain-related Catastrophizing thoughts scale. Acta fisiatr. 2008;15(1):31–6.
17. Castro MMC, Quarantini L, Batista-Neves S, Kraychete DC, Daltro C, Miranda-Scippa A. Validity of the hospital anxiety and depression scale in patients with chronic pain. Rev Bras Anestesiol. 2006;56(5):470–7. https://doi.org/10.1590/S0034-70942006000500005.
18. Shen T, You Y, Joseph C, Mirzaei M, Klistorner A, Graham SL, et al. BDNF polymorphism: a review of its diagnostic and clinical relevance in neurodegenerative disorders. Aging Dis. 2018;9(3):523–36. https://doi.org/10.14336/AD.2017.0717.
19. Tsai SJ. Critical issues in BDNF Val66Met genetic studies of neuropsychiatric disorders. Front Mol Neurosci. 2018;11:156. https://doi.org/10.3389/fnmol.2018.00156.
20. Lin CC, Huang TL. Brain-derived neurotrophic factor and mental disorders. Biom J. 2020;43(2):134–42. https://doi.org/10.1016/j.bj.2020.01.001.
21. Ursini G, Cavalleri T, Fazio L, Angrisano T, Iacovelli L, Porcelli A, et al. BDNF rs6265 methylation and genotype interact on risk for schizophrenia. Epigenetics. 2016;11(1):11–23. https://doi.org/10.1080/15592294.2015.1117736.
22. Berger SL. The complex language of chromatin regulation during transcription. Nature. 2007;447(7143):407–12. https://doi.org/10.1038/nature05915.
23. Kress M, Hüttenhofer A, Landry M, Kuner R, Favereaux A, Greenberg D, et al.

microRNAs in nociceptive circuits as predictors of future clinical applications. Front Mol Neurosci. 2013;6:33. https://doi.org/10.3389/fnmol.2013.00033.

24. Descalzi G, Ikegami D, Ushijima T, Nestler EJ, Zachariou V, Narita M. Epigenetic mechanisms of chronic pain. Trends Neurosci. 2015;38(4):237–46. https://doi.org/10.1016/j.tins.2015.02.001.
25. Tagliaferri SD, Miller CT, Owen PJ, Mitchell UH, Brisby H, Fitzgibbon B, et al. Domains of chronic low back pain and assessing treatment effectiveness: a clinical perspective. Pain Pract. 2020;20(2):211–25. https://doi.org/10.1111/papr.12846.
26. Heuch I, Hagen K, Heuch I, Nygaard Ø, Zwart JA. The impact of body mass index on the prevalence of low back pain: the HUNT study. Spine. 2010; 35(7):764–8. https://doi.org/10.1097/BRS.0b013e3181ba1531.
27. Goubert D, Oosterwijck JV, Meeus M, Danneels L. Structural changes of lumbar muscles in non-specific low back pain: a systematic review. Pain Phys. 2016;19(7):E985–E1000. 27676689.
28. Fortin M, Videman T, Gibbons LE, Battié MC. Paraspinal muscle morphology and composition: a 15-yr longitudinal magnetic resonance imaging study. Med Sci Sports Exerc. 2014;46(5):893–901.https://doi.org/10.1249/MSS.0000000000000179.
29. Yoshimoto T, Ochiai H, Shirasawa T, Nagahama S, Uehara A, Muramatsu J, et al. Clustering of lifestyle factors and its association with low back pain: a cross-sectional study of over 400,000 Japanese adults. J Pain Res. 2020;13: 1411–9. https://doi.org/10.2147/JPR.S247529.
30. Senba E, Kami K. A new aspect of chronic pain as a lifestyle-related disease. Neurobiol Pain. 2017;1:6–15. https://doi.org/10.1016/j.ynpai.2017.04.003.
31. Polli A, Ickmans K, Godderis L, Nijs J. When environment meets genetics: a clinical review of the epigenetics of pain, psychological factors, and physical activity. Arch Phys Med Rehabil. 2019;100(6):1153–61.https://doi.org/10.1016/j.apmr.2018.09.118.
32. Lubin FD, Roth TL, Sweatt JD. Epigenetic regulation of BDNF gene transcription in the consolidation of fear memory. J Neurosci. 2008;28(42): 10576–86. https://doi.org/10.1523/JNEUROSCI.1786-08.2008.
33. Rainville J, Smeets RJ, Bendix T, Tveito TH, Poiraudeau S, Indahl AJ. Fear-avoidance beliefs and pain avoidance in low back pain--translating research into clinical practice. Spine J. 2011;11(9):895–903. https://doi.org/10.1016/j.spinee.2011.08.006.
34. Sullivan MJ, Adams H, Rhodenizer T, Stanish WD. A psychosocial risk factor-targeted intervention for the prevention of chronic pain and disability following whiplash injury. Phys Ther. 2006;86(1):8–18. https://doi.org/10.1093/ptj/86.1.8.
35. Chapman CR, Tuckett RP, Song CW. Pain and stress in a systems perspective: reciprocal neural, endocrine, and immune interactions. J Pain. 2008;9(2):122–45. https://doi.org/10.1016/j.jpain.2007.09.006.
36. Clark JR, Nijs J, Yeowell G, Holmes P, Goodwin PC. Trait sensitivity, anxiety, and personality are predictive of central sensitization symptoms in patients with chronic low back pain. Pain Pract. 2019;19(8):800–10. https://doi.org/10.1111/papr.12809.
37. Clark JR, Yeowell G, Goodwin PC. Trait anxiety and sensory processing profile characteristics in patients with non-specific chronic low back pain and central sensitization - a pilot observational study. J Bodywork Mov Ther. 2018;22(4):909–16. https://doi.org/10.1016/j.jbmt.2017.11.007.
38. Jack K, McLean SM, Moffett JK, Gardiner E. Barriers to treatment adherence in physiotherapy outpatient clinics: a systematic review. Man Ther. 2010; 15(3):220–8. https://doi.org/10.1016/j.math.2009.12.004.
39. Nascimento PRC, Costa LOP. Prevalência da dor lombar no Brasil: uma revisão sistemática. Cad Saude Publica. 2015;31(6):1141–55. https://doi.org/10.1590/0102-311X00046114.
40. Buchbinder R, Tulder MV, Öberg B, Costa LM, Woolf A, Schoene M, et al. Low back pain: a call for action. Lancet. 2018;391(10137):2384–8. https://doi.org/10.1016/S0140-6736(18)30488-4.
41. Diatchenko L, Fillingim RB, Smith SB, Maixner W. The phenotypic and genetic signatures of common musculoskeletal pain conditions. Nat Rev Rheumatol. 2013;9(6):340–50. https://doi.org/10.1038/nrrheum.2013.43.
42. da Silveira Alves CF, Caumo W, Silvestri JM, Zortea M, Dos Santos VS, Cardoso DF, et al. Pain catastrophizing is associated with the Val66Met polymorphism of the brain-derived neurotrophic factor in fibromyalgia. Adv Rheumatol. 2020;60(1):39. https://doi.org/10.1186/s42358-020-00141-9.

12

Using urinary neutrophile gelatinase-associated lipocalin for prognosticate renal dysfunction in children with familial Mediterranean fever the study design

Sinem Can Oksay[1], Hasan Dursun[2,3*], Sebnem Tekin Neijmann[4] and Sami Hatipoglu[1]

Abstract

Background: The most important finding that affects the prognosis in Familial Mediterranean Fever is renal amyloidosis. The aim of the present study was to analyze neutrophil gelatinase-associated lipocalin levels in the urine, and to investigate whether it may be used as an early marker for renal involvement.

Methods: Forty attack-free children followed by diagnosis of Familial Mediterranean Fever with age range of 5 and 18 years, and 38 healthy children with similar ages and genders were enrolled into the study. Hemogram, sedimentation, C-reactive protein, urine analysis, creatinine in the spot urine, microalbumin and urinary neutrophil gelatinase-associated lipocalin levels were analyzed and evaluated statistically in the patients and controls.

Results: There was not any statistically significant difference between the patient and control groups for age, gender, height and body weight. Although there was not any clinical sign of attack in the patient group, sedimentation, C-reactive protein and fibrinogen levels were significantly higher than the control group ($p = 0.002$, $p = 0.023$, and $p = 0.006$, respectively). Similarly, urinary neutrophil gelatinase-associated lipocalin level and urinary creatinine ratio were significantly higher in the patient group ($p = 0.0001$, $p = 0.011$, respectively). We found a positive correlation between uNGAL level and uNGAL/uCr ratio and number of attacks per year in FMF patients ($r = 0.743$, $p = 0.001$ and $r = 0.516$, $p = 0.001$; respectively).

Conclusions: Detection of significantly higher levels of urinary neutrophil gelatinase-associated lipocalin level and urinary neutrophil gelatinase-associated lipocalin level to creatinine ratio were suggested as urinary neutrophil gelatinase-associated lipocalin level as a non-invasive marker for renal involvement better than microalbumin.

Keywords: Familial Mediterranean fever, Urinary neutrophil gelatinase-associated lipocalin

* Correspondence: dursunhs@yahoo.com
[2]Dr. Sadi Konuk Training and Research Hospital Department of Pediatric Nephrology, Health Science University, Istanbul, Turkey
[3]Okmeydani Training and Research Hospital Department of Pediatric Nephrology, Health Science University, Kaptan Paşa Mahallesi, Darülaceze Cad. No: 25 Okmeydani, 34384 Şişli/Istanbul, Turkey

Background

Familial Mediterranean Fever (FMF) is a recurrent disease with an autosomal recessive inheritance pattern, which is presented by fever for 12 to 72 h, attacks of abdominal, chest and joint pain. Family history is common in the progress of the disease; the most important factor in pathogenesis of the disease is pyrin dysfunction as a result of mutations on MEditerranean FeVer (MEFV) gene on the short arm of chromosome 16 [1–5].

Secondary amyloidosis is the most important and most common complication of FMF [3, 6, 7]. Despite the developments in diagnosis and treatment, FMF may progress to amyloidosis and subsequent renal failure. Amyloidosis manifests proteinuria at nephrotic limits and subsequent uremia, resulting with end-stage renal disease [8–10]. Some mutations on the MEFV gene, especially homozygote mutation of M694V were demonstrated to be associated with higher risk for amyloidosis [11–13]. Increase of certain acute phase markers such as C-reactive protein (CRP), serum amyloid A (SAA), erythrocyte sedimentation rate (ESR), and fibrinogen are detected [14–16]. Urinary microalbuminuria (uMA)/ urinary creatinine (uCr) is analyzed to detect AA amyloidosis in these patients earlier. It was demonstrated that uMA/uCr ratio is important for early detection of amyloidosis [17–20]. However, it is commonly accepted that more sensitive and specific markers are required in order to understand development and progression of nephropathy in patients with FMF.

Neutrophile gelatinase-associated lipocalcin (NGAL) is a member of lipocalin proteins. Members of this group are extracellular proteins which bind small and hydrophobic molecules, and play a role in cellular homeostasis [21, 22]. Urinary NGAL (uNGAL) is filtered by glomerules like other small lipocalin molecules. Almost all are absorbed through megalin receptors which are expressed in the brush border on proximal tubule, and uptaken through endocytosis. The level is eventually lower in the urine of healthy individuals. Previous studies indicated that uNGAL is a diagnostic marker in case of glomerular and tubular dysfunction [21–24]. It is accepted as an early predictive biological marker for acute renal injury and chronic renal diseases [25–27]. These findings suggest that uNGAL may be important for FMF patients in order to detect the renal disorder earlier to optimize the patient outcomes, and to achieve the recovery. The aim of the present study was to compare uNGAL and uMA levels as well as uNGAL/uCr and uMA/uCr rates for accurate and early prediction of amyloidosis which causes renal dysfunction in FMF patients, and to investigate whether uNGAL and uNGAL/uCr ratio may be used for disease monitoring.

Methods

Study design and participants

This study was performed on 40 attack-free patients who have referred Pediatric Nephrology Polyclinic of Bakırkoy Dr. Sadi Konuk Training and Research Hospital and diagnosed with FMF between February 2013 and August 2013 and 38 healthy volunteers with similar age and gender distribution. The patient group included 24 females and 16 males, whereas the control group included 22 females and 16 males. The study protocol was approved by local ethical committee of our hospital. The informed consent form was obtained from parent(s) of the patient following a detailed explanation about objectives and scope of the study in line with the principles of Helsinki Declaration of World Medical Association. All patients were receiving colchicine treatment. No patients resistant to colchicine were included in the study. None of our patients were receiving antiinterleukin-1 treatment.

Laboratory tests

Results of complete blood count, ESR, CRP, fibrinogen, SAA and urine analyses which have been performed on the patients enrolled during routine examination and tests were recorded from patient files. The initial and midstream urine samples were then collected from the patients for uNGAL, uMA and uCr analyses during referral. The urine samples taken into sterile containers were centrifuged at 4000 rpm for 10 min. The supernatant was stored at − 80 °C until the time of analysis. The analysis was performed through Enzyme-Linked Immunosorbent Assay (ELISA) after collection of all samples. The Lipocalin/2 NGAL ELISA kit (Aviscera Bioscıence, Inc. Santa Clara, CA), and sandwich enzyme immunoassay technique were used; results were evaluated in pg/mL. MA immunoturbidimetry [26] and spectrophotometric urinary Cr analysis were performed on same urine sample; results were evaluated in mg/dL. The patient and control groups were compared for uNGAL and uMA levels, uNGAL/uCr and uMA/uCr rates as well as other parameters.

Statistical analysis

Statistical analysis was performed through the statistical package SPSS software (Version 21.0, SPSS Inc. Chicago, IL, USA). If continuous variables were normal, they were defined as the mean ± standard deviation ($p > 0.05$ in Kolmogorov-Smirnov test or Shapira-Wilk ($n < 30$); and if the continuous variables were not normal, they were described as median. Comparisons between groups were applied by Student T test or OneWay ANOVA for normally distributed data; and Mann Whitney U test or Kruscall Wallis test were used for the data which have not distributed normally. The categorical variables between the groups were analyzed by the Chi-square test or Fisher Exc. test. Univariate analyses were performed by Spearman's correlation test. Receiver operating characteristic curves (ROC curves) were constructed and the areas under curve (AUC) as well as the sensitivity (sen.), and the specificity (spec.) were estimated. A multiple logistic regression analysis was used to determine the associations between measurements; dependent variable values of $p < 0.05$ were considered statistically significant.

Results

Demographic data and some laboratory tests results of the patients and controls were presented in Table 1. The patient group included 16 males and 24 females; the control group included 16 males and 22 females; and there was not any statistically significant difference in gender distribution ($p = 0.85$). Similarly, there was not any statistically significant difference between the patient and control groups for age, height, and body weight average ($p = 0.73$, $p = 0.68$, $p = 0.68$, respectively). The difference between systolic blood pressure (SBP) and diastolic blood pressure (DBP) averages of the patient and control groups was not statistically significant ($p > 0.05$).

There was not any statistically significant difference detected between average leukocyte, hemoglobin, hematocrit, and platelet levels in the patient and control groups ($p > 0.05$). However, the mean corpuscular volume (MCV) was lower whereas CRP, fibrinogen and ESR averages were significantly higher in the patient group when compared with the control group ($p = 0.01$, $p = 0.02$, $p = 0.002$ and $p = 0.006$, respectively). Spot uNGAL and uMA levels, and uNGAL/uCr and uMA/uCr rates were compared in the patients and controls. There was not any statistically significant difference observed in uMA level and uMA/uCr ratio of the patient and control groups ($p = 0.36$ and $p = 0.74$, respectively). However, uNGAL level and uNGAL/uCr ratio of FMF group was significantly higher than the control group ($p = 0.0001$ and $p = 0.01$, respectively).

The ROC analysis was performed to estimate diagnostic profile of uNGAL and uNGAL/uCr in order to detect renal injury in the patient group. There was not any statistically significant difference when ROC distribution of uNGAL for differential diagnosis of FMF, and the area under the ROC curve of uNGAl level and uNGAL/uCr ratio ($p = 0.0001$ and $p = 0.01$, Table 2, Fig. 1).

A logistic regression analysis was performed by adding the statistically significant parameters in the patient and control groups in order to investigate the risk factors that affect the patients. uNGAL ($p = 0.0001$) was

Table 1 Demographic data and laboratory findings in patients and controls

Parameters	Patients (n = 40) Mean ± SD	Controls (n = 38) Mean ± SD	p
Sex (boys/girls)	16/24	16/22	0.85
Age (year)	8.94 ± 3.73	9.21 ± 3.10	0.73
Height (cm)	130.15 ± 23.06	132.17 ± 20.12	0.68
Weight (kg)	31.21 ± 15.53	32.66 ± 14.97	0.68
SBP (mmHg)	102.25 ± 13.00	104.47 ± 11.14	0.42
DBP (mmHg)	63.13 ± 8.30	65.67 ± 8.48	0.19
Leukocyte (mm^3)	7.68 ± 4.03	6.73 ± 2.19	0.20
Hemoglobin (gr/dL)	11.99 ± 1.64	12.56 ± 1.03	0.07
Hematocrit (%)	37.38 ± 2.98	38.08 ± 2.83	0.29
*MCV (fL)	80.00 ± 5.40	83.60 ± 6.70	**0.01**
Platelet (mm^3)	302.356 ± 110.206	304.658 ± 59.945	0.91
*CRP (mg/dL)	2.60 ± 5.82	0.38 ± 0.79	**0.02**
*ESR (mm/h)	18.76 ± 13.98	10.18 ± 9.17	**0.002**
*Fibrinogen (mg/dL)	314.10 ± 67.89	273.79 ± 58.34	**0.006**
Urine findings	**Median (Min-Max)**	**Median (Min-Max)**	**P**
uMA (mg/dL)	20.14 (1.20–169.00)	14.08 (2.10–81.70)	0.34
*uNGAL (pg/mL)	2.1 (0.5–11.5)	0.9 (0.11–3.4)	**0.0001**
uCr (mg/dL)	71.95 (11.00–356.65)	98.53 (21.20–256.70)	0.06
uMA/uCr (mg/mg Cr)	0.35 (0.02–2.77)	0.19 (0.02–2.09)	0.13
*uNGAL/uCr (100 x pg/mg Cr)	3 (1–9)	1 (0.1–14)	**0.01**

SD Standard Deviation, *SBP* Systolic blood pressure, *DBP* Diastolic blood pressure, *MVC* Mean corpuscular volume, *CRP* C-reactive protein, *ESR* Erythrocyte sedimentation rate, *uMA* Urine microalbumine, *uNGAL* Urine neutrophil gelatinase-associated lipocalin, *uCr* Urine creatinine
*:$p < 0.05$

Table 2 The cut off, area under the curve (AUC), sensitivity and 1-specificity of uNGAL in patients with familial Mediterranean fever

Parameters	AUC (%95 CI)	*p*	Cutoff	Sensitivity (%95 CI)	1-Specificity (95% CI)
uNGAL	0.77 (0.67–0.88)	**0.0001**	1.12	70.0	68.2
uNGAL/uCr	0.78 (0.68–0.88)	**0.01**	1.80	72.5	68.4

CI Confidence interval, *uNGAL* Urine neutrophil gelatinase-associated lipocalin, *uCr* Urine creatinine

detected as an independent risk factor that affects FMF. Accordingly, uNGAL levels of the FMF patients are probably 3.38 times (1.74 to 6.57) as high as those of the control group (Table 3).

In this study, we examined the relationship between the number of attacks per year and the uNGAL and uMA in FMF patients. According to these results, a positive correlation was found between uNGAL and uNGAL/uCr and the number of attacks per year ($r = 0.743$, $p = 0.001$ and $r = 0.516$, $p = 0.001$; respectively) in children with FMF. On the other hand, no relationship was found between the annual number of attacks and uMA and uMA/uCr ($r = 0.230$, $p = 0.154$ and $r = 0.034$, $p = 0.835$; respectively) in FMF patients. The relations of uNGAL, uNGAL/uCr, uMA and uMA/Cr with number of attacks per year in FMF patients are shown in Tables 4

Discussion

In the present study, we detected higher uNGAL level as well as uNGAL/uCr ratio in FMF patients than the control group. In addition, we found a positive correlation between uNGAL level and uNGAL/uCr ratio and number of attacks per year in FMF patients. Fibrinogen, CRP and ESR levels which are significant acute phase reactants for diagnosis of FMF were detected significantly higher in the patient group even the patients were not at attack period. Furthermore, MCV was lower in the patient group than the control group. These findings indicate that a chronic inflammation also continues in FMF patients during attack-free period. Higher levels of spot uNGAL and uNGAL/uCr in the patient group than the control group may indicate that such chronic inflammation may be an early indicator for renal injury in the tubules and glomerules.

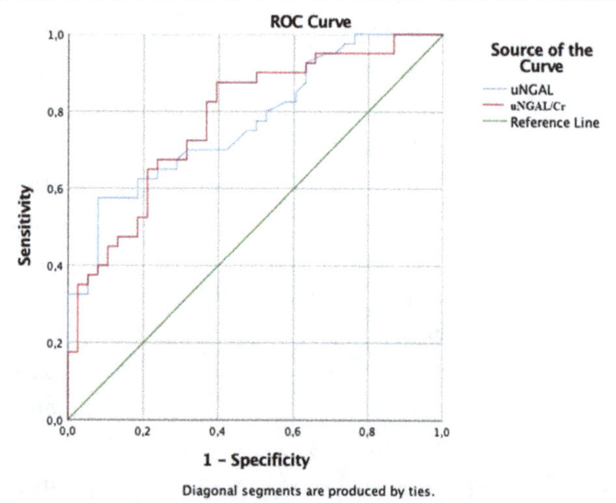

Fig. 1 Receiver operating characteristic curves for uNGAL and uNGAL/uCr in patients with Familial Mediterranean Fever

We analyzed only the urine and detected uNGAL level and uNGAL/uCr ratio in pediatric patients with FMF as compared to the healthy controls. There are a limited number of studies on the children in the literature. This study showed that renal amyloidosis should be monitored closely due to chronic inflammation in the children with FMF from early period. The increased risk in renal amyloidosis and acute inflammation attacks of serosal membrane is the most important outcome of FMF [1, 6, 7]. Amyloidosis actually appears in 50 to 60% of untreated patients, and may result with proteinuria, nephrotic syndrome, uremia, end-stage renal diseases, and death following subsequent steps [7, 28–30]. Routine urine analysis, urinary microalbuminuria and proteinuria are recommended for early diagnosis [31]. The diagnosis is confirmed by renal, rectal or abdominal fat biopsy [32]. However, like our study, microalbuminuria or proteinuria may not be detected in the early period. More sensitive and specific non-invasive tests are therefore needed. A previous study conducted on adult patients with FMF detected blood and urinary NGAL levels higher than the control group [33].

We detected CRP, ESH and SAA levels of our patients within normal reference ranges. These findings indicate

Table 3 Logistic regression analysis results in patients with familial Mediterranean fever

Parameters	Odds ratio	95% CI	*p*
Age (year)	1.07	0.87–1.32	0.50
Fibrinogen (mg/dL)	1.00	0.98–1.01	0.86
CRP (mg/dL)	1.45	0.86–2.44	0.17
uNGAL (pg/mL)	3.384	1.74–6.57	**0.0001**
ESR (mm/h)	1.03	0.944–1.128	0.49

CRP C-reactive protein, *uNGAL* Urine neutrophil gelatinase-associated lipocalin, *MVC* Mean corpuscular volume, *ESR* Erythrocyte sedimentation rate, *CI* Confidence interval
Data are expressed as odds ratio, 95% confidence interval and *P*-values for statistical significance

Table 4 The relations of uNGAL, uNGAL/uCr, uMA and uMA/Cr with number of attacks per year in familial Mediterranean fever patients

Parameters		Number of attacks per year
uNGAL	r	0.743
	p	**0.001**
uNGAL/uCr	r	0.516
	p	**0.001**
uMA	r	0.230
	p	0.154
uMA/uCr	r	0.034
	p	0.835

r: Correlation Coefficient
uNGAL Urine neutrophil gelatinase-associated lipocalin, *uCr* Urine creatinine, *uMA* Urine microalbumine

that the patients are attack-free; however, these levels in the patients were significantly higher than those in the control group. These results are significant to indicate persistence of a subacute chronic inflammation in these patients. As a result of this inflammation, uNGAL level and uNGAL/uCr ratio were elevated significantly through renal tubular and glomerular involvement. NGAL which is secreted from renal tubular cells secondarily to renal injury, is a protein from lipocalin family. Urinary biomarkers may be detected significantly higher from the first day of diagnosis for renal damage monitoring [34]. The important role of uNGAL was shown in pathophysiological process of chronic renal injury [26, 27]. Conventional biological markers which are used for early diagnosis of the renal injury provide positive results during late term; therefore, they may be used as early marker of acute and chronic renal injury in particular [35, 36]. Although uNGAL indicates the progression to chronic renal damage, the levels were detected elevated in correlation with serum creatinine level in the patients who had renal transplant within the first hour following cold ischemia; and it was shown that uNGAL may be important to predict the need for dialysis within the first week [37, 38].

There is a sustained need for markers which classifies the patients into risk categories that would establish the diagnosis earlier and prevent the adverse outcomes during clinical practice. The NGAL gene which meets most of these expectations was shown as the gene which is expressed most within a short period before creatinine elevation following ischemic and nephrotoxic injury [39, 40]. Inclusion of NGAL as a diagnostic biological marker into clinical use within a short period would make a great contribution to clinical benefits and development of new therapeutic approached.

In this study, we examined the relationship between the number of attacks per year and the uNGAL and uMA in FMF patients. According to these results, a positive correlation was found between uNGAL and uNGAL/uCr and the number of attacks per year. This pilot study is the first to examine the correlation between uNGAL and the number of attacks per year. For this reason, we believe that the results obtained are important. If our study is supported by a controlled study with a larger series, more precise results can be obtained.

Limitation of the present study is limited number of the patients. Furthermore, duration of the disease was very short in our patients. Majority of the patients were recently diagnosed. A further study that would include the patients who are followed-up for 5 years and more may provide significant results. Nevertheless, since the present study serves as the first study on the children about this topic, our outcomes are important.

Conclusion

In conclusion, uNGAL level and uNGAL/uCr ratio were detected higher in the pediatric patients with FMF when compared with the control group. In addition, we found a positive correlation between uNGAL level and uNGAL/uCr ratio and number of attacks per year in these children. The reason for higher levels of uNGAL during progress of other diseases is tubular injury-induced pattern of these diseases, and secretion of NGAL from proximal tubules. However, the disease may affect the glomerules during the progress; therefore, analysis of uNGAL levels may provide significant results, especially in the patients with poor control or lack of diagnosis. Further studies with larger series are required to establish the association between FMF and uNGAL.

Abbreviations

CRP: C-reactive protein; DBP: Diastolic blood pressure; ELISA: Enzyme-Linked Immunosorbent Assay; ESR: Erythrocyte sedimentation rate; FMF: Familial Mediterranean Fever; MCV: Mean corpuscular volume; MEFV: MEditerranean FeVer; SAA: Serum amyloid A; SBP: Systolic blood pressure; uCr: Urinary creatinine; uMA: Urinary microalbuminuria; uNGAL: Urinary neutrophile gelatinase-associated lipocalcin

Acknowledgements

We thank Cagla Sariturk (statistics specialist) for statistical support.

Authors' contributions

HD and SH design to the study and evaluated the laboratory findings. SCO collected patient data and wrote the article. STN made the blood analysis. The author(s) read and approved the final manuscript.

Author details

[1]Dr. Sadi Konuk Training and Research Hospital Department of Pediatrics, Health Science University, Istanbul, Turkey. [2]Dr. Sadi Konuk Training and Research Hospital Department of Pediatric Nephrology, Health Science University, Istanbul, Turkey. Okmeydani Training and Research Hospital Department of Pediatric Nephrology, Health Science University, Kaptan Paşa

Mahallesi, Darülaceze Cad. No: 25 Okmeydani, 34384 Şişli/Istanbul, Turkey.
[4]Dr. Sadi Konuk Training and Research Hospital Department of Biochemistry, Health Science University, Istanbul, Turkey.

References

1. Ben-Chetrit E, Levy M. Familial Mediterranean fever. Lancet. 1998;351(9103): 659–64. https://doi.org/10.1016/S0140-6736(97)09408-7.
2. Ozdogan H, Ugurlu S. familial Mediterranean fever. Presse Med. 2019;48(1): e61–76. https://doi.org/10.1016/j.lpm.2018.08.014.
3. Sohar E, Gafni J, Pras M, Heller H. Familial Mediterranean fever. A survey of 470 cases and review of the literature. Am J Med. 1967;43(2):227–53. https://doi.org/10.1016/0002-9343(67)90167-2.
4. Alghamdi M. Familial Mediterranean fever, review of the literature. Clin Rheumatol. 2017;36(8):1707–13. https://doi.org/10.1007/s10067-017-3715-5
5. Booty MG, Chae JJ, Masters SL, Remmers EF, Barham B, le JM, et al. Familial Mediterranean fever with a single MEFV mutation: where is the second hit? Arthiritis Rheum. 2009;60(6):1851–61. https://doi.org/10.1002/art.24569.
6. Konstantopoulos K, Michael S, Kanta A, et al. Renal amyloidosis as a first manifestation of familial Mediterranean fever. Scand J Rheumatol. 2000;29: 129–30.
7. Heller H, Sohar E, Gafnı J, Heller J. Amyloidosis in familial Mediterranean fever. An independent genetically determined character. Arch Intern Med. 1961;107(4):539–50. https://doi.org/10.1001/archinte.1961.03620040065007
8. Saatci U, Ozen S, Ozdemir S, et al. Familial Mediterranean fever in children: report of a large series and discussions of the risk and prognostic factors of amyloidosis. Eur J Pediatr. 1997;156(8):619–23. https://doi.org/10.1007/s004310050677.
9. Touitou I, Sarkisian T, Medlej-Hashim M, et al. International Study Group for phenotype-genotype correlation in familial Mediterranean fever. Country as the primary risk factor for renal amyloidosis in familial Mediterranean fever. Arthritis Rheum. 2007;56:1706–12.
10. Kasifoglu T, Bilge SY, Sari I, et al. Amyloidosis and its related factors in Turkish patients with familial Mediterranean fever: a multicenter study. Rheumatology. 2014;53:741–5.
11. Akpolat T, Özkaya O, Özen S. Homozygous M694V as a risk factorfor amyloidosis in Turkish FMF patients. Gene. 2012;492(1):285–9. https://doi.org/10.1016/j.gene.2011.10.012.
12. Livneh A, Langevitz P, Shinar Y, Zaks N, Kastner DL, Pras M, et al. MEFV mutation analysis in patients suffering from amyloidosis of familial Mediterranean fever. Amyloid. 1999;6(1):1–6. https://doi.org/10.3109/13506129908993281.
13. Shohat M, Magal N, Shohat T, Chen X, Dagan T, Mimouni A, et al. Phenotype-genotype correlation in familial Mediterranean fever: evidence for an association between Met694Val and amyloidosis. Eur J Hum Genet. 1999;7(3):287–92. https://doi.org/10.1038/sj.ejhg.5200303.
14. Stankovic Stojanovic K, Hentgen V, Fellahi S, Georgin-Lavialle S, Amselem S, Grateau G, et al. Concordance between CRP and SAA in familial Mediterranean fever during attack free period: a study of 218 patients. Clin Biochem. 2017; 50(4-5):206–9. https://doi.org/10.1016/j.clinbiochem.2016.11.008.
15. Erer B, Demirkaya E, Ozen S, Kallinich T. What is the best acute phase reactant for familial Mediterranean fever follow-upandits role in the prediction of complications? A systematic review. Rheumatol Int. 2016;36(4): 483–7. https://doi.org/10.1007/s00296-015-3413-z.
16. Anton PA, Targan SR, Vigna SR, Durham M, Schwabe AD, Shanahan F. Enhanced neutrophil chemiluminescence in familial Mediterranean fever. J Clin Immunol. 1988;8(2):148–56. https://doi.org/10.1007/BF00917903.
17. Saatci U, Ozdemir S, Ozen S, Bakkaloglu A. Serum concentration and urinary excretion of beta 2-microglobulin and microalbuminuria in familial Mediterranean fever. Arch Dis Child. 1994;70(1):27–9. https://doi.org/10.1136/adc.70.1.27.
18. Baskin E, Saatci U. Microalbuminuria in the course of familial Mediterranean fever. Nephrol Dial Transplant. 2004;19(10):2678. https://doi.org/10.1093/ndt/gfh285.
19. Ergüven M, Emeksiz C, Deveci M, Ozlü SG. Relation between microalbuminuria and gene mutations in familial Mediterranean fever. Turk J Pediatr. 2008;50(4):326–30.
20. Uslu AU, Aydin B, Icagasıoglu IS, et al. The relationship among the level of serum amyloid A, high-density lipoprotein and microalbuminuria in patients with familial Mediterranean fever. J Clin Lab Anal. 2016;30(6):1003–8. https://doi.org/10.1002/jcla.21971
21. Devarajan P. Neutrophil gelatinase-associated lipocalin (NGAL): a new marker of kidney disease. Scand J Clin Lab Investig Suppl. 2008;241:89–94. https://doi.org/10.1080/00365510802150158.
22. Schmidt-Ott KM, Mori K, Li JY, Kalandadze A, Cohen DJ, Devarajan P, et al. Review dual action of neutrophil gelatinase-associated lipocalin. J Am Soc Nephrol. 2007;18(2):407–13. https://doi.org/10.1681/ASN.2006080882.
23. Devarajan P. Biomarkers for the early detection of acute kidney injury. Curr Opin Pediatr. 2011;23(2):194–200. https://doi.org/10.1097/MOP.0b013e328343f4dd.
24. Bolignano D, Coppolino G, Lacquaniti A, Nicocia G, Buemi M. Pathological and prognostic value of urinary neutrophil gelatinase associated lipocalin in macroproteinuric patients with worsening renal function. Kidney Blood Press Res. 2008;31(4):274–9. https://doi.org/10.1159/000151665.
25. Bolignano D, Lacquaniti A, Coppolino G, et al. Neutrophil gelatinase-associated lipocalin (NGAL) and progression of chronic kidney disease. Clin J Am Soc Nephrol. 2009;4(2):337–44. https://doi.org/10.2215/CJN.03530708.
26. Nishida M, Kawakatsu H, Okumura Y, Hamaoka K. Serum and urinary neutrophil gelatinase-associated lipocalin levels in children with chronic renal diseases. Pediatr Int. 2010;52(4):563–8. https://doi.org/10.1111/j.1442-200X.2010.03067.x.
27. Bolignano D, Lacquaniti A, Coppolino G, Campo S, Arena A, Buemi M. Neutrophil gelatinase-associated lipocalin reflects the severity of renal impairment in subjects affected by chronic kidney disease. Kidney Blood Press Res. 2008;31(4):255–8. https://doi.org/10.1159/000143726.
28. Bolignano D, Cappolino G, Campo S, et al. Urinary neutrophil gelatinase-associated lipocalin (NGAL) is associated with severity of renal isease in proteinuric patients. Nephrol Dial Transplant. 2008;23:414–6.
29. Meijer E, Boertien WE, Nauta FL, et al. Association of urinary biomarkers with disease severity in patients with autosomal dominant polycystic kidney disease: a cross-sectional analysis. Am J Kidney Dis. 2010;56(5):883–95. https://doi.org/10.1053/j.ajkd.2010.06.023.
30. Mori K, Nakao K. Neutrophil gelatinase-associated lipocalin as the real-time indicator of active kidney damage. Kidney Int. 2007;71(10):967–70. https://doi.org/10.1038/sj.ki.5002165.
31. Assadi FK. Quantitation of microalbuminuria using random urine samples. Pediatr Nephrol. 2002;17(2):107–10. https://doi.org/10.1007/s00467-001-0762-5.
32. Röcken C, Shakespeare A. Pathology, diagnosis and pathogenesis of AA amyloidosis. Virchows Arch. 2002;440(2):111–22. https://doi.org/10.1007/s00428-001-0582-9.
33. Deveci K, Korkmaz S, Senel S, Deveci H, Sancakdar E, Uslu AU, et al. Do neutrophil gelatinase-associated lipocalin and interleukin-18 predict renal dysfunction in patients with familial Mediterranean fever and amyloidosis? Ren Fail. 2014;36(3):339–44. https://doi.org/10.3109/0886022X.2013.865486.
34. Hall IE, Coca SG, Perazella MA, Eko UU, Luciano RL, Peter PR, et al. Risk of poor outcomes with novel and traditional biomarkers at clinical AKI diagnosis. Clin J Am Soc Nephrol. 2011;6(12):2740–9. https://doi.org/10.2215/CJN.04960511.
35. Guo L, Zhu B, Yuan H, Zhao W. Evaluation of serum neutrophil gelatinase-associated lipocalin in older patients with chronic kidney disease. Aging Med. 2020;3:32–9.
36. Fuchs TC, Frick K, Emde B, Czasch S, von Landenberg F, Hewitt P. Evaluation of novel acute urinary rat kidney toxicity biomarker for subacute toxicity studies in preclinical trials. Toxicol Pathol. 2012;40(7):1031–48. https://doi.org/10.1177/0192623312444618.
37. Bolignano D, Donato V, Coppolino G, Campo S, Buemi A, Lacquaniti A, et al. Neutrophil gelatinase-associated lipocalin (NGAL) as a marker of kidney damage. Am J Kidney Dis. 2008;52(3):595–605. https://doi.org/10.1053/j.ajkd.2008.01.020.
38. Cappuccilli M, Capelli I, Comai G, Cianciolo G, La Manna G. Neutrophil gelatinase associated lipocalin as a biomarker of allograft function after renal transplantation: evaluation of the current status and future insights. Artif Organs. 2018;42(1):8–14. https://doi.org/10.1111/aor.13039.
39. Cai L, Rubin J, Han W, Venge P, Xu S. The origin of multiple molecular forms in urine of HNL/ NGAL. Clin J Am Soc Nephrol. 2010;5(12):2229–35. https://doi.org/10.2215/CJN.00980110.
40. Ronco C, Legrand M, Goldstein SL, et al. Neutrophil gelatinase-associated lipocalin: ready for routine clinical use? An international perspective. Blood Purif. 2014;37:271–85.

13

Sacroiliitis in children and adolescents with familial Mediterranean fever

Hülya Kaçmaz[1], Esin Aldemir[2], Ayşe Tanatar[3], Şerife Gül Karadağ[4], Mustafa Çakan[5], Hafize Emine Sönmez[6] and Nuray Aktay Ayaz[3*]

Abstract

Background: Familial Mediterranean fever (FMF) is an autoinflammatory disease characterized by recurrent episodes of fever and serositis. Sacroiliitis can be observed in some FMF patients. This study aimed to compare the demographic, clinical, and laboratory findings, and treatment in children with FMF and sacroiliitis, and children with juvenile spondyloarthropathy (JSpA).

Methods: In total, 1687 pediatric FMF patients that were followed-up between May 2010 and June 2020 were evaluated retrospectively. Among them, those with sacroiliitis ($n = 63$) were included in the study and compared to patients with JSpA ($n = 102$).

Results: The study included 63 FMF patients with sacroiliitis (38 males [60.3%] and 25 females [39.7%]) with a mean age of 15.2 ± 4.1 years. Mean age at symptom onset was 7.2 ± 5.05 years and mean age at diagnosis was 9.74 ± 4.67 years. The most common mutation in the FMF patients was *M694V/M694V* ($n = 22$). Patients were diagnosed with sacroiliitis with a mean of 12 months (range: 6–36 months) after the diagnosis of FMF. Among the FMF patients, 28 (44.4%) had enthesitis, 23 (36.5%) had heel pain, and 11 (17.4%) had low back pain. The study also included 102 JSpA patients (90 males [88.2%] and 12 females [11.8%]). Mean age of patients with JSpA was 16.1 ± 2.8 years. As compared to 102 JSpA patients, patients with FMF and sacroiliitis had higher acute phase reactants, whereas HLA-B27 positivity rate was lower. In addition, axial involvement rate was higher in the JSpA patients.

Conclusion: Sacroiliitis is a common co-morbidity in FMF patients. The phenotypic features of these patients are different from patients with JSpA.

Keywords: Familial Mediterranean fever, Enthesitis-related arthritis, Spondyloarthropathy, Sacroiliitis, Childhood

Introduction

Familial Mediterranean fever (FMF) is an autoinflammatory disease characterized by self-limited recurrent febrile attacks and polyserositis accompanied by elevated acute phase reactants. Joint involvement is one of the most common features during the disease course and about 75% of patients have arthritis during FMF attacks. Acute recurrent monoarthritis is the most common form of musculoskeletal involvement in FMF patients, whereas about 5% of FMF patients can develop sacroiliitis [1]. The increased frequency of sacroiliitis have been reported among FMF patients. Patients with FMF and sacroiliitis usually present with unilateral or bilateral sacroiliitis, recurrent enthesitis, and inflammatory back or neck pain [1].

Sacroiliac involvement in FMF patients can resemble spondyloarthropathy (SpA); however, in patients with FMF and sacroiliitis, the presence of HLA-B27 or spinal involvement is unusual, whereas SpA is a group of seronegative arthritis type characterized by enthesitis, asymmetrical oligoarthritis of the lower extremities, axial involvement, HLA-B27 positivity, and age at onset < 16 years. However, it is still controversial whether sacroiliitis is a part of FMF or it is related with the coexistence

* Correspondence: nurayaktay@gmail.com
[3]Department of Pediatric Rheumatology, Istanbul University Medical School, Istanbul, Turkey

of two diseases; FMF and SpA. Revealing the differences and similarities between these two diseases may help clinicians to clarify this controversy. Therefore; the present study aimed to determine the differences between FMF patients with sacroiliitis, and patients with juvenile SpA (JSpA).

Materials and methods

The files of 1687 FMF patients and 548 JIA patients that were followed-up by the pediatric rheumatology outpatient clinic between May 2010 and June 2020 were retrospectively reviewed. Among 1687 FMF patients, those with concurrent sacroiliitis were included in the study ($n = 63$, group 1). Furthermore, among 548 JIA patients, those with JSpA were also included in the study ($n = 102$, group 2). Patients having psoriasis and inflammatory bowel disease or a follow-up period of less than 6 months or missing data were excluded.

FMF was diagnosed according to pediatric FMF diagnostic criteria [2] and JSpA was diagnosed according to ILAR criteria [3].

Demographic findings (age, gender, age at diagnosis, and family history of HLA-B27-associated disease or FMF), clinical findings (fever, abdominal pain, nausea, vomiting, diarrhea, constipation, chest pain, duration of attacks, joint pain, joint swelling, muscle pain, prolonged febrile myalgia, erysipelas-like erythema, enthesitis, waist and hip pain, heel pain, and morning stiffness), and laboratory findings (complete blood count, the erythrocyte sedimentation rate [ESR], C-reactive protein [CRP], anti-nuclear antigen [ANA], HLA-B27, and *MEFV* gene results) were retrospectively obtained from the patients' files.

The frequency of FMF attacks, disease severity scores, use of colchicine, and colchicine resistance were evaluated. Treatments were also documented from medical files. The resistance to colchicine treatment was defined as experiencing ≥1 attack per month despite receiving the maximally tolerated dose for ≥6 months.

Disease severity was determined via the Pras score, which was readjusted according to the colchicine dose [4, 5].

MRI was performed using a 1.5 T (T) device. Active sacroiliitis was determined via MRI according to Assessment in Spondyloarthritis International Society (ASAS) criteria. Groups 1 and 2 were compared in terms of demographic findings, clinical and laboratory findings, and treatment.

The study protocol was approved by the local ethics committee (Approval no. KAEK/2020.06.69).

Statistical analysis

Statistical analysis was performed using IBM SPSS Statistics for Windows v.21 (IBM Corp., Armonk, NY). The study variables were investigated using visual (histogram and probability plots) and analytic methods (Kolmogorov-Smirnov and Shapiro-Wilk's tests) to determine the normality of their distribution. Descriptive analyses are presented as percentage, mean, standard deviation, median, and range, as appropriate. Categorical parameters were compared with the Chi-square test or Fisher test when appropriate. The Student's T test was used to compare normally distributed variables between the 2 groups. The Mann-Whitney U test was used to compare non-normally distributed variables between the 2 groups. The level of statistical significance was set at $P < 0.05$.

Results

Among 1687 FMF patients that were followed-up by the pediatric rheumatology outpatient clinic, 63 had concurrent sacroiliitis (group 1). The most common mutation was *M694V/M694V* ($n = 22$). Moreover, 44 FMF patients had ≥1 *M694V* mutations (Table 1). Mean duration of follow-up was 60.9 ± 40 months. The median colchicine dose was 3 mg d^{-1} (range: 2–3 mg d^{-1}). The median monthly FMF attack frequency was 1 (range: 0–2). The median disease severity score was 9 (range: 7–12). According to the Pras severity score, 1 (1.6%) of the FMF patients was classified as mild, 39 (61.9%) as moderate, and 23 (36.5%) as severe.

The FMF patients were diagnosed with sacroiliitis with a mean of 12 months (range: 6–36 months) after being diagnosed with FMF. In all, 28 (44.4%) of the FMF patients had enthesitis, 23 (36.5%) had heel pain, and 11 (17.4%) had lower back pain. Upon physical examination sacroiliac joint tenderness was detected in 26 (42%) patients. MRI findings of sacroiliac joints were compatible with unilateral sacroiliitis in 2 of the FMF patients and bilateral sacroiliitis in 61. Among group I, 32 patients fulfilled the classification criteria for JSpA. In total, 15

Table 1 Demographical and clinical findings of patients with familial Mediterranean fever (FMF)

Findings	Number of patients
Female/Male	25/38
The mean age of patients, years	15.1 ± 4.1
The mean age at symptom onset, years	7.2 ± 5.05
The mean age at diagnosis, years	9.7 ± 4.6
The mean duration of disease, years	7.4 ± 5.3
The frequency of consanguineous marriage, n (%)	24 (38.1)
The history of FMF in family	22 (34.9)
The history of FMF in siblings	10 (15.9)
Recurrent fever, n (%)	35 (55.6)
Abdominal pain, n (%)	38 (60.3)
Chest pain, n (%)	15 (23.8)
Exertional leg pain, n (%)	22 (34.9)
Erysipelas-like erythema (ELE), n (%)	19 (30.2)

FMF patients received anti-TNF (adalimumab: $n = 6$; etanercept: $n = 9$) and 6 patients were treated with tocilizumab. At the time of study, all patients were inactive both clinically and laboratory means.

The study also included 102 JSpA patients (group 2), of which 90 (88.2%) were male and 12 (11.8%) were female. Mean age in group 2 was 16.1 ± 2.8 years and mean age at diagnosis of JSpA was 13.2 ± 2.6 years. Mean diagnostic delay was 8.3 ± 6.1 months. In all, 4 (3.9%) of the JSpA patients had anterior uveitis. ANA test results were positive in 13 (12.7%) patients and HLA-B27 positivity was noted in 51 (50%). Ankylosis developed in 4 (3,9%) patients, as follows: both ankles ($n = 1$); right ankle (n = 1); left ankle ($n = 2$). Among the JSpA patients, 24 (23.5%) received methotrexate and 87 (85.7%) received salazopyrin. Biological therapy was administered to 32 (27.1%) patients, as follows: etanercept: $n = 23$; adalimumab: $n = 9$. None of the patients in group II carried *MEFV* mutations.

Acute phase reactants were higher (CRP; 14.4 versus 4.6, $P < 0.001$ and ESR; 32 versus 16, $P < 0.001$) and HLA-B27 positivity rate was lower in group 1 than in group 2 (6.3% versus 50%, $P < 0.001$). Moreover, axial involvement was not observed in group 1, but was noted in 4.9% of the patients in group 2 ($P = 0.07$) (Table 2). The biological treatment rate in group 1 was 33.3% ($n = 21$), versus 31.3% ($n = 32$) in group 2 ($P = 0.79$). Only anti-TNF drugs were used as biological agents in group 2, whereas 15 of the patients in group 1 were treated with anti-TNF drugs and 6 with anti-interleukin 6 (tocilizumab).

Discussion

Musculoskeletal symptoms are very common in patients with FMF. Joint swelling in FMF patients usually occurs in the form of acute transient monoarthritis affecting the ankles or knees; however, some patients can also have chronic arthritis affecting the hips or small joints. The presence of *M694V* mutation is associated with musculoskeletal symptoms [6]. Inflammatory back or hip pain can occur in FMF patients with sacroiliac joint involvement. Generally, such patients are negative for HLA-B27 antigen and spinal involvement is rare. The frequency of sacroiliitis is higher in Turkish and Jewish FMF patients than in those of other ethnicities [7, 8]; however, sacroiliac joint involvement is relatively rare in children. Earlier adult FMF studies noted that the frequency of sacroiliitis is 0.4–10.5% [7–10]. In addition, HLA-B27 antigen is generally negative, but positive cases are also reported, although rarely. In the present study concomitant sacroiliitis was noted in 63 (3.7%) of 1687 pediatric FMF patients, of which only 4 were HLA-B27 antigen positive. Moreover, 44 of the patients had ≥1 M694V mutations.

Langevitz et al. [9] evaluated 3000 adult FMF patients living in Israel and reported that the frequency of sacroiliitis was 0.4% and that 11 patients had seronegative SpA, of which 9 were male and 2 were female with mean age at diagnosis of 32.4 ± 7.1 years. These 11 patients were followed-up with the diagnosis of FMF for a mean 27.4 ± 5.1 years. They also reported that all of these 11 patients had inflammatory back pain, and neck pain ($n = 4$), bilateral or unilateral stage 3–4 sacroiliitis ($n = 7$), bilateral stage 2 sacroiliitis ($n = 4$), monoarthritis ($n = 5$), oligoarthritis ($n = 6$), enthesitis ($n = 6$), and heel pain ($n = 7$). HLA-B27 antigen was negative in all of them [9]. In the present study sacroiliitis was noted in 3.7% ($n = 63$) of 1687 FMF patients. Patients were diagnosed with sacroiliitis with a mean of 12 months (range 6–36 months) following diagnosis of FMF; 28 of these patients had enthesitis and 11 had lower back pain.

Table 2 Comparison of Group 1 and Group II patients

Findings	Group I ($n = 63$)	Group II ($n = 102$)	*P* value
Gender (Female/Male), n (%)	25/38 (39.7)/ (60.3)	12/90 (11.8)/ (88.2)	< 0.001
Enthesitis, n (%)	28 (44.4)	36 (35.2)	0.18
Heel pain, n (%)	23 (36.5)	42 (41.1)	0.62
Low back pain, n (%)	11 (17.4)	48 (47.0)	< 0.001
Ankylosis, n (%)	0 (0)	5 (4.9)	0.07
Positivity of HLA-B27, n (%)	4 (6.3)	51 (50)	< 0.001
Leukocyte count, ($\times 10^3/mm^3$)	9800 (7200–12,000)	9720 (6800–11,800)	0.33
CRP[a] (mg/L) (normal range:0–5)	14.4 (0.8–142)	4.6 (0.1–137)	< 0.001
ESR[a](mm/hour) (normal range:0–20)	32 (20–120)	16 (1–112)	< 0.001
Methotrexate, n (%)	19 (30.1)	24 (23.5)	0.22
Salazopyrin, n (%)	46 (73.1)	87 (85.2)	0.06
Biologic drugs, n (%)	21 (33.3)	32 (31.3)	0.79

CRP C-reactive protein, *ESR* erythrocyte sedimentation rate, *HLA-B27* Human- leucocyte antigen-B27 [a] These values are the values at the time of diagnosis of spondyloarthropathy

Why sacroiliitis occurs in FMF patients remains a matter of debate; however, a family history of SpA in some patients suggests a genetic relationship. Akar et al. [11] reported an increased risk of sacroiliitis in adult patients with FMF and their families (the risk ratio is 3.3 [95% CI: 2–5] in first-degree relatives and 2.9 [95% CI: 1.3–6.4] in individuals with FMF). Of the 63 FMF patients with sacroiliitis in the present study, 22 had a family history of FMF, but none had a family history of SpA.

Sacroiliitis has also been reported in pediatric FMF patients. Sonmez et al. [12] compared 15 children diagnosed with FMF and sacroiliitis, and 30 juvenile SpA patients, observing that the FMF patients with sacroiliitis had higher inflammatory markers, whereas the frequency of enthesitis, axial involvement, and HLA-B27 antigen positivity was lower. Aydın et al. [13] analyzed 650 children with FMF and reported that 17 (2.6%) had sacroiliitis, of which 90% carried the *M694V* mutation. Özdel et al. [14] compared 18 children with FMF and sacroiliitis, and 38 children diagnosed with JSpA, noting that there was no difference between the 2 groups in HLA-B27 antigen positivity, family history, clinical findings, enthesitis, or treatment. In the present study the patients with FMF and sacroiliitis had higher acute phase reactants and a lower HLA-B27 antigen positivity rate, as well as no axial involvement. In addition, there wasn't a significant difference between groups 1 and 2 in terms of the presence of enthesitis.

There is no standard treatment for FMF associated with sacroiliitis. Sonmez et al. [12] reported treating all such patients with non-steroidal anti-inflammatory drugs, and that 9 patients were treated with methotrexate, 9 with sulfasalazine, and 10 with anti-TNF (etanercept). Aydın et al. [13] reported that of 17 patients diagnosed with FMF and sacroiliitis, 14 were treated with non-steroidal anti-inflammatory drugs in addition to colchicine, 10 received sulfasalazine, and 7 received biological drugs. Özdel et al. [14]] compared 18 children with FMF and sacroiliitis, and 38 children diagnosed with JSpA, reporting that there was no difference between the 2 groups in terms of treatment. Cherqaoui et al. [15] observed that patients diagnosed with FMF and JSpA required fewer non-steroidal anti-inflammatory drugs and anti-TNF drugs than patients with other JSpA. In the present study anti-TNF drugs were given to 15 of the FMF patients with sacroiliitis (adalimumab: $n = 6$; etanercept: $n = 9$) in addition to colchicine, and 6 patients were using tocilizumab. Moreover, the biological drug use rate did not differ significantly between groups 1 and 2, but the preferred biological therapy varied. Tocilizumab failed to achieve remission in the adult patients with spondyloarthritis [16]. However, previous studies have reported successful results with tocilizumab in FMF patients [17, 18]. In presented study, all 6 patients with FMF and sacroiliitis receiving tocilizumab achieved remission in terms of FMF and sacroilliitis. This suggests that FMF and sacroillitis has different pathogenetic mechanisms than JSpA.

The limitation of the present study is its retrospective design, whereas the large number of patients included is a strength.

Conclusion

To the best of our knowledge the present study is the largest such study to date, highlighting the association between FMF disease and sacroiliitis. These patients may show different phenotype than classical JSpA patients. Further delineation of the clinical and laboratory findings in pediatric FMF patients with sacroiliitis will facilitate easier diagnosis and prevent delays in treatment. Although clinical differences are revealed, studies on etiopathogenesis are needed to show the main differences of these two diseases.

Acknowledgments

None.

Authors' contributions

HK conceptualized and designed the study, drafted the initial manuscript, and had full access to all the data in the study; EA, AT, SGK, MÇ, HES and NAA designed the study, conducted the data analyses, drafted the initial manuscript, and had full access to all the data in the study. All authors reviewed and revised the manuscript and approved the final version of the manuscript.

Author details

[1]Department of Pediatric Rheumatology, University of Health Sciences, Kanuni Sultan Süleyman Research and Training Hospital, Istanbul, Turkey. [2]Department of Pediatric Rheumatology, University of Health Sciences, Başakşehir Çam ve Sakura City Hospital, Istanbul, Turkey. [3]Department of Pediatric Rheumatology, Istanbul University Medical School, Istanbul, Turkey. [4]Department of Pediatric Rheumatology, Sadi Konuk Research and Training Hospital, Istanbul, Turkey. [5]Department of Pediatric Rheumatology, University of Health Sciences, Zeynep Kamil Research and Training Hospital, Istanbul, Turkey. [6]Department of Pediatric Rheumatology, Kocaeli University, Istanbul, Turkey.

References

1. Younes M, Kahn MF, Meyer O. Hip involvement in patients with familial Mediterranean fever. A review of ten cases. Joint Bone Spine. 2002;69(6): 560–5. https://doi.org/10.1016/S1297-319X(02)00452-9.
2. Yalcinkaya F, Ozen S, Ozcakar ZB, Aktay N, Cakar N, Duzova A, et al. A new set of criteria for the diagnosis of familial Mediterranean fever in childhood. Rheumatology (Oxford). 2009;48(4):395–8. https://doi.org/10.1093/rheumatology/ken509.
3. Petty RE, Southwood TR, Manners P, Baum J, Glass DN, Goldenberg J, et al. International league of associations for rheumatology classification of juvenile idiopathic arthritis: second revision, Edmonton, 2001. J Rheumatol. 2004;31(2):390–2.
4. Ozen S, Aktay N, Lainka E, Duzova A, Bakkaloglu A, Kallinich T. Disease severity in children and adolescents with familial Mediterranean fever: a comparative study to explore environmental effects on a monogenic disease. Ann Rheum Dis. 2009;68(2):246–8. https://doi.org/10.1136/ard.2008.092031.
5. Pras E, Livneh A, Balow JE, Pras E, Kastner DL, Pras M, et al. Clinical

differences between north African and Iraqi Jews with familial Mediterranean fever. Am J Med Genet. 1998;75(2):216–9. https://doi.org/10.1002/(SICI)1096-8628(19980113)75:2<216::AID-AJMG20>3.0.CO;2-R.

6. Akkoc N, Gul A. Familial Mediterranean fever and seronegative arthritis. Curr Rheumatol Rep. 2011;13(5):388–94. https://doi.org/10.1007/s11926-011-0191-9.
7. Cefle A, Kamali S, Sayarlioglu M, Inanc M, Ocal L, Aral O, et al. A comparison of clinical findings of familial Mediterranean fever patients with and without amyloidosis. Rheumatol Int. 2005;25(6):442–6. https://doi.org/10.1007/s00296-004-0471-z.
8. Kasifoglu T, Calisir C, Cansu DU, Korkmaz C. The frequency of sacroiliitis in familial Mediterranean fever and the role of HLA-B27 and MEFV mutations in the development of sacroiliitis. Clin Rheumatol. 2009;28(1):41–6. https://doi.org/10.1007/s10067-008-0980-3.
9. Langevitz P, Livneh A, Zemer D, Shemer J, Pras M. Seronegative spondyloarthropathy in familial Mediterranean fever. Semin Arthritis Rheum. 1997;27(2):67–72. https://doi.org/10.1016/S0049-0172(97)80007-8.
10. Tunca M, Akar S, Onen F, Ozdogan H, Kasapcopur O, Yalcinkaya F, et al. Familial Mediterranean fever (FMF) in Turkey: results of a nationwide multicenter study. Medicine (Baltimore). 2005;84:1–11.
11. Akar S, Soysal O, Balci A, Solmaz D, Gerdan V, Onen F, et al. High prevalence of spondyloarthritis and ankylosing spondylitis among familial Mediterranean fever patients and their first-degree relatives: further evidence for the connection. Arthritis Res Ther. 2013;15:R21.
12. Sonmez HE, Batu ED, Demir S, Bilginer Y, Ozen S. Comparison of patients with familial Mediterranean fever accompanied with sacroiliitis and patients with juvenile spondyloarthropathy. Clin Exp Rheumatol. 2017;108:124–7.
13. Aydin F, Ozcakar ZB, Cakar N, Celikel E, Uncu N, Celikel Acar B, et al. Sacroiliitis in children with familial Mediterranean fever. J Clin Rheumatol. 2019;25(2):69–73. https://doi.org/10.1097/RHU.0000000000000770.
14. Ozdel S, Baglan E, Cakici EK, Yazilitas F, Gur G, Celikkaya E, et al. Similarities between pediatric FMF patients with sacroiliitis and pediatric juvenile spondyloarthropathy patients with sacroiliitis: a preliminary study. Acta Clin Belg. 2020:1–6. https://doi.org/10.1080/17843286.2020.1724450.
15. Cherqaoui B, Rossi-Semerano L, Georgin-Lavialle S, Dusser P, Galeotti C, Piram M, et al. Boundaries between familial Mediterranean fever and juvenile spondyloarthritis: analysis of three French retrospective cohorts. Joint Bone Spine. 2018;85(6):733–9. https://doi.org/10.1016/j.jbspin.2018.01.010.
16. Sieper J, Porter-Brown B, Thompson L, Harari O, Dougados M. Assessment of short-term symptomatic efficacy of tocilizumab in ankylosing spondylitis: results of randomised, placebo-controlled trials. Ann Rheum Dis. 2014;73(1):95–100. https://doi.org/10.1136/annrheumdis-2013-203559.
17. Kuemmerle-Deschner JB, Gautam R, George AT, Raza S, Lomax KG, Hur P. A systematic literature review of efficacy, effectiveness and safety of biologic therapies for treatment of familial Mediterranean fever. Rheumatology (Oxford). 2020;59(10):2711–24. https://doi.org/10.1093/rheumatology/keaa205.
18. Umeda M, Aramaki T, Fujikawa K, Iwamoto N, Ichinose K, Terada K, et al. Tocilizumab is effective in a familial Mediterranean fever patient complicated with histologically proven recurrent fasciitis and myositis. Int J Rheum Dis. 2017;20(11):1868–71. https://doi.org/10.1111/1756-185X.12776.

14

Vasculitis damage index in Behçet's disease

Fatema T. Elgengehy[1*], Sherif M. Gamal[1], Nesreen Sobhy[1], Ibrahem Siam[2], Ahmed M. Soliman[3], Ghada W. Elhady[4] and Tamer A. Gheita[1]

Abstract

Background: Vasculitis damage index (VDI) is a validated damage index for systemic vasculitis, and as Behçet's disease is considered one of systemic vascular disease we aimed to study the relationship of the vasculitis damage index to clinical manifestations and comorbidity in patients with Behçet's disease (BD) to determine if VDI could be used to assess damage in patients with BD.

Methods: A total of 109 patients with BD were recruited from the Rheumatology Department (outpatient and inpatient clinic), Cairo University Hospitals. All patients were subjected to full history taking, clinical examination, and routine laboratory investigations. Disease activity was assessed by the BD current activity form, and the VDI was calculated in all patients. The relationship of the VDI to the disease clinical manifestations was studied. Mann–Whitney and Kruskal Wallis tests were used to estimate differences in quantitative variables. Spearman correlation test was used to test for correlation between quantitative variables.

Results: In the current study, the VDI ranged from 1 to 10, with a mean of 3.5 ± 1.8. It was significantly associated with total thrombosis ($P = 0.022$); total neurological manifestations ($P = 0.000$), especially stroke and cranial nerve affection; uveitis ($P = 0.005$); avascular necrosis (AVN) ($P = 0.015$); osteoporosis ($P = 0.01$); impaired vision ($P < 0.0001$); cataract ($P < 0.0001$); and diabetes ($P = 0.012$). Generally, immunosuppressive treatment was significantly associated with VDI ($P = 0.039$), especially cyclophosphamide ($P < 0.0001$), biological agent ($P = 0.008$), chlorambucil ($P = 0.003$), and anticoagulant ($P = 0.02$). VDI was also significantly correlated with age ($P = 0.033$), disease duration ($P = 0.029$), and duration of eye involvement ($P = 0.003$).

Conclusion: VDI is significantly associated with most disease parameters of BD, except for parameters such as mucocutaneous manifestations and uncomplicated venous thrombosis; however, further studies may be needed to establish BD-specific damage index.

Keywords: Vasculitis damage index, Behçet's disease, Egyptian Patients

Background

Behçet's disease (BD) is a multisystem, inflammatory, autoimmune disease with unknown etiology and pathogenesis and unpredictable prognosis [1, 2]. BD is classified among systemic vasculitides [3]. Vascular involvement is a common finding in BD, which is significantly associated with higher morbidity and mortality rates, and may affect up to 40% of patients with BD, mostly in the form of deep venous thrombosis (DVT) and superficial thrombophlebitis [4–6]. Arterial vascular involvement is less frequent than venous affection in BD; however, the prognosis is poorer in such cases [7]. Furthermore, recent data also verified the presence of accelerated classical subclinical arterial damage, such as arteriosclerosis, even in patients without overt vascular complications and may be complementary to that of vasculitis [1].

The prognosis for a patient with systemic vasculitis has improved with treatment [8, 9]. However, the long-term outlook may be associated with accumulation of damage, from recurrent flares or treatment [9, 10 Careful differentiation between activity and damage is mandatory to prevent unnecessary exposure to cytotoxic medications. Damage significantly influences both long-

* Correspondence: fatematalaat1980@yahoo.com
[1]Rheumatology and Rehabilitation Department, Cairo University, Cairo, Egypt

term prognosis and quality of life, so systemic recording of damage may be helpful in improving treatment decision and predicting disease outcomes [1, 10].

A well-established validated damage index, "vasculitis damage index" (VDI) [11], is currently the most widely used assessment tool for damage in vasculitis. It is based on a score derived from individual items from disease onset and comprises 64 items (grouped into 11 organ-based systems). The items were originally selected by consensus among experienced physicians. Damage was defined by three key characteristics: irreversibility, presence for > 3 months, and attribution of the lesion to vasculitis or its therapy. Each item was not weighted; therefore, all items contribute equally to the score. The VDI has been used to demonstrate that irreversible damage occurs early in the disease course and has a significant effect on subsequent morbidity and mortality. Multi-organ involvement within 2 years is associated with an increased risk of death [12].

The Outcome Measures in Rheumatology (OMERACT) has defined the core set domain of outcome measures for BD, and concluded that both measures of disease activity and damage should be included, as separate and complementary entities, into the core outcome set for BD [13]. However, no BD damage index had been developed until 2020, when Piga et al. published the first BD damage index (BODI) and validated it through several steps, one of which was the correlation with VDI, and they concluded that pending further validation still required [14]. Thus, this study aimed to evaluate the relationship of the VDI to clinical manifestations and comorbidities in patients with BD. Our study may be a preliminary study to assess if VDI is suitable tool for damage assessment in patients with BD.

Patients and methods

This cross-sectional study included 109 adult patients with BD (98 men and 11 women [8.9:1]). Patients were recruited consecutively (with exclusion of juvenile onset BD patients), from 2016 to 2018, from the Rheumatology Department (inpatient and outpatient clinic) of Cairo University Hospitals, Egypt. All patients met the criteria of the International Study Group for BD [3]. Patients were subjected to full history taking, thorough clinical examination and all clinical manifestations were assessed if ever happened in the disease course, either acute or chronic or both. Routine laboratory tests and relevant medications used were recorded. The treatment protocol of our patients was generally in accordance with 2008 and 2018 EULAR recommendations [15, 16], with few modifications due to financial issues or special case situations.

In the present study, disease activity was assessed for all patients by BD current activity form (BDCAF) by filling the items of the BDCAF according to the information provided by the patients and current medical reports [17], while VDI was also calculated for each patient at the time of recruitment [11]. A comparative and correlative study of the VDI of our patients was conducted with respect to different disease parameters. It is to be noted that medical records of Behçet's patients who died during the period of the study were reviewed for the previously mentioned data. The study was performed in accordance with the Declaration of Helsinki and approved by the local ethical committee. Informed consent was obtained from all patients before their enrollment in the study.

Statistical analysis

Data were processed and analyzed using the Statistical Package for the Social Sciences (SPSS) software version 15 for Windows (SPSS Inc., Chicago, Illinois, USA). For quantitative variables, median (minimum, maximum, inter quartile range (IQR), or mean (±SD) were used. Frequency and percentage were presented for qualitative variables. Mann–Whitney and Kruskal Wallis tests were used to estimate differences in quantitative variables. Spearman correlation test was used to test for correlation between quantitative variables. A P-value < 0.05 indicated statistical significance.

Results

In the current study, the age of our patients ranged from 18 to 58 years, with a mean of 35.3 ± 8 years. Moreover, 98 patients were male, and 11 were female (8.9:1). Oral ulcers were reported in 94.5% of patients, genital ulcers in 85.3%, uveitis in 69.7%, skin lesions in 39.4%, and vascular involvement in 50.5%. Demographic and clinical data of our patients are shown in Table 1. Medications received by patients with BD are shown in Table 2.

VDI in the current study ranged from 1 to 10, with a mean of 3.5 ± 1.8, and was significantly associated with major organ damage including; total thrombosis, total neurological manifestations (especially stroke and cranial nerve affection), eye manifestations (uveitis, visual impairment, cataract), and disease-related complications or associated comorbidities (avascular necrosis [AVN], osteoporosis, and diabetes). The use of immunosuppressive drugs in general was significantly associated with VDI, especially cyclophosphamide, biological agent, chlorambucil, and anticoagulant. VDI was also significantly correlated with age, disease duration ($P = 0.029$), and duration of eye involvement. Details of association of VDI to different disease variables are shown in Tables 3 and 4. Correlation of VDI score with clinical variables is shown in Table 5.

Discussion

BD is a chronic autoimmune systemic vasculitis with an obscure pathogenesis [18]. Vasculitis of BD can involve

Table 1 Demographic and clinical data of patients with BD

Parameter	Patients with BD (*n* = 109)
Age, mean ± SD (range)	35.3 ± 8 (18–58) years
Sex, male:female	98:11 (8.9:1)
Disease duration, median, minimum, maximum, IQR	9,1, 38, 8.5 years
Delay in diagnosis, median, minimum, maximum, IQR	12, 0.2, 216, 48 months
BDCAF grades 0/1/2/3	50/45/11/3
Oral ulcers, n(%)	103 (94.5)
Genital ulcers, n(%)	93 (85.3)
Skin lesions, n(%)	43 (39.4)
Eye (uveitis), n(%)	76(69.7)
Duration of eye affection, mean ± SD (range)	86.7 ± 60.1(2–264) months
Impaired vision, n(%)	62(56.9)
Blindness, n(%)	12(11)
Cataract, n(%)	40(36.7)
Vascular involvement, n(%)	55 (50.5)
DVT, n(%)	29 (26.6)
DVT (no. of attacks), n(%)	Once 9 (8.3) or twice 20 (18.3)
Thrombosis (arterial/venous), n(%)	52 (47.7)
Thrombosis (no. of attacks), n(%)	Once 27 (24.8) or twice 25 (22.9)
Aneurysms, n(%)	14 (12.8)
Neurological involvement, n(%)	19 (17.4)
Cranial nerve affection, n(%)	12 (11)
Ataxia, n(%)	3 (2.8)
Coma, n(%)	1 (0.9)
Stroke, n(%)	9 (8.3)
Arthritis, n(%)	12 (11)
AVN, n(%)	4 (3.7)
Osteoporosis, n(%)	7 (6.4)
Diabetes, n(%)	8 (7.3)
Mortality, n(%)	8 (7.3)
VDI	3.5 ± 1.8 (1–10)

BD Behçet's disease, *BDCAF* BD current activity form, *DVT* Deep venous thrombosis, *AVN* Avascular necrosis, *VDI* Vasculitis damage index

Table 2 Medications received by patients with Behçet's disease

Medications	Patients with BD (n = 109)
Cyclophosphamide, n (%)	61 (56)
Azathioprine, n (%)	62 (56.9)
Cyclosporine A, n (%)	39 (35.8)
Biologic therapy, n (%)	22 (20.2)
Colchicine, n (%)	2 (1.8)
MMF, n (%)	1 (0.9)
Chlorambucil, n (%)	3 (2.8)
Leflunomide, n (%)	1 (0.9)
Anticoagulants, n (%)	40 (36.7)

BD Behçet's disease, *MMF* Mycophenolate mofetil

any type and size of vessels, which explains why the disease has the ability of multi-systemic involvement [19], which could lead to serious morbidity and mortality [18].

In conditions associated with systemic vasculitis, a comprehensive assessment of disease severity should include measurements of disease activity, damage, and functional status. Damage develops as a consequence of recurrent or persistent active disease or its treatment and is defined as the accumulation of non-healing scars that are unlikely to respond to immunosuppressive therapy [20]. Therefore, a damage index is needed to quantify damage, aid in the separation of damage from disease activity, and rationalize selection of therapy.

In the current study, the male/female ratio was quite high (8.9:1). This may be similar to some previous studies conducted on patients with BD in Egypt [21, 22]. In addition, our university is a tertiary referral hospital, receiving severe cases including vascular involvement, which has a higher frequency of male patients [23].

Thrombosis is the most frequent vascular manifestation in BD and an important factor of poor prognosis [24]. A study performed by Gerco et al. in 2018 revealed that the major causes of morbidity and mortality rates in BD result from ocular, major vascular, and neurological involvement [25].

Amigo et al. reported that thrombotic events that are considered the hallmark of antiphospholipid syndrome may cause irreversible damage from the onset of the disease. In our opinion, this is also applicable for BD and may explain the association of thrombosis and VDI [26].

In addition, most neurological manifestations and part of the total thromboses are caused by arterial affection, which was found to be associated with greater mortality rate (13.5% in patients with BD with arterial lesions compared to 3.6% in those without arterial involvement) [27].

The association of VDI with uveitis and its complication may also be predictable, if we consider that ocular inflammation develops in approximately 70% of patients and refractory ocular inflammation that may lead to blindness is common in those not responding well to systemic corticosteroids combined with other immunosuppressive agents observed in patients with BD [28].

Osteoporosis, AVN and diabetes; these specific damage items are shared by different damage indices as SLICC for lupus [29] and even VDI itself because they commonly result from high cumulative doses of glucocorticoids used for the treatment of different manifestations

Table 3 Comparison of Vasculitis Damage Index (VDI) with respect to demographic and clinical manifestations

	VDI score		
	Minimun-Maximum	Median (IQR)	*P*-value
Sex			
Male	1–10	3 (2)	0.1*
Female	1–7	5 (2)	
Oral ulcers			
Yes	1–10	3 (3)	0.21*
No	1–3	3 (1)	
Genital ulcers			
Yes	1–10	3 (3)	0.487*
No	1–8	3 (2)	
Other skin lesions			
Yes	1–8	3 (3)	0.197*
No	1–10	3 (2)	
Vascular involvement			
Yes	1–10	4 (3)	0.073*
No	1–7	3 (2)	
DVT attacks			
Yes	1–8	4 (3)	0.566*
No	1–10	3 (2)	
Arterial or venous thrombosis			
Yes	1–10	4 (3)	**0.022***
No	1–8	3 (2)	
Aneurysm			
Yes	1–8	3 (2)	0.539*
No	1–10	3 (2)	
Neurological affection			
Yes	3–10	5 (2)	**< 0.0001***
No	1–8	3 (2)	
Cranial nerve affection			
Yes	5–10	6 (3)	**< 0.0001***
No	1–8	3 (2)	
Ataxia			
Yes	4–7	4***	0.102*
No	1–10	5 (2)	
Stroke			
Yes	3–6	4 (1)	**0.014***
No	1–10	3 (2)	
Arthritis			
Yes	1–8	4 (1)	0.741*
No	1–10	3 (2)	
AVN			
Yes	3–10	7 (7)	**0.015***
No	1–8	3 (2)	
Osteoporosis			
Yes	3–10	7 (7)	**0.01***
No	1–8	4 (1)	
Uveitis			
Yes	1–10	4 (3)	**0.005***
No	1–8	3 (2)	
Vision			
Normal	1–8	2 (1)	**< 0.0001****
Impaired	1–7	3 (2)	
Blindness	2–10	5 (5)	
Cataract			
No involvement	1–8	2 (2)	**< 0.0001****
Single eye involvement	3–10	5 (4)	
Both eye involvement	2–7	4 (2)	
Diabetes			
Yes	3–10	4 (4)	**0.012***
No	1–8	3 (2)	

*Mann–Whitney test, **Kruskal–Wallis test, *** no IQR is calculated; as only 3 patients had ataxia. *VDI* Vasculitis damage index, *BD* Behçet's disease, *DVT* Deep venous thrombosis, *AVN* Avascular necrosis

of rheumatic diseases thus it is not surprising to find an association between these damage items and VDI.

Systemic immunosuppressive and biological agents are the standard therapy for severe organ involvement in BD [30–32], and the goal of management is early treatment to avoid recurrences and irreversible damage to the vital organs [33]. As other autoimmune diseases, medications used may be associated with serious side effects and damage [31, 34, 35]. In our study, the use of immunosuppressive drugs in general was significantly associated with VDI, especially cyclophosphamide, infliximab, and chlorambucil, in addition to anticoagulant, while the use of other medications that may be used in BD for milder presentation, such as colchicine and azathioprine, was not significantly associated with VDI. In our opinion, although such medications may improve survival and disease outcomes, they should be reserved for severe aggressive disease manifestations, as these medications may show some serious side effects, increasing the damage; thus, the association of immunosuppressive drug use and VDI could be expected, also from another point of view such medications may be used to treat active, aggressive disease, which itself may be associated with increased damage.

Table 4 Comparison of Vasculitis Damage Index (VDI) with respect to the medication received

	VDI score		
	Minimun-Maximum	Median (IQR)	*P*-value
Immunosuppressive drugs			
Yes	1–10	3 (2)	**0.039***
No	1–4	3.5 (2)	
CYC			
Yes	1–10	4 (3)	**< 0.0001***
No	1–7	2.5 (1)	
AZA			
Yes	1–10	3 (3)	0.294*
No	1–8	3 (2)	
CSA			
Yes	1–10	3 (2)	0.874*
No	1–8	3 (3)	
Biological			
Yes	1–10	4(2)	**0.008***
No	1–8	3 (2)	
Colchicine			
Yes	2–2	2**	0.16*
No	1–10	3 (2)	
Chlorambucil			
Yes	7–10	8**	**0.003***
No	1–8	3 (2)	
Anticoagulant			
Yes	1–10	4(4)	**0.02***
No	1–7	3 (2)	

*Mann–Whitney test, **no IQR is calculated; as the number of patients who recieved the drug was less than 4. *CYC* Cyclophosphamide, *AZA* Azathioprine, *CSA* Cyclosporine A

Table 5 Correlation of the Vasculitis Damage Index (VDI) score with some patients´ demographic and clinical variables

Variable	VDI in patients with BD ($n = 109$)	
	[a]r	*P
Delay in diagnosis	0.02	0.84
BDCAF	0.15	0.13
Age	0.2	**0.03**
Disease duration	0.21	**0.03**
Stroke score	0.09	0.8
Duration of eye affection	0.34	**0.003**

[a]Spearman correlation coefficient. *P is significant at < 0.05. *VDI* Vasculitis damage index, *BD* Behçet's disease, *BDCAF* BD current activity form

It seems expected that longer disease duration and duration of eye involvement may be associated with increased damage, which is the case in our study, as VDI was significantly correlated with disease duration and eye involvement. However, the correlation between VDI and age ($P = 0.033$), may contradict the decreased mortality rate in patients with BD aged > 35 years reported by Saadoun et al. [36], In our opinion this decline in mortality after age of 35, may raise an important point, that elderly onset BD patients may show milder disease manifestations as some elderly onset lupus, which is appoint that may require further studies.

In this study, we found that VDI is correlated with most aggressive disease manifestations of BD. However, some damage found in patients with BD may not be covered by VDI, especially damage related to genital ulcers or venous occlusion, e.g., Budd Chiari syndrome, vena caval thrombosis, and cerebral venous sinus thrombosis. Moreover, the development of venous thrombosis (unless complicated) or recurrent venous thrombosis is excluded in the VDI. In contrast, some items mentioned in VDI may not be of value in patients with BD, such as alopecia and proteinuria. Thus, according to the aforementioned reasons, in our opinion, BD modified specific VDI version as that studied by Piga et al. 2020 and including many modified items of VDI [14], may be needed for better assessment of damage in patients with BD, which must be assessed in further prospective, large scale, longitudinal studies.

Among strengths of our study is that, it is one of the pioneer studies in attempt to evaluate Damage index for BD. On the other hand, study limitations include: we did not assess the inter-rater agreement by evaluating Cohen's kappa and the interclass correlation coefficient (ICC), we also did not correlate VDI with the number of flares, cumulative corticosteroid doses, or delay in immunosuppressive therapy.

Vasculitis is a main pathologic finding in BD, and damage index is required in most rheumatic diseases to quantify damage, aid in the separation of damage from disease activity, and rationalize selection of therapy. Fortunately; a recent damage index for Behçet's disease has been validated "Behçet's syndrome overall damage index (BODI)" most items of which, has been derived from VDI, however further validation is needed for such damage index to be established as concluded by their authors.

Conclusions

VDI is significantly associated with most disease parameters of BD, except for parameters such as mucocutaneous manifestations and uncomplicated venous thrombosis; however, further studies may be needed to establish and validate VDI derived BD-specific damage index.

Acknowledgements

Non applicable.

Authors' contributions

All authors have participated sufficiently in this work. The authors read and approved the final manuscript.

Author details

Rheumatology and Rehabilitation Department, Cairo University, Cairo, Egypt. Internal Medicine Department, National Research Center, Cairo, Egypt. Dermatology and venereology Department, National Research Center, Cairo, Egypt. [4]Public Health Department, Cairo University, Cairo, Egypt.

References

1. Protogerou AD, Nasothimiou EG, Sfikakis PP, Tzioufas AG. Non-invasive vascular biomarkers in patients with Behçet's disease: review of the data and future perspectives. Clin Exp Rheumatol. 2017;35 Suppl 108(6):100–7.
2. Schirmer M, Calamia KT, Direskeneli H. Ninth international conference on Behçet's disease, Seoul, Korea, May 27-29, 2000. J Rheumatol. 2001;28(3): 636–9.
3. Davatchi F, Assaad-Khalil S, Calamia K, Crook JE, Sadeghi-Abdollahi B, Schirmer M, et al. The international criteria for Behçet's disease (ICBD): a collaborative study of 27 countries on the sensitivity and specificity of the new criteria. J Eur Acad Dermatol Venereol. 2014;28:338–47.
4. Emmi G, Bettiol A, Silvestri E, Di Scala G, Becatti M, Fiorillo C, et al. Vascular Behçet's syndrome: an update. Intern Emerg Med. 2019;14(5):645–52. https://doi.org/10.1007/s11739-018-1991-y.
5. Desbois AC, Wechsler B, Cluzel P, Helft G, Boutin D, Piette JC, et al. Cardiovascular involvement in Behçet's disease. Rev Med Interne. 2014;35(2): 103–11. https://doi.org/10.1016/j.revmed.2013.12.002.
6. Alibaz-Oner F, Direskeneli H. Management of vascular Behcet's disease. Int J Rheum Dis. 2019;22:105–8. https://doi.org/10.1111/1756-185X.13298.
7. Ketari Jamoussi S, Chaaba H, Ben Dhaou B, Boussema F, Kochbati S, Cherif O, et al. Arterial involvement in Behcet's disease: a series of 7 cases. Tunis Med. 2009;87(9):583–8.
8. Jayne D. Challenges in the management of microscopic polyangiitis: past, present and future. Curr Opin Rheumatol. 2008;20(1):3–9. https://doi.org/10.1097/BOR.0b013e3282f370d1.
9. Mukhtyar C, Flossmann O, Hellmich B, Bacon P, Cid M, Cohen-Tervaert JW, et al. Outcomes from studies of anti-neutrophil cytoplasm antibody associated vasculitis: a systematic review by the European league against rheumatism systemic vasculitis task force. Ann Rheum Dis. 2008;67(7):1004–10. https://doi.org/10.1136/ard.2007.071936.
10. Seo P, Luqmani RA, Flossmann O, Hellmich B, Herlyn K, Hoffman GS, et al. The future of damage assessment in vasculitis. J Rheumatol. 2007;34(6): 1357–71.
11. Exley AR, Bacon PA, Luqmani RA, Kitas GD, Gordon C, Savage CO, et al. Development and initial validation of the vasculitis damage index for the standardized clinical assessment of damage in the systemic vasculitides. Arthritis Rheum. 1997;40(2):371–80. https://doi.org/10.1002/art.1780400222.
12. Watts RA, Scott DG. Recent developments in the classification and assessment of vasculitis. Best Pract Res Clin Rheumatol. 2009;23(3):429–43. https://doi.org/10.1016/j.berh.2008.12.004.
13. Piga M. Behçet's Disease Overall Damage Index (BODI). https://clinicaltrials.gov/ct2/show/NCT03803462
14. Piga M, Floris A, Espinosa G, et al. Development and preliminary validation of the Behçet's syndrome overall damage index (BODI). RMD Open. 2020;6: e001192. https://doi.org/10.1136/rmdopen-2020-001192.
15. Hatemi G, Christensen R, Bang D, Bodaghi B, Celik AF, Fortune F, et al. 2018 update of the EULAR recommendations for the management of Behçet's syndrome. Ann Rheum Dis. 2018;77:808–18. https://doi.org/10.1136/annrheumdis-2018-213225.
16. Hatemi G, Silman A, Bang D, Bodaghi B, Chamberlain AM, Gul A, et al. EULAR recommendations for the management of Behçet disease. Ann Rheum Dis. 2008;67(12):1656–62. https://doi.org/10.1136/ard.2007.080432 Epub 2008 Jan 31.
17. Lawton G, Bhakta BB, Chamberlain MA, Tennant A. The Behçet's disease activity index. Rheumatology. 2004;43(1):73–8. https://doi.org/10.1093/rheumatology/keg453.
18. Zayed HS, Medhat BM, Seif EM. Evaluation of treatment adherence in patients with Behçet's disease: its relation to disease manifestations, patients' beliefs about medications, and quality of life. Clin Rheumatol. 2019; 38(3):761–8. https://doi.org/10.1007/s10067-018-4344-3.
19. Kural-Seyahi E, Fresko I, Seyahi N, Ozyazgan Y, Mat C, Hamuryudan V, et al. The long-term mortality and morbidity of Behçet syndrome: a 2-decade outcome survey of 387 patients followed at a dedicated center. Medicine (Baltimore). 2003;82(1):60–76. https://doi.org/10.1097/00005792-200301000-00006.
20. Silveira LH. Damage assessment in systemic vasculitis. Curr Rheumatol Rep. 2008;10(6):436–41. https://doi.org/10.1007/s11926-008-0071-0.
21. Attia DHS, Abdel Noor RA. Severe Behçet's disease equally affects both genders in Egyptian patients: a multicentre retrospective follow-up study. Reumatismo. 2019;71(4):218–25.
22. El-Garf A, Abdo M, Alkemary A, Mohamed S. Behçet's disease patterns and subsets in a cohort of Egyptian patients. Egypt Rheumatol. 2019;14:135–8. https://doi.org/10.1016/j.ejr.2018.05.006.
23. Cansu DU, Kaşifoğlu T, Korkmaz C. Do clinical findings of Behçet's disease vary by gender?: a single-center experience from 329 patients. Eur J Rheumatol. 2016;3(4):157–60. https://doi.org/10.5152/eurjrheum.2016.038.
24. Wu X, Li G, Huang X, et al. Behcet's disease complicated with thrombosis. A report of 93 Chinese cases. Medicine. 2014;93(28):e263. https://doi.org/10.1097/MD.0000000000000263.
25. Greco A, De Virgilio A, Ralli M, Ciofalo A, Mancini P, Attanasio G, et al. Behçet's disease: new insights into pathophysiology, clinical features and treatment options. Autoimmun Rev. 2018;17(6):567–75. https://doi.org/10.1016/j.autrev.2017.12.006.
26. Amigo MC, Goycochea-Robles MV, Espinosa-Cuervo G, Medina G, Barragán-Garfias JA, Vargas A, et al. Development and initial validation of a damage index (DIAPS) in patients with thrombotic antiphospholipid syndrome (APS). Lupus. 2015;24(9):927–34. https://doi.org/10.1177/0961203315576858.
27. Saadoun D, Asli B, Wechsler B, Houman H, Geri G, Desseaux K, et al. Long-term outcome of arterial lesions in Behçet disease: a series of 101 patients. Medicine. 2012;91(1):18–24. https://doi.org/10.1097/MD.0b013e3182428126.
28. Yang P, Huang G, Du L, Ye Z, Hu K, Wang C, et al. Long-term efficacy and safety of interferon alpha-2a in the treatment of Chinese patients with Behçet's uveitis not responding to conventional therapy. Ocul Immunol Inflamm. 2019;27(1):7–14. https://doi.org/10.1080/09273948.2017.1384026.
29. Gladman D, Ginzler E, Goldsmith C, Fortin P, Liang M, Urowitz M, et al. The development and initial validation of the systemic lupus international collaborating clinics/American College of Rheumatology damage index for systemic lupus erythematosus. Arthritis Rheum. 1996;39(3):363–9. https://doi.org/10.1002/art.1780390303.
30. Celiker H, Kazokoglu H, Direskeneli H. Conventional immunosuppressive therapy in severe Behcet's uveitis: the switch rate to the biological agents. BMC Ophthalmol. 2018;18(1):261. https://doi.org/10.1186/s12886-018-0929-5.
31. Zaghetto JM, Yamamoto MM, Souza MB, Silva FT, Hirata CE, Olivalves E, et al. Chlorambucil and cyclosporine a in Brazilian patients with Behçet's disease uveitis: a retrospective study. Arq Bras Oftalmol. 2010;73(1):40–6. https://doi.org/10.1590/S0004-27492010000100007.
32. Goker B, Goker H. Current therapy for Behçet's disease. Am J Ther. 2002;9(5): 465–70. https://doi.org/10.1097/00045391-200209000-00015.
33. Kaklamani VG, Kaklamanis PG. Treatment of Behçet's disease--an update. Semin Arthritis Rheum. 2001;30(5):299–312. https://doi.org/10.1053/sarh.2001.19819.
34. Hsu CY, Lin MS, Su YJ, Cheng TT, Lin YS, Chen YC, et al. Cumulative immunosuppressant exposure is associated with diversified cancer risk among 14 832 patients with systemic lupus erythematosus: a nested case-control study. Rheumatology (Oxford). 2017;56(4):620–8. https://doi.org/10.1093/rheumatology/kew457.
35. Caza T, Oaks Z, Perl A. Interplay of infections, autoimmunity, and immunosuppression in systemic lupus erythematosus. Int Rev Immunol. 2014;33(4):330–63. https://doi.org/10.3109/08830185.2013.863305.
36. Saadoun D, Wechsler B, Desseaux K, Le Thi HD, Amoura Z, Resche-Rigon M, et al. Mortality in Behçet's disease. Arthritis Rheum. 2010;62(9):2806–12. https://doi.org/10.1002/art.27568.

15

Relationship of the sacral slope with early gait derangements in robust older women

Leda Magalhaes Oliveira[1], Suely Roizenblatt[2*], Flavio Duarte Silva[3], Arnaldo Roizenblatt[4], Artur Rocha Correa Fernandes[3] and Vera Lucia Szejnfeld[1]

Abstract

Background: Trunk pelvic dissociation is fundamental to the compensatory mechanism for muscle weakness during body bending. We carried out an early investigation of gait changes in a sample of community-dwelling women ≥60 years without gait complaints. The primary objective was to correlate spine and pelvic angles with performance tests and accelerometry parameters. The secondary objective was to correlate performance tests with accelerometry.

Methods: In this cross-sectional study, 54 community-dwelling women ≥60 years were subjected to Falls Efficacy Scale-International (FES-I), performance tests (Berg Balance Scale, Timed Up and Go, and Gait analysis), and radiographic analysis of sagittal alignment (Thoracic and Lumbar Cobb, Pelvic Incidence, Sacral Slope, and Pelvic Tilt angles). Gait speed was assessed in a 10-m comfortable walk, and accelerometry parameters were obtained in a 30-m walk distance.

Results: The sample, aged 72 ± 6 years, exhibited moderate correlation between Sacral Slope and Step Length (+ 0.615). Sacral Slope weakly correlated with FES-I (− 0.339), Berg Balance Scale (+ 0.367), and with further accelerometry data in the AP plane: RMS, (+ 0.439) and Stride Regularity (+ 0.475), $p < 0.05$, all. Lumbar Cobb weakly correlated with the following accelerometry data in the AP plane: Step Length (+ 0.405), RMS, (+ 0.392), and Stride Regularity (+ 0.345), $p < 0.05$, all. Additionally, Stride Regularity in AP moderately correlated with FES-I (0,561, $p < 0.05$), among other weak correlations between performance tests and accelerometry data in AP.

Conclusions: Early alterations in Sacral Slope and gait abnormalities in the AP plane may provide understanding of the early gait changes in robust older women.

Keywords: Gait; disability, Spinal curvatures, Pelvis, Aging

Background

With ageing, a compensatory mechanism to the alignment derangement between pelvis and trunk occurs as a deliberate strategy to overcome the decrease in muscle strength [1]. Since the walking function requires integrity and fine-tuning of various body systems, the study of gait can reveal early changes in functional performance [2, 3]. With the loss of strength, decrease in deceleration control of the upper segments of the trunk in relation to the lower ones occurs particularly in the anteroposterior (AP) plane [1]. The control of the shoulder to head acceleration is less effective in older women than in men, suggesting a strain in the ability to exploit the cervical joints to attenuate the AP acceleration [4]. Furthermore, instead of using the ankle muscles to maintain balance, there is a greater demand from the muscles around the hips and thoracolumbar region [1, 5, 6].

As posture tends to flexion, the progressive forward displacement of the center of mass (CM) near the stability limit requires compensation to maintain gait speed [7]. The kinematics analysis of the pelvis and lower extremities using a 3-dimensional video-based motion

* Correspondence: suely.roizenblatt@unifesp.br
[2]Department of Internal Medicine, Universidade Federal de Sao Paulo (UNIFESP), Rua Angelina Maffei Vita 670. CEP:01455070, Sao Paulo, SP, Brazil

system has shown that the retroversion of the pelvis is the resulting compensation for the increased kyphosis acquired over time. Studies on the role of the sagittal alignment in gait have confirmed that compensation mechanisms of increased kyphosis in the elderly include a sequence of events, such as posterior pelvic tilting, increase in hip extension, then knee flexion and increase ankle dorsiflexion [8]. A study of the sagittal alignment and gait speed influences on falls of middle-aged and older males has shown that falls in the previous year was associated with the reduction in lumbar lordosis, sacral slope, and decrease of the gait speed [9].

When accelerometers were incorporated into clinical practice as an instrumental method to objectively detect small changes in the functioning of postural control in older adults [10], there was a progress in the assessment of gait adaptive mechanisms that compensate for changes in posture. The advantage of these portable devices is the possibility of recording spontaneous movements out of the laboratory environment. For review on the advantages of accelerometers as a method of early detection of alterations in balance in older people see Leirós-Rodríguez et al., 2019 [11]. Very few studies have used accelerometers to access the gait responses to the body's forward displacement of the CM in older adults in a free-living context. Groot et al., demonstrated that the correcting responses result in an increase in the risk of falling due to lower stability of the gait, and a more irregular trunk acceleration [12]. Lack of coordination linking acceleration variability between the trunk and feet in a constrained gait have been demonstrated by accelerometry, even in healthy older fallers, when subjected to a protocol of gait analysis in a treadmill with variable speed [13].

Considering the value of early physical ability improvement on the prevention of falls in older adults [14], and the lack of studies on the association of sagittal alignment and accelerometry analysis of gait, this study was conducted to investigate the correlation of the spine and pelvis alignment with changes in accelerometer-based gait parameters in asymptomatic women aged 60 years or older. The primary objective was to evaluate the correlation between spine and pelvic angles in performance tests and accelerometry parameters. The secondary objective was to study the correlation of performance tests and accelerometry.

Methods

Participants

In this cross-sectional study of a sample of women aged 60 years or older, who were physically active and independent from assistance or assistive tools, were consecutively recruited from the Open University of the Third Age of the XXXXXXXX. Inclusion criteria comprised good cognitive condition (MiniMental State Examination (MMSE) score > 24 [15], Body Mass Index below 30 kg/m^2, and robustness [16]. Exclusion criteria comprised the reporting of falls in the previous year, complaints of back pain or impaired gait, ≥ 7 points in the Clinical-Functional Vulnerability Index (IVCF-20) [16], scoliosis Cobb angle > 20°; skeletal abnormalities, neurological or musculoskeletal disabilities that interfered with gait; uncontrolled diabetes mellitus; alcoholism; history of spine surgery, and fractures or prosthesis implants in the lower limbs.

The research was approved by the Ethical Committee of XXXX (#824.155), and written informed consent was obtained from each participant after the explanation of the objective and methodology of the study. During the first visit, participants answered questionnaires regarding cognitive condition, vulnerability, falls, and self-reported *exercise* adherence. The answers were evaluated by a rheumatologist (XX) and in case of eligibility for the study, the participants were sent to radiological evaluation of the sagittal balance, carried out by a trained radiologist (XX). In a second visit, performance tests and accelerometry recordings were conducted by a trained physical therapist (XXX).

Questionnaires

The IVCF-20 was used to assess vulnerability. The IVCF-20 is a 20 question multidimensional inventory that covers aspects of the elderly's health conditions, which includes age, health self-perception, functional disabilities, cognition, mood, mobility, communication, and multiple comorbidities. The maximum score is 40 points and the higher the value obtained, higher is the elderly's risk for clinical-functional vulnerability. In our study, robustness was defined for scores < 7 as reported for the Brazilian elderly [16].

Cross-cultural adaptation of the Falls Efficacy Scale-International (FES-I) for Brazilians was used to assess the fear of falling during the previous year. This 16-question inventory inquiring "how concerned are you about the possibility of falling" is rated as not at all, somewhat, fairly, and very concerned. The total score ranges from 16 to 64 points, being the higher values indicative of higher concern about falling [17].

Self-reported exercise adherence was assessed by the weekly frequency of reported aerobic or resistance training exercises in the previous month. According to the answers, subjects were considered as highly active (physical exercises at least 3 days a week), moderate (at least once a week) and inactive (less than once a week).

Performance tests

Participants were subjected to two sessions of a 10-m walk at a comfortable speed, which was measured in meters/second. The tests were performed on a level and clear 30-m corridor, with 1.5-m space for acceleration and deceleration, and without encouraging words. Gait speed between 0.90–1.42 m/s has been considered adequate for the walking economy during the ageing process [18, 19]. Berg Balance Scale validated to Brazilian Portuguese [20] was used to assess functional balance performance; and was based on 14 questions with answers ranging from 0 to 4 points. Total scores of 0 to 20 represent balance impairment, of 21 to 40 indicate acceptable balance, and of 41 to 56, good balance [21].

Timed Up-and-Go (TUG) was also carried out for functional performance. Participants, wearing their usual footwear, were seated on a standard chair with solid seat, with their backs supported by a flat backrest, and their arms supported by armrests. At the evaluator's instruction, they had to stand up, walk a 3 m-distance in a straight line, in a comfortable speed, cross a mark on the floor, then turn around 180°, walk back, and sit down again. There was one practice session immediately before the test session was performed. The evaluator initiated the chronometer at the moment the participants stood up, and stopped it only when they were seating on the chair with their arms and back supported again. TUG values over 12.47 s are considered as predictive of falls for the Brazilian older adults [22]..

Radiological evaluation

For Pelvic Incidence, complete overlap between the femoral heads was required. Sagittal images were obtained with subjects in the orthostatic position, with upper limbs flexed, hands on the shoulders in 30° flexion, knees extended, and looking straight ahead. The image scope was from the cervical spine to the femoral heads, and the distance from source-to-film was 2.3 m [23].

Thoracic Cobb angle was computed as the angle formed between the two straight lines that were orthogonal to the upper endplate of T4 to the endplate of T12. For Lumbar Cobb the reference points were the upper endplate of L1 to the lower endplate of L5 [24]. Thoracic Cobb mean values for older Brazilian women are 43.1° ± 13.6°, and for the Lumbar Cobb, – 41.7° ± 11.9° [25].

Pelvic Incidence angle was defined by a line drawn from the center of the femoral heads to the midpoint of the sacral endplate, and a line perpendicular to the center of the sacral endplate. Pelvic Tilt was defined as the angle subtended by a vertical reference line originating from the center of the femoral head and the midpoint of the sacral endplate. Sacral Slope was defined as the angle subtended by a horizontal reference line and the sacral endplate line. The reported mean reference values for Brazilians, older than 60 years were: Pelvic Incidence angle of 50.9° ± 6.6°, Sacral Slope of 37.4° ± 5.1°, and Pelvic Tilt of 13.8° ± 5° [26].

Accelerometry

We used the MiniMod DynaPort™ (McRoberts, Netherlands) with a signal acquisition frequency of 100 Hz, in a range of variation of ±2 g in a 30-m walking trial [27]. The device was attached to a belt that was placed firmly at the point behind the spinal process of L3. This point is easily located and it is convenient for global measure of walking parameters, due to its proximity to the CM in the upright stance and during walking [28, 29]. Gait was assessed in a 30-m walk distance held at comfortable speed, with a 1.5-m space for acceleration and deceleration, and without encouraging words.

Data was collected by MiniMod Acquire (MIRA™; McRoberts, Netherlands) and processed using iGait, which is an open-source software from MatLab™ environment [30]. After alignment correction, gait data extracted in the temporal domain included: Stride Regularity, Gait Symmetry, Root Mean Square (RMS) value in the anteroposterior (AP), vertical (V), and medio-lateral (ML) planes. The square root values of the three planes were normalized to the average value of square root/RMS. Step and Stride Regularities were defined as the correlation between the original acceleration signal and the acceleration signal phase shifted to the average step and stride time, respectively [28–30]. Gait Symmetry was defined as the difference between the consistency of strides and steps in the accelerometer waveforms. Step Length was calculated dividing the 30-m walk distance by the number of peaks of acceleration detected by the accelerometer during the foot contact with the ground.

Statistical analysis

A sample of 38 elderly women allowed detection of a correlation of 0.44 or more between radiographic and accelerometer-derived data with an alpha of 0.05 and power of 80% [31].

Mean and standard deviation (SD) were used for data with parametric distribution whereas median and interquartile range (IQR) were used for the non-parametric data. The Spearman's rank correlation coefficient was used to calculate correlations between the angles of the spine and pelvis with clinical, functional and accelerometer-derived parameters.

Multivariate regression was used to evaluate the existing association of age with radiological and accelerometer-derived data of normal distribution. Independent variables tested were age, height, weight, Thoracic Cobb, Lumbar Cobb, Sacral Slope, Pelvic Tilt, whereas the dependent variables tested were, RMS, Step Length, Stride Regularity and Gait Symmetry in all planes. Data were tabulated and analyzed using SPSS Statistics for Windows, Version 22.0, IBM Corp and the significance was set at 5%.

Results

The sample of 54 women, aged 60 years and older, who met inclusion criteria and agreed to participate in the protocol was selected among 220 volunteers (Fig. 1).

The characteristics of the sample are described in Table 1. In comparison to what has been reported for Brazilians older than 60 years [26], we observed an increase in the following pelvic angles mean ± SD: Pelvic Incidence (50.9° ± 6.6° vs. 57.9° ± 11.5°), Pelvic Tilt (13.8 ± 5° vs. 17.4 ± 8.0°) and Sacral Slope (37.4° ± 5.1° vs. 40.4° ± 7.8°). In comparison to the literature on older women [25], there was an increase in mean ± SD Thoracic Cobb (43.1° ± 13.6° vs. 47.4° ± 9.7°) and Lumbar Cobb (− 41.7° ± 11.9° vs. -46.3° ± 7.5°).

Regarding self-reported *exercise* adherence, 21 (38.8%) of the women were considered as inactive, 27 (50.0%) as active, and 6 (11.1%) as highly active. Even though report of falls in the previous year was one of the exclusion criteria, 30 participants (55.5%) scored above 23 in FES-I, which has been associated with the adoption of strategies to avoid falls [17].

In the performance tests, 43 (79.6%) of the subjects presented TUG values below the predictive cut-off for falls for older Brazilians, which corresponds to 12.47 s [22]. As shown in Table 1, the median TUG value was 9.4 with IQR of 2.2. The median Berg Balance Scale score was 50 with IQR of 4, and a minimum score of 37 [20]. Two participants (3.7%) scored between 20 and 41, which is considered an acceptable balance. Mean ± SD comfortable gait speed obtained in the 10-m walk test was 1.10 ± 0.19 m/s and the one obtained by accelerometry was 1.09 ± 0.19, with a correlation r_S of 0.679, (p < 0.01) between them. Comfortable gait speed in the 10-m walk test negatively correlated with TUG (− 0.620; p < 0.01) and with Thoracic Cobb (− 0.341; p < 0.05).

Table 1 Sample characteristics

N = 54	Mean or *Median*	SD or *IQR*	Minimum	Maximum
Age (years)	72.33	6.14	61.00	85.00
Height (m)	151.52	6.21	140.00	165.00
Weight (kg)	59.82	8.97	44.00	80.00
MMSE	*26.48*	*4.04*	*24.00*	*30.00*
FES-I (median [IQR])	*24.00*	*7.25*	*17.00*	*45.00*
Berg scale (median [IQR])	*50.00*	*4.00*	*37.00*	*56.00*
TUG (sec) (median [IQR])	*9.43*	*2.20*	*6.57*	*15.45*
Gait speed (m/sec)	1.10	0.19	0.57	1.54
Thoracic Cobb (degrees)	47.43	9.67	17.00	62.00
Lumbar Cobb (degrees)	46.31	7.54	19.00	55.00
Pelvic Incidence (degrees)	57.91	11.46	39.40	85.78
Sacral Slope (degrees)	40.41	7.79	30.17	49.41
Pelvic Tilt (degrees)	17.42	8.03	0.00	46.00

Comfortable gait speed in 10-m gait test
SD standard deviation, *IQR* interquartile range, *MMSE* MiniMental State Examination, *FES-I* Fall Efficacy Scale –International, *TUG* Timed up and Go

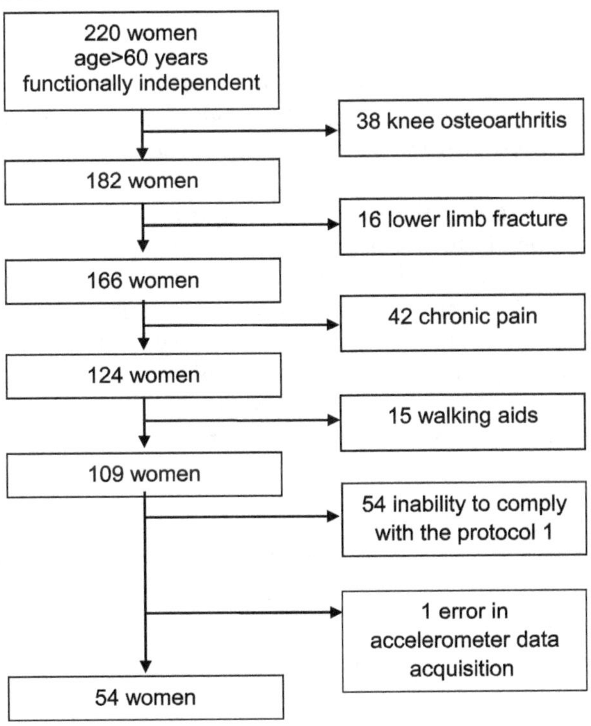

Fig. 1 Inclusion of participants in the study

Correlations of spine and pelvis angles were assessed with FES-I, performance tests, and with accelerometer-derived data. Significant findings are shown in Tables 2 and 3, respectively. Complementarily, significant correlations of FES-I and performance tests with accelerometer-derived data were found in the AP plane are (Table 4). Mean ± SD values of the accelerometer-derived parameters that presented significant correlations with sagittal alignment data (Table 3) and performance tests (Table 4) were: RMS (0.17 ± 0.04, range 0.06–0.25 g), Step Length (0.59 ± 0.08, range 0.34–0.73 m), Stride Regularity (0.81 ± 0.10 range 0.61–0.90), and Gait Symmetry (6.04 ± 3.04, range 0.3–0.97). Pelvic Tilt angle and accelerometer-derived variables in the ML and V planes were not included in the Tables due to the lack of correlation with the other parameters.

In the multiple regression analysis, age accounted for 12.3% of the variance of RMS in AP and the overall regression model was F (1,53) = 7.43, p = 0.009, R^2 coefficient of 12.3, with a positive independent contribution of age (unstandardized beta coefficient of 0.002). In addition, there was a slight correlation of age with RMS in AP (− 0.351; p < 0.01).

Table 2 Correlations of spine and pelvis angles with FES-I and performance tests

N = 54	Thoracic Cobb	Lumbar Cobb	Pelvic Incidence	Sacral Slope
Gait speed	−0.341*	−0.130	− 0.139	0.178
FES-I	+ 0.242	+ 0.199	+ 0,149	−0.339*
TUG (sec)	+ 0.341*	−0.030	−0.039	+ 0.178
Berg Balance Scale	+ 0.197	+ 0.187	+ 0.269	+ 0.367**

Comfortable gait speed in 10-m gait test
FES –I Fall Efficacy Scale – International, *TUG* Timed Up and Go
Spearman correlations: * $p < 0.05$, ** $p < 0.01$

Discussion

This study was proposed to provide new information on the relationship between radiographic measures of spinal alignment and parameters of gait extracted from accelerometry in robust, community-dwelling women aged 60 years and older. The results revealed that Sacral Slope, rather than Lumbar Cobb, positively correlated with Step Length and weakly with RMS and Stride Regularity in the AP plane. Furthermore, weak correlations of Sacral Slope were obtained with FES-I and Berg Balance Scale. The underlying implications of such correlations, albeit weak, need to be reported.

During walking, the tendency is to choose a gait speed that optimizes the body movement and minimizes the energy cost per distance. Walking faster or slower requires more energy and increases the magnitude of speed variation due to gait instability [32]. The gait speed of our sample was within the expected range for a comfortable gait speed in a 10-m walk by robust women between 60 and 79 years [18, 33]. The association of age with slowing of temporal gait measurements still remains controversial [34–36]. It has been suggested that a "cautious gait" pattern, is a marker of an underlying pathology and not an age-related process [37]. While low walking speed has a negative effect on stability, short Step Length has a positive effect on it [18].

Kerrigan et al., 2001 observed that in a group of robust older adults (10 men and 13 women) with similar mean age of our sample, fallers presented a shorter Step Length than non-fallers (0.49 ± 0.08 m vs, 0.61 ± 0.06 m). The Step Length mean value obtained in our group of non-faller older women was 0.59 ± 0.08 m. The slight difference may be attributed to the inclusion of men in their sample [3]. Even though we only included non-faller older women in our research, FES-I median score of 25 indicates their substantial fear of falling [17]. In TUG test, 79.6% of the sample exhibited values below 12.47 s, which has been considered as a predictive cut-off for falls for older Brazilians [22]. The finding of negative correlations between FES-I and TUG with Step Length supports the hypothesis that shortening of the Step Length corresponds to a postural adaptation to increase time spent in double support for maintenance of balance [34, 38]. Postural control and balance are important aspects of gait stability and are necessary to reduce the chances of falling [39].

Hyperkyphosis has been considered as the earliest body posture change throughout ageing, both in healthy women [6] and men [40]. The impact of the forward displacement of the CM on gait, related to a hyperkyphotic posture, was confirmed in the present study by the negative correlation between Thoracic Cobb and Gait Speed in the 10-m walk test, and with the positive correlation with TUG. For the maintenance of the sagittal alignment, thoracic kyphosis compensation by retroversion of the pelvis and sacral verticalization would be expected when Pelvic Incidence allows the CM projection not to exceed the base of support [41]. The stress that hyperkyphosis poses to the gait yields in decline in the walking economy [18].

Furthermore, the pelvic *three-dimensional* movement corresponds to a kinematic mechanism that maintains the efficient translation of the CM and pelvic anteversion-retroversion movement influence on the Step Length [42]. How reduction in pelvic rotation contributes to the "cautious gait" in older adults still *remains* unknown. The negative correlation between FES-I and Sacral Slope, albeit weak, suggests that the fear of

Table 3 Correlations of spine and the pelvis angles with accelerometer-derived data in the anteroposterior plane

N = 54	Thoracic Cobb	Lumbar Cobb	Pelvic Incidence	Sacral Slope
RMS	+ 0.017	+ 0.392**	+ 0.318*	+ 0.439**
Step Length	+ 0.124	+ 0.405**	+ 0.430**	+ 0.615**
Stride Regularity	+ 0.091	+ 0.345*	+ 0.260	+ 0.475**
Gait symmetry	+ 0.107	−0.102	− 0.248	−0.150

RMS Root Mean Square of acceleration during walking (center of mass displacement)
Spearman correlations: * $p < 0.05$, ** $p < 0.01$

Table 4 Correlations of accelerometer-derived data in the anteroposterior plane with FES-I and performance tests

$N = 54$	RMS	Step Length	Stride Regularity	Gait symmetry
Gait speed	0.236	0.035	0.118	0.005
FES-I	+ 0.407**	−0.414**	+ 0.561**	−0.318*
TUG (sec)	+ 0.313*	−0,367*	+ 0.381 *	−0.489**
Berg Balance Scale	+ 0.103	+ 0.249	+ 0.105	−0.031

Comfortable gait speed in 10-m gait test
RMS Root Mean Square of acceleration during walking (center of mass displacement), *FES –I* Fall Efficacy Scale – International, *TUG* Timed Up and Go
Spearman correlations: * $p < 0.05$, ** $p < 0.01$

falling was greater in those with a verticalized sacrum. The retroversion of the pelvis and the sacrum verticalization impose a maximum hip extension impairing the ankle push-off reaction, with a negative effect on the displacement of the CM which oscillates back and forth from the support base during walking [3, 12, 43].

In our sample of older women, without gait complaints, there was an increase in the expected mean value of Pelvic Incidence and Sacral Slope [26]. Notwithstanding, a Sacral Slope between 35° and 45°, as obtained in our sample, is described as representative of a healthy balanced spine [44]. Pelvic Incidence values below 44° are related to a decrease in Sacral Slope and flattening of Lumbar Lordosis, whereas values above 62° have the opposite effect. Sacral Slope is the key parameter contributing to the sagittal curvature. The degree of the Sacral Slope determines the position of the lumbar spine, since the sacral plateau forms the base of the spine and therefore may provide the possibility of balance [45]. Lower Pelvic Incidence results in lower Sacral Slope and lower degree of Lumbar Lordosis [46]. Even though this relationship is independent of the ageing process, parameters of the sagittal alignment of the spine and pelvis should be taken into account in studies of gait even for the robust older adults.

The detrimental effect of sagittal imbalance on gait performance has been evidenced by Miyazaki et al., in a sample of asymptomatic older men with an age range similar to our sample [40]. Our finding of a positive Berg Balance Scale correlation with Pelvic Incidence and Sacral Slope, although weak, is in line with the positive effect of high Pelvic Incidence and Sacral Slope on balance. The Berg Balance Scale was originally developed to assess the functional performance of balance through functional tasks that require equilibrium in older people. The weak correlation that we obtained might be attributed to the discrepancy between the static characteristic of most tasks assessed by Berg Balance Scale and the dynamic nature of walking [47].

The correlation of our sagittal alignment data with accelerometer-derived gait parameters suggests early difficulty in controlling the displacement of the CM in the AP plane, Ideally, a perfect sagittal alignment occurs when the body weight is positioned along a line slightly behind the rotation axis of the two femoral heads. Low values of Sacral Slope and Lumbar Cobb angles limit the pelvis movements, what result in an inefficient balance control [48], as shown in our study by the negative correlation of Sacral Slope with FES-I and positive correlation with Step Length. Further positive correlations, albeit weak, are in line with this finding, such as Pelvic Incidence and Lumbar Lordosis correlation with Step Length and RMS in AP, and Sacral Slope with both RMS and Stride Regularity in AP.

Early alterations found in AP plane result in a loss in propulsion and braking phases of gait in older women with preserved mobility, suggesting a correlation between shortening of Step Length and gait destabilization [2, 29]. Considering that the major component of gait occurs in the AP plane, it becomes necessary to increase the effort at this plane to keep the progression of the gait [49].. Increased fear of falling requires more energy consumption to support the AP displacement due to the increase in step rate. Shortening of the Step Length is associated with a decline in the walking economy and irregular body acceleration in the AP plane, which is the major component of gait [18, 32]. Our data shows negative correlation of FES-I with Step Length, but a positive correlation of FES-I with Stride Regularity in AP, suggesting preservation of the functional ability to control the step sequence. The increase in energy required to sustain the walking forward is reflected by the positive correlation of FES-I with RMS in AP plane. Acceleration RMS estimates the magnitude of the variation of the gravitational potential energy of the CM that is exchanged for forward kinetic energy. The increase in energy consumption can be expressed as an increase in RMS [50].

Age related decline in walking economy is associated with the adoption of an increased gait rate and progressive irregular body acceleration in the horizontal plane. A higher gait rate is a consequence of the shortening of the Step Length which characterizes an unstable walking [18]. The negative correlations of both FES-I and TUG with Gait Symmetry in AP suggest that impaired Gait Symmetry might also be a predictor of future falls [51]. The value of TUG remains in the fact that it corresponds to the challenge in the energy required to adopt different postures and change of directions.

Our data shows the impact of the insufficient compensation of the sagittal alignment by the upper or lower body segments on the gait pattern [45], even in robust older women, However, there are several limitations in this study. First, the cross-sectional design and consecutive sampling prevent generalization of our findings.

However, our decision to enroll every single participant who met inclusion criteria until the sample size was reached was based on the higher reliability of the results than we would get with subjects chosen the by the investigator's convenience sampling. This way, our results can be considered as useful guidelines for future studies. Second, since a longitudinal design is better suited for studies on the gait pattern in older adults, we intend to follow this sample of robust older women over time in order to detect the turning point when gait changes become symptomatic. Third, many of the correlations we found were not strong. Subtle gait changes that increase the risk of falls might not have been accurately recorded. A longitudinal study will enable confirmation of the relevance of the findings with weaker correlations, which are already supported by the literature. Fourth, potential measurement errors in the Cobb angle may be attributed to the variation within and between observers due to the poor visualization of the vertebral body limits; that are covered by overlying tissue densities, the presence of transition vertebra, variations related to the minor rotation of the subject between examinations, and the variation in the same subject. Lack of accuracy is more relevant for smaller angles (< 10°), which was not the case for the present study.

Even with these limitations, our results support the hypothesis that there is a correlation between the spine and pelvic angles with the performance tests and accelerometry parameters. Sacral Slope and Lumbar Cobb positively correlate with Step Length. Further weak correlations of sagittal alignment were obtained with accelerometry-derived parameters, however considering the complexity of the walking mechanics that influence gait, we would not expect that any single correlation would be particularly high in robust older women. The contribution of the Sacral Slope on impact absorption and variability of trunk movements during gait deserves further elucidation.

Conclusions

While we expected preserved walking conditions, gait alterations in the AP plane were detected and were correlated to lower Sacral Slope and Lumbar Lordosis. Our results have a possible application in the understanding of the early changes in the postural control during gait in robust older women.

Aknowledgments The authors thank all subjects who participated in this study and Associacao Fundo de Incentivo a Pesquisa for providing the accelerometer devices that were used in this research.

Abbreviations

AP: Anteroposterior; CM: Center of mass; FES-I: Falls Efficacy Scale-International; IQR: Interquartile range; MMSE: MiniMental State Examination; IVCF-20: Clinical-Functional Vulnerability Index; RMS: Root mean square; SD: Standard deviation; TUG: Timed Up-and-Go

Authors' contributions

LMO: Participated in the in the elaboration of the research, data discussion and the article writing. Collection and data discussion and the article writing. SR: Participated in the study data collection, statistical analysis and the article writing. FDS and ARCF: Participated in the design and execution of the radiological evaluation of the participants, analyzed and interpreted the results and contributed in data discussion. AR: performed statistical analysis, drafted and critically revised the manuscript. VLS: Participated in the data discussion and the article writing. The authors read and approved the final version of the manuscript.

Author details

[1]Rheumatology Division, Universidade Federal de Sao Paulo (UNIFESP), São Paulo, Brazil. [2]Department of Internal Medicine, Universidade Federal de Sao Paulo (UNIFESP), Rua Angelina Maffei Vita 670. CEP:01455070, Sao Paulo, SP, Brazil. [3]Department of Diagnostic Imaging, Universidade Federal de Sao Paulo (UNIFESP), São Paulo, Brazil. [4]Medical Student Universidade Federal de Sao Paulo (UNIFESP), São Paulo, Brazil.

References

1. Van Emmerik RE, McDermott WJ, Haddad JM, Van Wegen EE. Age-related changes in upper body adaptation to walking speed in human locomotion. Gait Posture. 2005;22(3):233–9. https://doi.org/10.1016/j.gaitpost.2004.09.006
2. Winter DA, Patla AE, Frank JS, Walt SE. Biomechanical walking pattern changes in the fit and healthy elderly. Phys Ther. 1990;70(6):340–7. https://doi.org/10.1093/ptj/70.6.340.
3. Kerrigan DC, Lee LW, Collins JJ, Riley PO, Lipsitz LA. Reduced hip extension during walking: healthy elderly and fallers versus young adults. Arch Phys Med Rehabil. 2001;82(1):26–30. https://doi.org/10.1053/apmr.2001.18584.
4. Mazza C, Iosa M, Picerno P, Cappozzo A. Control of the upper body accelerations in young and elderly women during level walking. J Neuroeng Rehabil. 2008;5(1):30. https://doi.org/10.1186/1743-0003-5-30.
5. Daly RM, Rosengren BE, Alwis G, Ahlborg HG, Sernbo I, Karlsson MK. Gender specific age-related changes in bone density, muscle strength and functional performance in the elderly: a-10 year prospective population-based study. BMC Geriatr. 2013;13(1):71. https://doi.org/10.1186/1471-2318-13-71.
6. Drzal-Grabiec J, Snela S, Rykala J, Podgorska J, Banas A. Changes in the body posture of women occurring with age. BMC Geriatr. 2013;13(1):108. https://doi.org/10.1186/1471-2318-13-108.
7. Sinaki M, Brey RH, Hughes CA, Larson DR, Kaufman KR. Balance disorder and increased risk of falls in osteoporosis and kyphosis: significance of kyphotic posture and muscle strength. Osteoporos Int. 2005;16(8):1004–10. https://doi.org/10.1007/s00198-004-1791-2.
8. Le Huec JC, Charosky S, Barrey C, Rigal J, Aunoble S. Sagittal imbalance cascade for simple degenerative spine and consequences: algorithm of decision for appropriate treatment. Eur Spine J. 2011;20(Suppl 5):699–703. https://doi.org/10.1007/s00586-011-1938-8.
9. Imagama S, Ito Z, Wakao N, Seki T, Hirano K, Muramoto A, et al. Influence of spinal sagittal alignment, body balance, muscle strength, and physical ability on falling of middle-aged and elderly males. Eur Spine J. 2013;22(6): 1346–53. https://doi.org/10.1007/s00586-013-2721-9.
10. Culhane KM, O'Connor M, Lyons D, Lyons GM. Accelerometers in rehabilitation medicine for older adults. Age Ageing. 2005;34(6):556–60. https://doi.org/10.1093/ageing/afi192.
11. Leirós-Rodríguez R, García-Soidán JL, Romo-Pérez V. Analyzing the Use of Accelerometers as a Method of Early Diagnosis of Alterations in Balance in Elderly People: A Systematic Review. Sensors (Basel). 2019;19:3883. https://doi.org/10.3390/s19183883.
12. de Groot MH, van der Jagt-Willems HC, van Campen JP, Lems WF, Beijnen JH, Lamoth CJ. A flexed posture in elderly patients is associated with impairments in postural control during walking. Gait Posture. 2014;39(2): 767–72. https://doi.org/10.1016/j.gaitpost.2013.10.015.
13. Craig JJ, Bruetsch AP, Huisinga JM. Coordination of trunk and foot

acceleration during gait is affected by walking velocity and fall history in elderly adults. Aging Clin Exp Res. 2019;31(7):943–50. https://doi.org/10.1007/s40520-018-1036-4.

14. Imagama S, Hasegawa Y, Matsuyama Y, Sakai Y, Ito Z, Hamajima N, et al. Influence of sagittal balance and physical ability associated with exercise on quality of life in middle-aged and elderly people. Arch Osteoporos. 2011; 6(1-2):13–20. https://doi.org/10.1007/s11657-011-0052-1.
15. Bertolucci PH, Brucki SM, Campacci SR, Juliano Y. The Mini-Mental State Examination in a general population: impact of educational status. Arq Neuropsiquiatr. 1994;52(1):1–7. https://doi.org/10.1590/S0004-282X1994000100001.
16. Moraes EN, Carmo JA, Moraes FL, Azevedo RS, Machado CJ, Montilla DE. Clinical-functional vulnerability Index-20 (IVCF-20): rapid recognition of frail older adults. Rev Saude Publica. 2016;50(0):81. https://doi.org/10.1590/s1518-8787.2016050006963.
17. Camargos FF, Dias RC, Dias JM, Freire MT. Cross-cultural adaptation and evaluation of the psychometmianric properties of the falls efficacy scale-international among elderly Brazilians (FES-I-BRAZIL). Rev Bras Fis. 2010;14(3): 237–43. https://doi.org/10.1590/S1413-35552010000300010.
18. Valenti G, Bonomi AG, Westerterp KR. Body acceleration as indicator for walking economy in an ageing population. PLoS One. 2015;10(10):e0141431. https://doi.org/10.1371/journal.pone.0141431.
19. Schrack JA, Zipunnikov V, Simonsick EM, Studenski S, Ferrucci L. Rising Energetic Cost of Walking Predicts Gait Speed Decline With Aging. J Gerontol A Biol Sci Med Sci. 71:947–53. https://doi.org/10.1093/gerona/glw002.
20. Miyamoto ST, Lombardi Junior I, Berg KO, Ramos LR, Natour J. Brazilian version of the Berg balance scale. Braz J Med Biol Res. 2004;37(9):1411–21. https://doi.org/10.1590/S0100-879X2004000900017.
21. Berg KO, Maki BE, Williams JL, Holliday PJ, Wood-Dauphine SL. Clinical and laboratory measures of postural balance in an elderly population. Arch Phys Med Rehabil. 1992;73(11):1073–80.
22. Alexandre TS, Meira DM, Rico NC, Mizuta SK. Accuracy of timed up and go test for screening risk of falls among community-dwelling elderly. Rev Bras Fis. 2012;16(5):381–8. https://doi.org/10.1590/S1413-35552012005000041.
23. Mac-Thiong JM, Roussouly P, Berthonnaud E, Guigui P. Sagittal parameters of global spinal balance: normative values from a prospective cohort of seven hundred nine Caucasian asymptomatic adults. Spine (Phila Pa 1976). 2010;35:E1193–8. https://doi.org/10.1097/BRS.0b013e3181e50808.
24. Furlanetto TS, Sedrez JA, Candotti CT, Loss JF. Reference values for cobb angles when evaluating the spine in the sagittal plane: a systematic review with meta-analysis. Motricidade. 2018;14(2-3):115–28. https://doi.org/10.6063/motricidade.10890.
25. Gasparotto LPR, Falsarella GR, Coimbra AMV. Lumbar spine angular measures in older people: comparison between two radiographic analysis strategies. Fisioter Pesqui [online]. 2016;23(4):388–93. https://doi.org/10.1590/1809-2950/15932723042016.
26. Pratali RR, Nasreddine MA, Diebo B, Oliveira C, Lafage V. Normal values for sagittal spinal alignment: a study of Brazilian subjects. Clinics (Sao Paulo). 2018;73:e647. https://doi.org/10.6061/clinics/2018/e647.
27. Van Hees VT, Slootmaker SM, De Groot G, Van Mechelen W, Van Lummel RC. Reproducibility of a triaxial seismic accelerometer (DynaPort). Med Sci Sports Exerc. 2009;41(4):810–7. https://doi.org/10.1249/MSS.0b013e31818ff636.
28. Kobayashi H, Kakihana W, Kimura T. Combined effects of age and gender on gait symmetry and regularity assessed by autocorrelation of trunk acceleration. J Neuroeng Rehabil. 2014;11(1):109. https://doi.org/10.1186/1743-0003-11-109.
29. Kobsar D, Olson C, Paranjape R, Barden JM. The validity of gait variability and fractal dynamics obtained from a single, body-fixed triaxial accelerometer. J Appl Biomech. 2014;30(2):343–7. https://doi.org/10.1123/jab.2013-0107.
30. Yang M, Zheng H, Wang H, McClean S, Newell D. iGAIT: an interactive accelerometer based gait analysis system. Comput Methods Prog Biomed. 2012;108(2):715–23. https://doi.org/10.1016/j.cmpb.2012.04.004.
31. Hulley SB, Cummings SR, Browner WS, Grady D, Newman TB. Designing clinical research : an epidemiologic approach. 4th ed. Philadelphia: Lippincott Williams & Wilkins; 2013. Appendix 6C, page 79. ISBN-10: 0781722187, ISBN-13: 978–0781722186
32. Kavanagh JJ. Lower trunk motion and speed-dependence during walking. J Neuroeng Rehabil. 2009;6(1):9. https://doi.org/10.1186/1743-0003-6-9.
33. Brodie MA, Coppens MJ, Ejupi A, Gschwind YJ, Annegarn J, Schoene D, et al. Comparison between clinical gait and daily-life gait assessments of fall risk in older people. Geriatr Gerontol Int. 2017;17(11):2274–82. https://doi.org/10.1111/ggi.12979.
34. Callisaya ML, Blizzard L, McGinley JL, Srikanth VK. Risk of falls in older people during fast-walking--the TASCOG study. Gait Posture. 2012;36(3):510–5. https://doi.org/10.1016/j.gaitpost.2012.05.003.
35. Zijlstra A, de Bruin ED, Bruins N, Zijlstra W. The step length-frequency relationship in physically active community-dwelling older women. Eur J Appl Physiol. 2008;104(3):427–34. https://doi.org/10.1007/s00421-008-0795-6.
36. Park JH, Mancini M, Carlson-Kuhta P, Nutt JG, Horak FB. Quantifying effects of age on balance and gait with inertial sensors in community-dwelling healthy adults. Exp Gerontol. 2016;85:48–58. https://doi.org/10.1016/j.exger.2016.09.018.
37. Giladi N, Herman T, Reider-Groswasser II, Gurevich T, Hausdorff JM. Clinical characteristics of elderly patients with a cautious gait of unknown origin. J Neurol. 2005;252(3):300–6. https://doi.org/10.1007/s00415-005-0641-2.
38. Osoba MY, Rao AK, Agrawal SK, Lalwani AK. Balance and gait in the elderly: a contemporary review. Laryngoscope Investig Otolaryngol. 2019;4(1):143–53. https://doi.org/10.1002/lio2.252.
39. Mak TCT, Young WR, Chan DCL, Wong TWL. Gait stability in older adults during level-ground walking: the Attentional focus approach. J Gerontol B Psychol Sci Soc Sci. 2020;75:274–81. https://doi.org/10.1093/geronb/gby115.
40. Miyazaki J, Murata S, Horie J, Uematsu A, Hortobágyi T, Suzuki S. Lumbar lordosis angle (LLA) and leg strength predict walking ability in elderly males. Arch Gerontol Geriatr. 2013;56(1):141–7. https://doi.org/10.1016/j.archger.2012.09.004.
41. Dar G, Peleg S, Masharawi Y, et al. Sacroiliac joint bridging: demographical and anatomical aspects. Spine (Phila Pa 1976). 2005;30:E429–32. https://doi.org/10.1097/01.brs.0000172232.32082.e0.
42. Gimmon Y, Riemer R, Rashed H, Shapiro A, Debi R, Kurz I, et al. Age-related differences in pelvic and trunk motion and gait adaptability at different walking speeds. J Electromyogr Kinesiol. 2015;25(5):791–9. https://doi.org/10.1016/j.jelekin.2015.05.003.
43. McAndrew Young PM, Dingwell JB. Voluntary changes in step width and step length during human walking affect dynamic margins of stability. Gait Posture. 2012;36(2):219–24. https://doi.org/10.1016/j.gaitpost.2012.02.020.
44. Harding IJ. Understanding sagittal balance with a clinical perspective. Eur J Phys Rehabil Med. 2009;45(4):571–82 PMID: 20032917.
45. Boulay C, Tardieu C, Hecquet J, Benaim C, Mouilleseaux B, Marty C, et al. Sagittal alignment of spine and pelvis regulated by pelvic incidence: standard values and prediction of lordosis. Eur Spine J. 2006;15(4):415–22. https://doi.org/10.1007/s00586-005-0984-5.
46. Le Huec JC, Aunoble S, Philippe L, Nicolas P. Pelvic parameters: origin and significance. Eur Spine J. 2011;20(Suppl 5):564–71. https://doi.org/10.1007/s00586-011-1940-1.
47. Laratta JL, Glassman SD, Atanda AA, Dimar JR, Gum JL, Crawford III CH, et al. The Berg balance scale for assessing dynamic stability and balance in the adult spinal deformity (ASD) population. J Spine Surg. 2019;5(4):451–6. https://doi.org/10.21037/jss.2019.09.15.
48. Bae JS, Jang JS, Lee SH, Kim JU. Radiological analysis of lumbar degenerative kyphosis in relation to pelvic incidence. Spine J. 2012;12(11): 1045–51. https://doi.org/10.1016/j.spinee.2012.10.011.
49. van Schooten KS, Pijnappels M, Rispens SM, Elders PJ, Lips P, van Dieën JH. Ambulatory fall-risk assessment: amount and quality of daily-life gait predict falls in older adults. J Gerontol A Biol Sci Med Sci. 2015;70(5):608–15. https://doi.org/10.1093/gerona/glu225.
50. Sekine M, Tamura T, Yoshida M, Suda Y, Kimura Y, Miyoshi H, et al. A gait abnormality measure based on root mean square of trunk acceleration. J Neuroeng Rehabil. 2013;10(1):118. https://doi.org/10.1186/1743-0003-10-118.
51. Mignardot JB, Deschamps T, Barrey E, Auvinet B, Berrut G, Cornu C, et al. Gait disturbances as specific predictive markers of the first fall onset in elderly people: a two-year prospective observational study. Front Aging Neurosci. 2014;6:22. https://doi.org/10.3389/fnagi.2014.00022.

16

Influenza and pneumococcal vaccination coverage in Latin American patients with systemic lupus erythematosus

Edson Hernán Chiganer*, Bruno Camargo Ochi and Carmen Flora Lessa

Abstract

Background: Infections are a major cause of morbidity and mortality in systemic lupus (SLE). Vaccination would be an effective method to reduce infection rate. Coverage for influenza and pneumococcus appears to be low in Latin America. The objective of this study was to evaluate vaccination coverage for influenza and pneumococcus in Latin America, causes of non-vaccination and to compare it with European patients.

Methods: A survey was conducted through social networks targeting Latin American lupus patients. A self-report was used to assess the demographics, risk factors for pneumonia, vaccination status, and causes of non-vaccination. The same method was used for European patients. We used binary logistic regression to identify factors associated with pneumococcal and influenza vaccination.

Results: There were 1130 participants from Latin America. Among them, 97% were women with an average of 37.9 years (SD: 11.3) and 46.5% had more than 7 years of disease duration. Two or more risk factors for pneumonia were found in 64.9%. Coverage for influenza and pneumococcal was 42.7 and 25% respectively, being lower than in Europe. Tetanus coverage was the most important predictor for receiving influenza and pneumococcal vaccination. Lack of prescription was the most common cause of non-application (64.6%).

Conclusions: Vaccination coverage for influenza and pneumonia is low in Latin America, especially compared to Europe. It is necessary to make specialists aware of their role in vaccine control and to implement measures to improve coordination between them and general practitioners.

Keywords: Systemic lupus erythematosus, Vaccination coverage, Influenza vaccine, Pneumococcal vaccine, Latin America

Introduction

Infections are a major cause of morbidity and mortality in systemic lupus erythematosus (SLE) [1]. Nearly half of deaths from infections are attributed to pneumonia [2]. Patients with SLE are at increased risk of infection due to several factors such as the underlying condition [3], disease activity [4, 5] and the use of immunosuppressive agents [6], although some treatments such as hydroxychloroquine may decrease this risk [7]. Vaccination would be an effective method to decrease morbidity and mortality from infections in SLE.

The European League Against Rheumatism (EULAR) recommends that vaccination against influenza (flu) and pneumococcus should be strongly considered for most adult patients with SLE, in particular those treated with immunosuppressive therapy or who have other medical conditions of high-risk for pneumonia (e.g., chronic bronchitis) [8]. Both vaccines have acceptable

* Correspondence: edsonchiganer@gmail.com
Department of Immunology and Histocompatibility Unity, Carlos G Durand Hospital, Díaz Vélez Avenue, 5044, C1405DCS Buenos Aires, Argentina

immunogenicity and are safe in these patients [9–11]. These vaccines should preferably be administered during inactive disease but may also be considered for use in patients with active disease [8].

SLE coverage for influenza and pneumococcus does not exceed 60% in many countries [12, 13]. The main reasons for non-vaccination are lack of recommendation from their treating physician or rejection by patients [13–16]. The use of prednisone at doses ≥7.5 mg and high age are predictors of receiving these vaccines [16].

There are few works on this subject in Latin America. A recent study conducted in Brazil [13] showed that the percentage of influenza vaccination in patients with SLE is less than 50%. In order to implement policies on vaccination in this population, it is necessary to know the scope of this problem at the regional level. For this reason, the authors decided to carry out this study.

The main objective of this study was to assess the degree of influenza and pneumococcal vaccination coverage in SLE patients in Latin America and to identify causes and predictors of non-vaccination. The secondary objective was to compare these data with those of European patients.

Methods

The survey was conducted using a self-administered questionnaire and disseminated through social networks, mainly Facebook. To avoid diagnostic bias, it was disseminated only through SLE associations and patient groups on Facebook. The questionnaire included questions to assess the demographics, risk factors for pneumonia, vaccination status, and causes for non-vaccination. For the composition of the questionnaire, validated questionnaires in Spanish [17, 18], English [19–22], Portuguese [23–25], French [26, 27] and Italian [28] were used as a basis. Once the final questionnaire was composed, it was translated into these five languages. Before publishing the survey, the questionnaires were shown to the patient associations to check their comprehension and to evaluate possible linguistic differences (e.g. between Latin Spanish and Spanish).

Data collection began in October 2018 and ended in November 2019. For the sample calculation, the number of patients with SLE in Latin America was estimated at 422400. This value arises from an average prevalence of SLE of 66 per 10,000 inhabitants [29] for a population of approximately 640 million [30]. The Pan American Health Organization (PAHO) in 2017 reported that the level of influenza vaccination coverage ranged from 32% (Uruguay) to 100% (Panama) and in older adults and from 55% (Argentina) to 100% (Mexico) in patients with chronic diseases [31]. Thus, a 50% coverage level was chosen for the sample calculation, with a 3% error. The calculated sample, using the finite population correction, was 1064.

Case ascertainment and variables included in database

Participants over 18 years of age with a diagnosis of SLE who consented to participate and had completed the questionnaire in full were included. The survey was completely anonymous. To avoid duplicates, participants were asked to enter an email address without the domain. No duplicates were found.

Demographic data were collected on gender, date of birth, and country of residence. The general risk factors for pneumonia evaluated were: diabetes, smoking, and chronic cardiac, respiratory and renal pathologies. Diagnosis of diabetes was evaluated with a simple question: "Have you ever been told by a doctor that you have diabetes or do you take medication for diabetes? To assess smoking status (including cigarettes, cigars and pipes), they were asked whether they smoked currently, had quit less than or more than 6 months ago, or had never smoked. For the purposes of the study, smokers were defined as those who currently smoked or had quit less than six months ago. Chronic heart disease was evaluated with a simple question: "Have you ever been told by a doctor that you have a heart disease like valve disease, ischemic heart disease or heart failure, or do you take medication for the heart?" Similarly, chronic respiratory and renal diseases were evaluated with these questions: "Has a doctor ever told you that you have a respiratory illness such as asthma, chronic bronchitis, or COPD, or do you use inhalers?" and "Has a doctor ever told you that you have a renal disease such as kidney failure, or do you need to do dialysis?" All the questions mentioned above were closed-ended. For the purposes of this work, age over 50 years was considered a risk factor for pneumonia [32].

Vaccination status was assessed using two questions adapted from a validated self-report [19]: "Did you receive the flu vaccine this year" and "Did you receive at least one dose of pneumonia vaccine" Given that tetanus vaccination is widely distributed throughout the world in all age groups, we asked about its coverage to assess the overall vaccination rate in the region. To assess causes of non-vaccination, participants were asked to choose one or more of the following options: "Not indicated by doctor", "not available", "related to costs / problems with health insurance coverage", "vaccination refusal" and "others".

SLE-specific data were collected on duration of illness, current use of immunosuppressors and hydroxychloroquine, use of corticosteroids, and average monthly dose. For the purposes of this work, SLE activity was defined as self-reference of flare-ups occurred < 6 months ago [33] diagnosed by a doctor.

Statistical analysis

Continuous variables were summarized using mean, standard deviation (SD) and range, and analyzed with the Student-t-test. Categorical variables were expressed as numbers, percentages and analyzed with the chi-squared test.

We used binary logistic regression to identify factors associated with pneumococcal and influenza vaccination. Variables that were significant in the univariate analysis ($p < 0.10$) were included in the adjusted model. Odds ratio (OR) and adjusted OR with 95% confidence intervals (95% CI) was reported. Statistical significance was set at p value < 0.05 (2-tailed). Factors proposed for the analysis were: age > 50 years, diabetes, smoking, chronic cardiac/respiratory/renal disease, SLE activity, disease duration > 7 years, current use of immunosuppressors and use of ≥7.5 mg prednisone or equivalent, and a history of tetanus vaccination.

Analyses were conducted using Stata version 12.0 and Epidat version 3.1.

Results

Latin America

In total there were 1196 participants from Latin America. Sixty six were excluded because they did not meet inclusion criteria. Seven countries contributed more than 50 patients each, constituting 87.2% of the sample: Argentina, Mexico, Brazil, Chile, Peru, Colombia and Uruguay. Demographic data, risk factors for pneumonia, and SLE-specific information are shown in Table 1. Most of the patients were women under 40 years, with more than 5 years of disease duration. More than 60% had two or more risk factors for pneumonia, the most frequent being the use of immunosuppressors and corticosteroids, and SLE activity. Hydroxychloroquine use exceeded 50% in the entire region, reaching almost 90% in some countries.

Data on vaccination coverage are shown in Table 2. Overall, coverage for influenza and pneumonia did not exceed 50 and 25% respectively. These vaccination rates were consistent with coverage for tetanus, which did not exceed 50%. However, the vaccination coverage rate was found to be highly heterogeneous among the countries of the region. While in Argentina coverage for influenza and pneumococcus reached 65 and 55% respectively, in Mexico it was less than 20%. The most frequent (> 60%) reported cause of non-vaccination in all countries was lack of prescription or medical recommendation. Issues related to availability or cost of vaccines were less than 13% of the causes of non-vaccination.

Considering that vaccination is recommended in patients receiving immunosuppressants and/or prednisone

Table 1 Demographics, risk factors for pneumonia, and SLE-specific data of Latin American patients*

	Argentina (265)	Mexico (214)	Brazil (190)	Chile (99)	Peru (96)	Colombia (63)	Uruguay (59)	All patients (1130) **
Age, years (SD)	39.7 (10.9)	36.2 (11.1)	36.7 (10.4)	37.4 (11.3)	37.7 (10.6)	37.8 (13.7)	44 (12.5)	37.9 (11.3)
Female	260 (98.1)	209 (97.7)	186 (97.9)	95 (96)	91 (94.8)	60 (95.2)	59 (100)	1096 (97)
Patients > 50 years	51 (19.2)	24 (11.2)	25 (13.2)	15 (15.2)	12 (12.5)	12 (19)	18 (30.5)	171 (15.1)
Disease duration, years (range)	7 (0–40)	6 (0–39)	6 (0–32)	5 (0–32)	5 (0–34)	5 (1–28)	8 (1–30)	6 (0–40)
Disease duration > 7 years	126 (47.5)	106 (49.5)	92 (48.4)	86 (86.9)	44 (45.8)	31 (49.2)	29 (49.1)	525 (46.5)
Immunosuppressors [a]	226 (85.3)	193 (90.2)	151 (79.5)	81 (81.8)	86 (89.6)	56 (63)	49 (83.1)	972 (86)
SLE activity [b]	153 (58)	111 (51.9)	142 (74.7)	56 (56.6)	48 (50)	42 (66.7)	39 (66.1)	674 (59.6)
Corticosteroid use [c]	91 (34.9)	67 (32.4)	105 (55.9)	44 (46.3)	36 (50)	29 (48.3)	22 (39,3)	445 (40.5)
Hydroxychloroquine	236 (89.1)	114 (53.3)	138 (72.6)	86 (86.9)	76 (79.2)	48 (76.2)	49 (83.1)	858 (75.9)
Smoking [d]	64 (24.2)	31 (14.5)	25 (13.2)	29 (29.3)	9 (9.4)	15 (23.8)	25 (42.4)	209 (18.5)
Chronic renal disease	52 (19.6)	34 (15.9)	39 (20.5)	17 (17.2)	19 (19,8)	17 (27)	8 (13.6)	202 (17.9)
Chronic respiratory disease	25 (9.4)	26 (12.1)	18 (9.5)	15 (15.2)	19 (19.8)	8 (12.7)	13 (22)	149 (13.2)
Chronic cardiac disease	24 (9.1)	14 (6.5)	20 (10.5)	8 (9.1)	12 (12.5)	9 (14.3)	12 (20.3)	110 (9.7)
Diabetes	11 (4.2)	13 (6.1)	11 (5.8)	10 (10.1)	6 (6.3)	8 (12.7)	6 (10.2)	72 (6.4)
> 1 risk factors for pneumonia [e]	176 (66.4)	129 (60.3)	150 (78.9)	72 (72.7)	57 (59,4)	46 (73)	45 (76.3)	733 (64.9)

* Except where indicated otherwise, values are the number (%) of patients. SD: Standard deviation, SLE: Systemic Lupus Erythematosus

** Other participating countries: Costa Rica (31 patients), Bolivia (24 patients), Puerto Rico (22 patients), Guatemala (12 patients), Venezuela (11 patients), Ecuador (9 patients), Paraguay (9 patients), Honduras (7 patients), El Salvador (6 patients), Nicaragua (6 patients), Panama (3 patients), Dominican Republic (2 patients), Cuba (2 patients)

[a]Not including corticosteroids and hydroxychloroquine

[b]SLE activity was defined as the presence of flares-up diagnosed by a doctor during the previous 6 months

[c]Corticosteroid use was defined as use of prednisone ≥7.5 mg daily or equivalent during the last month

[d]Smoking was defined as currently smoking or having quit < 6 months ago

[e]Risk factors for pneumonia assessed were: age > 50 years, diabetes, current use of immunosuppressors, daily dose of prednisone > 7.5 mg or equivalent during the last month, SLE activity, and the coexistence of chronic cardiac, respiratory or renal disease

Table 2 Vaccine coverage and reasons for non-vaccination of Latin American patients*

	Argentina (265)	Mexico (214)	Brazil (190)	Chile (99)	Peru (96)	Colombia (63)	Uruguay (59)	All patients (1130)
Influenza	178 (67.2)	38 (17.8)	114 (60)	51 (51.5)	21 (21.9)	15 (23.8)	19 (32.2)	482 (42.7)
Pneumococcal	146 (55.1)	23 (10.7)	41 (21.6)	14 (14.1)	9 (9.4)	8 (12.7)	14 (23.7)	282 (25)
Influenza and pneumococcal	128 (48.3)	11 (5.1)	35 (18.4)	10 (10.1)	6 (6.3)	5 (7.9)	9 (15.3)	222 (19.6)
Tetanus	129 (48.7)	61 (28.5)	87 (45.8)	9 (9.1)	21 (21.9)	18 (28.6)	50 (84.7)	424 (37.5)
No influenza and no pneumococcal	69 (26)	164 (76.6)	70 (36.8)	44 (44.4)	72 (75)	45 (71.4)	35 (59.3)	588 (52)
Incomplete vaccination[a]	194 (73.2)	205 (95.8)	165 (86.8)	96 (97)	93 (96.9)	61 (96.8)	53 (89.8)	998 (88.3)
Lack of medical prescription [b]	126 (64.9)	135 (63.1)	104 (63)	73 (76)	65 (69.9)	48 (78.7)	27 (50.9)	645 (64.6)
Rejection by patients [b]	26 (13.4)	29 (14.1)	15 (9.1)	9 (9.4)	16 (17.2)	1 (1.6)	15 (28.3)	127 (12.7)
Not available/ cost issues [b]	18 (9.3)	13 (6.3)	21 (12.7)	9 (9.4)	12 (12.9)	5 (8.2)	1 (1.9)	113 (11.3)
Others [b]	28 (14.4)	36 (17.6)	31 (18.8)	13 (13.5)	7 (7.5)	9 (14.8)	10 (18.9)	164 (16.4)

* Except where indicated otherwise, values are the number (%) of patients
[a]Includes those who reported not having received at least one of the vaccines (influenza, pneumonia or tetanus)
[b]The percentage was calculated using the number of non-vaccinated as the denominator

≥7.5 mg (or equivalent), this subgroup was analyzed. A total of 1015 (89.6%) met this condition. Of them, 437 (43%) and 259 (25.2%) received the influenza and pneumococcal vaccines respectively. In addition, we analyzed vaccination coverage among not immunosuppressed (115 patients, 10.2%). Of them, 45 (39.1%) and 23 (20%) reported having received the influenza and pneumococcal vaccines respectively. No differences were found regarding vaccination coverage between both groups (influenza coverage: 43% vs 39.1%, *p*-value: 0.42 and pneumococcal coverage: 25.2% vs 20%, *p*-value: 0.20).

Europe

There were 794 participants from Europe. Fifty were excluded because they did not meet inclusion criteria. The majority of patients (95% of the total) were from Spain, Portugal, United Kingdom/Ireland, France and Italy. Data on demographics, risk factors for pneumonia and specific for SLE are shown in Table 3. Like the Latin American participants, the majority were young women with more than 5 years of SLE diagnosis. Almost 75% had two or more risk factors for pneumonia, the most frequent being the use of immunosuppressors / corticosteroids and the activity of SLE. Remarkably, approximately 30% reported being a smoker. Hydroxychloroquine use did not exceed 73% in any of the countries.

Information on vaccination coverage is shown in Table 4. Influenza coverage in the region only reached 49.3%, while for pneumonia it did not exceed 37%. Along the same lines, tetanus coverage was less than 50%. Similar to what was found in Latin America, marked differences were observed between the countries with respect to the vaccination rate. Lack of a medical prescription was the most frequent cause of non-vaccination, although almost 20% did not get vaccinated because of refusal.

As with Latin American patients, vaccine coverage was analyzed in immunosuppressed patients (549, 73.5%) and those who were not (198, 26.5%). Coverage rates for influenza and pneumococcus for immunosuppressed were 53% (291/549) and 39.7% (218/549) respectively, while for non-immunosuppressed were 38.9% (77/198) and 27.8% (55/198). Unlike Latin America, a significant difference was found in the vaccination rate, being greater in immunosuppressed (influenza vaccine: 53% vs 38.9%, *p*-value: 0.000; and pneumococcal vaccine: 39.7% vs 27.8%, *p*-value: 0.003).

Comparison between Latin America and Europe

Comparison between the two regions is shown in Table 5. Statistically significant differences were observed in most of the variables compared although in general they did not reach 10%. Regarding demographics, risk factors for pneumonia and SLE-specific data, the most remarkable differences were average age, mean disease duration, immunosuppressors and hydroxychloroquine use, and the percentage of risk factors. Latin American patients were 5 years younger on average, with shorter mean disease duration, higher percentage of use of immunosuppressors and hydroxychloroquine, while European patients presented a higher percentage of risk factors for pneumonia, the high percentage of smokers being remarkable. In terms of vaccination coverage, Latin American patients had lower coverage for pneumococcus and tetanus, and a higher percentage of unvaccinated patients for both influenza and pneumococcus. Furthermore, vaccination rate in immunosuppressed patients was found to be higher in Europe (influenza coverage: 43% vs 53%, *p*-value: 0.000; and pneumococcal coverage: 25.2% vs 39.7%, *p*-value: 0.000). The most frequent reported cause of non-vaccination in both regions was

Table 3 Demographics, risk factors for pneumonia, and SLE-specific data of European patients *

	Spain (232)	Portugal (184)	UK/Ireland (151)	France (82)	Italy (59)	All patients (744)**
Age, years (SD)	43 (11.1)	42,1 (10.1)	44.5 (11.6)	40,3 (11.2)	42.8 (10.1)	42.7 (11)
Female	220 (94.8)	179 (97.3)	144 (95.4)	79 (96.3)	56 (94.9)	711 (95.6)
Patients > 50 years	60 (25.9)	37 (20.1)	42 (27.8)	13 (15.9)	13 (22)	174 (23.4)
Disease duration, years (range)	10 (1–39)	10 (0–34)	9 (0.5–41)	5 (1–31)	10 (1–37)	9 (0–41)
Disease duration > 7 years	141 (60.8)	109 (59.2)	86 (57)	38 (46.3)	37 (62.7)	426 (57.2)
Immunosuppressors [a]	173 (74.6)	135 (73.4)	102 (67.5)	67 (81.7)	43 (72.9)	546 (73.4)
SLE activity [b]	119 (51.3)	94 (51.1)	88 (58.3)	45 (54.9)	30 (50.8)	395 (53.1)
Corticosteroid use [c]	70 (30.2)	81 (44)	40 (26.5)	26 (31.7)	23 (39)	249 (33.5)
Hydroxychloroquine	152 (65.5)	129 (70.1)	109 (72.2)	44 (53.7)	31 (52.5)	492 (66.1)
Smoking [d]	70 (30.2)	61 (33.2)	29 (19.2)	29 (35.4)	22 (37.3)	219 (29.4)
Chronic renal disease	42 (18.1)	16 (8.7)	17 (11.3)	8 (9.8)	14 (23.7)	104 (14)
Chronic respiratory disease	35 (15.1)	22 (12)	33 (21.9)	18 (22)	9 (15.3)	124 (16.7)
Chronic cardiac disease	22 (9.5)	18 (9.8)	8 (5.3)	4 (4.9)	6 (10.2)	64 (8.6)
Diabetes	6 (2.6)	6 (3.3)	3 (2.0)	2 (2.4)	2 (3.4)	20 (2.7)
> 1 risk factors for pneumonia [e]	172 (74.1)	140 (76.1)	113 (74.8)	57 (69.5)	47 (79.7)	556 (74.7)

* Except where indicated otherwise, values are the number (%) of patients. SD: Standard deviation, SLE: Systemic Lupus Erythematosus
** Other participating countries: Belgium (12 patients), Netherlands (6 patients), Luxembourg (4 patients), Denmark (3 patients), Germany (2 patients), Greece (2 patients), Switzerland (2 patients), Andorra (1 patient), Croatia (1 patient), Cyprus (1 patient), Iceland (1 patient), Norway (1 patient)
[a]Not including corticosteroids and hydroxychloroquine
[b]SLE activity was defined as the presence of flares-up diagnosed by a doctor during the previous 6 months
[c]Corticosteroid use was defined as use of prednisone ≥7.5 mg daily or equivalent during the last month
[d]Smoking was defined as currently smoking or having quit < 6 months ago
[e]Risk factors for pneumonia assessed were: age > 50 years, diabetes, current use of immunosuppressors, daily dose of prednisone > 7.5 mg or equivalent during the last month, SLE activity, and the coexistence of chronic cardiac, respiratory or renal disease

lack of medical prescription, with no statistically significant difference between the two regions. Statistically significant differences, although small, were observed in the percentage of non-vaccination due to cost/accessibility, being more frequent in Latin America, while in Europe refusal to be vaccinated was more frequent.

Factors associated with vaccination coverage

Latin America

Analysis of the factors associated with vaccination coverage is shown in Table 6. Initial analysis found that history of chronic renal disease, age > 50 years, and tetanus coverage were associated with vaccination. The multivariate analysis showed that all three factors mentioned

Table 4 Vaccine coverage and reasons for non-vaccination of European patients*

	Spain (232)	Portugal (184)	UK/Ireland (151)	France (82)	Italy (59)	All patients (744)
Influenza	116 (50)	79 (42.9)	112 (74.2)	26 (31.7)	13 (22)	367 (49.3)
Pneumococcal	72 (31)	53 (28.8)	74 (49)	47 (57.3)	8 (13.6)	271 (36.4)
Influenza and pneumococcal	59 (25.4)	38 (20.7)	69 (45.7)	21 (25.6)	5 (8.5)	202 (27.2)
Tetanus	84 (36.2)	123 (66.8)	66 (43.7)	53 (64.6)	18 (30.5)	366 (49.2)
No influenza and no pneumococcal	103 (44.4)	90 (48.9)	34 (22.5)	30 (36.6)	37 (62.7)	308 (41.4)
Incomplete vaccination [a]	202 (87.1)	174 (94.6)	113 (74.8)	67 (81.7)	56 (94.9)	620 (83.3)
Lack of medical prescription [b]	143 (70.8)	99 (56.9)	76 (67.3)	25 (37.3)	34 (60.7)	392 (63.2)
Rejection by patients [b]	26 (12.9)	25 (14.4)	17 (15)	27 (40.3)	12 (21.4)	114 (18.4)
Not available/ cost issues [b]	7 (3.5)	5 (2.9)	10 (8.8)	3 (4.5)	1 (1.8)	26 (4.2)
Others [b]	34 (16.8)	29 (16.7)	15 (13.3)	15 (22.4)	9 (16.1)	110 (17.7)

* Except where indicated otherwise, values are the number (%) of patients
** Other participating countries: Belgium (12 patients), Netherlands (6 patients), Luxembourg (4 patients), Denmark (3 patients), Germany (2 patients), Greece (2 patients), Switzerland (2 patients), Andorra (1 patient), Croatia (1 patient), Cyprus (1 patient), Iceland (1 patient), Norway (1 patient)
[a]Includes those who reported not having received at least one of the vaccines (influenza, pneumonia or tetanus)
[b]The percentage was calculated using the number of non-vaccinated as the denominator

Table 5 Comparison between Latin American and European patients *

	Latin America (1130)	Europe (744)	Difference (95% CI)	*P* Value
Age, years (SD)	37.9 (11.3)	42.7 (11)	4.8 (3.8–5.9)	< 0.001
Female	1096 (97)	711 (95.6)	1.4 (−0.3–3,4)	0.13
Patients > 50 years	171 (15.1)	174 (23.4)	8.2 (4.6–12)	< 0.001
Disease duration > 7 years	525 (46.5)	426 (57.2)	10.8 (6.2–15.3)	< 0.001
Immunosuppressors [a]	972 (86)	546 (73.4)	12.6 (8.9–16.4)	< 0.001
SLE activity [b]	674 (59.6)	395 (53.1)	6.6 (2.0–11.1)	0.004
Corticosteroid use [c]	445 (39.4)	249 (33.5)	5.9 (1.5–10.3)	0.009
Hydroxychloroquine	858 (75.9)	492 (66.1)	9.8 (5.6–14.0)	< 0.001
Smoking [d]	209 (18.5)	219 (29.4)	10.9 (7–14.9)	< 0.001
Chronic renal disease	202 (17.9)	104 (14)	3.9 (0.5–7.2)	0.02
Chronic respiratory disease	149 (13.2)	124 (16.7)	3.5 (0.2–6.9)	0.04
Chronic cardiac disease	110 (9.7)	64 (8.6)	1.13 (−1.6–3.7)	0.39
Diabetes	72 (6.4)	20 (2.7)	3.7 (1.8–5.5)	< 0.001
> 1 risk factors for pneumonia [e]	733 (64.9)	556 (74.7)	9.9 (5.6–14.0)	< 0.001
Influenza	482 (42.7)	367 (49.3)	6.7 (2.1–11.3)	0.005
Pneumococcal	282 (25)	271 (36.4)	11.5 (7.2–15.7)	< 0.001
Influenza and pneumococcal	222 (19.6)	202 (27.2)	7.5 (3.6–11.5)	< 0.001
Tetanus	424 (37.5)	366 (49.2)	11.7 (7.1–16.2)	< 0.001
No influenza and no pneumococcal	588 (52)	308 (41.4)	10.6 (6.0–15.2)	< 0.001
Incomplete vaccination [f]	998 (88.3)	620 (83.3)	5.0 (1.8–8.3)	0.002
Lack of medical prescription [g]	645 (64.6)	392 (63.2)	1.4 (−3.4–6.2)	0.06
Rejection by patients [g]	127 (12.7)	114 (18.4)	5.7 (2.1–9.4)	0.007
Not available/ cost issues [g]	113 (11.3)	26 (4.2)	7.1 (4.5–9.6)	< 0.001
Others [g]	164 (16.4)	110 (17.7)	1.3 (−5.2–2.4)	0.90

* Except where indicated otherwise, values are the number (%) of patients. SD: Standard deviation, SLE: Systemic Lupus Erythematosus

[a]Not including corticosteroids and hydroxychloroquine

[b]SLE activity was defined as the presence of flares-up diagnosed by a doctor during the previous 6 months

[c]Corticosteroid use was defined as use of prednisone ≥7.5 mg daily or equivalent during the last month

[d]Smoking was defined as currently smoking or having quit < 6 months ago

[e]Risk factors for pneumonia assessed were: age > 50 years, diabetes, current use of immunosuppressors, daily dose of prednisone > 7.5 mg or equivalent during the last month, SLE activity, and the coexistence of chronic cardiac, respiratory or renal disease

[f]Includes those who reported not having received at least one of the vaccines (flu, pneumonia or tetanus)

[g]The percentage was calculated using the number of non-vaccinated as the denominator

were positively associated with influenza coverage (chronic renal disease: OR = 1.38, 95% CI = 1.01–1.88,*p* value = 0.044; age > 50 years: OR = 1.70, 95% CI = 1.22–2.37, *p* value = 0.002; and tetanus coverage: OR = 2.25, 95% CI = 1.75–2.88, *p* value < 0.001) and pneumococcal (chronic kidney disease: OR = 2. 30, 95% CI = 1.63–3.35, *p* value < 0.001; age > 50 years: OR = 1.67, 95% CI = 1.15–2.42, *p* value = 0.007; and tetanus coverage: OR = 3.79, 95% CI = 2.85–5.05, *p* value < 0.001). Thus, tetanus coverage was the most important factor associated with coverage of both vaccines.

Europe

The analysis is shown in Table 6. The univariate analysis found an association between history of chronic respiratory disease, smoking, use of immunosuppressors, age > 50 years, and tetanus coverage with vaccination coverage. Multivariate analysis showed that immunosuppression and tetanus coverage were positively associated with influenza coverage (OR = 1.97, 95% CI = 1.40–2.77.*p* value < 0.001and OR = 1.54, 95% CI = 1.14–2.07.*p* value = 0. 005 respectively) and pneumococcus (OR = 1.85, 95% CI = 1.27–2. 70. *p* value 0.001 and OR 3.91, 95% CI 2.83–5.40.*p* value < 0.001 respectively), while smoking was negatively associated with both (coverage for influenza: OR 0.55, 95% CI 0.39–0.76, *p* value < 0.001; and coverage for pneumococcus: OR = 0.67, 95% CI = 0.47–0.96, *p* value = 0.029). Multivariate analysis also showed that age > 50 years was positively associated with coverage for influenza (OR = 2.37, 95% CI = 1.65–3.41, *p* value < 0.001), while history of chronic respiratory disease was associated with coverage for pneumococcus (OR = 1.86,

Table 6 Factors associated with vaccination coverage*

	Influenza coverage				Pneumococcal coverage			
	Initial analysis		Adjusted model [a]		Initial analysis		Adjusted model [a]	
	OR (95% CI)	*p* value	OR (95% CI)	*p* value	OR (95% CI)	*p* value	OR (95% CI)	*p* value
Latin America								
Chronic renal disease	1.30 (0.96–1.77)	0.089	1.38 (1.01–1.88)	0.044	2.00 (1.44–2.77)	< 0.001	2.30 (1.63–3.35)	< 0.001
Age > 50 years	1.69 (1.22–2.35)	0.001	1.70 (1.22–2.37)	0.002	1.63 (1.15–2.32)	0.006	1.67 (1.15–2.42)	0.007
Tetanus coverage	2.24 (1.75–2.86)	< 0.001	2.25 (1.75–2.88)	< 0.001	3.62 (2.74–4.80)	< 0.001	3.79 (2.85–5.05)	< 0.001
Europe								
Chronic respiratory disease	NS [d]	NS [d]			1.73 (1.18–2.56)	0.006	1.86 (1.23–2.82)	< 0.001
Smoking [b]	0.57 (0.42–0.79)	0.001	0.55 (0.39–0.76)	< 0.001	0.72 (0.52–1.01)	0.058	0.67 (0.47–0.96)	0.029
Immunosuppressors [c]	1.77 (1.27–2.47)	0.001	1.97 (1.40–2.77)	< 0.001	1.71 (1.20–2.44)	0.003	1.85 (1.27–2. 70)	< 0.001
Age > 50 years	2.16 (1.53–3.08)	< 0.001	2.37 (1.65–3.41)	< 0.001	NS [d]	NS [d]		
Tetanus coverage	1.45 (1.08–1.93)	0.012	1.54 (1.14–2.07)	0.005	3.74 (2.72–5.14)	< 0.001	3.91 (2.83–5.40)	< 0.001

* Statistical significance was set at p value < 0.05

[a]Only variables that were significant in the univariate analysis ($p < 0.10$) were included

[b]Smoking was defined as currently smoking or having quit < 6 months ago

[c]Not including corticosteroids and hydroxychloroquine

[d]Not significant

95% CI = 1.23–2.82, *p* value = 0.003). As in Latin America, tetanus coverage was an important factor associated with vaccination.

Discussion

To our knowledge, this is the first study on influenza and pneumococcus coverage in SLE with focus on Latin America. We note that the coverage of influenza and pneumococcus in Latin America is very low, especially for the latter. Only Argentina had coverage for influenza and pneumococcus > 50%, while Brazil and Chile only reached this percentage for influenza coverage. The percentage of patients who received both vaccines did not exceed 50% in any country. These results are not surprising when compared to tetanus coverage which is widely used in Latin America These findings are similar to a study on influenza coverage in a cohort of lupus patients from Brazil, with a value of 46% [13].

As expected, vaccination rate, especially for pneumococcus, was lower than in Europe. Furthermore, there were no significant differences in the reported vaccination rate of immunosuppressed and non-immunosuppressed patients. This is noteworthy considering the strong recommendation for vaccination against influenza and pneumococcus in immunosuppressed patients with SLE. This finding contrasts with Europe, where immunosuppressed patients reported the highest rate of vaccination.

Difference in coverage between Latin American countries has been noted before and has no single explanation. According to reports from the Pan American Health Organization [34], coverage for diphtheria vaccine ranged from 64% in Venezuela to 96% in Chile during 2018. A recent systematic review [35] found that the main barriers to vaccination reported were adverse socioeconomic factors, a low level of education, lack of awareness of diseases and their vaccines, religious and cultural beliefs. Thus, the different health policies, socioeconomic level and the culture of the countries could be the cause of this great discrepancy. However, our study showed that the percentage of non-vaccination that could be attributed to these causes did not exceed 35%.

Contrary to expectations, cost or accessibility issues were not the main causes of non-vaccination, but rather lack of medical prescription in both Latin America and Europe as previously reported [13–16]. These findings are in line with several studies conducted on the subject. A study in Germany showed that less than 8 and 60% of rheumatologists and general practitioners (GP), respectively, monitored the vaccination status of lupus patients [16]. Similarly, in a survey conducted in Ireland, it was found that 50% of rheumatologists did not evaluate vaccination coverage of patients and less than 45% did so before indicating immunosuppression [36]. Causes for lack of indication for vaccination may include lack of knowledge about vaccination recommendations and concerns about vaccine safety in immunosuppressed hosts [15]. However, several studies suggest that an important cause would be the perceived responsibility of specialists regarding their role in preventive health care. In the Irish work mentioned above, it was observed that more than half of the rheumatologists considered that the responsibility for vaccination was the domain of the GP [36]. Similarly, a survey of rheumatologists on screening for hyperlipidemia in rheumatoid arthritis (RA) showed that the majority did not regard this practice as their responsibility [37]. In the same line, a study on preventive care of risk factors for cardiovascular disease in RA showed that, although most rheumatologists are aware of the increased risk in these patients, they rarely identify or act to modify them [38]. Thus, patients who are only seen by specialists are less likely to be vaccinated [39]. This would explain the differences in vaccination coverage among Latin American countries: those countries with a good primary care system will have a higher vaccination rate. Similarly, those European countries with a better primary care system are those that would present the highest vaccination rates for pneumococcus and influenza in the region. On the other hand, GP may not be aware of the need for lupus patients to be vaccinated against pneumococcus and influenza, regardless of patient age [15].

For the aforementioned, it is necessary to involve the specialist in vaccination control. Several measures can be useful to improve vaccination control without significantly overloading patient care time. Placing vaccination reminders in specialized care centers has proven to be a cost-effective measure to improve the vaccination rate in patients with rheumatic disease [40]. Automatic reminders in digital medical records would also be another useful measure [12], although not all care centers in Latin America have this technology. For these measures to be useful, it is essential that the specialist and the GP work together, sharing responsibility for the primary prevention of the patient with rheumatic disease.

This study has several limitations. First, the final questionnaire used, in each of the language versions, was a modified and unvalidated version of other questionnaires. Second, self-reported data may overestimate or underestimate true vaccination coverage due primarily to recall bias [19, 41]. Third, diagnosis of SLE was self-referred and could not be verified in a medical record. Fourth, to avoid the respondent's burden we tried to make the questionnaire as short and simple as possible [42]. Socioeconomic situation was evaluated with a single question within the causes of non-vaccination and SLE activity was assessed with a short question rather than using long questionnaires (eg, SLAQ [43]). However, this oversimplification could produce a significant information bias. Fifth, as only those who use the internet and especially social networks participate, there is an important selection bias. Finally, the participation of some countries in the region was low, probably due to the lack of interest of patients in participating. This implies that the sample could be non-representative.

Conclusion

In conclusion, our work shows that there is poor coverage for pneumococcus and influenza in Latin America, especially compared to regions such as Europe, the main cause being the lack of medical prescription. Health policies are needed that improve coordination between specialists and GPs as well as raise awareness about the importance of preventive health care for lupus patients.

Supplementary Information

Additional file 1. Spanish version of the survey questionnaire.
Additional file 2. English version of the survey questionnaire.
Additional file 3. French version of the survey questionnaire.
Additional file 4. Italian version of the survey questionnaire.
Additional file 5. Portuguese version of the survey questionnaire.

Acknowledgements

The authors are grateful to the Argentinean Lupus Association ALUA , especially its president Teresa Cattoni; the Uruguayan Lupus Association "AdeLUr"; the Chilean Lupus Association; the Spanish Lupus Federation "Felupus", especially Pilar Pazos Casal; to the Madrid Association of Lupus Patients and Friends "AMELYA"; to the Malaga Lupus and Autoimmune Association; to Lupus UK and especially to Paul Howard; to the Lupus Foundation of America and especially to Dr. Karin Tse; and to all the social network groups and patients who collaborated on this work.

Authors , contributions

ECH and BCO participated in study design and data collection. ECH participated in data analysis. ECH, BCO and CFL participated in drafting of the manuscript. All authors have read and approved the final manuscript.

References

1. Cervera R, Khamashta MA, Font J, Sebastiani GD, Gil A, Lavilla P, et al. Morbidity and mortality in systemic lupus erythematosus during a 10-year period: a comparison of early and late manifestations in a cohort of 1,000 patients. Medicine (Baltimore). 2003;82(5):299–308. https://doi.org/10.1097/01.md.0000091181.93122.55.
2. Bernatsky S, Boivin JF, Joseph L, Manzi S, Ginzler E, Gladman DD, et al. Mortality in systemic lupus erythematosus. Arthritis Rheum. 2006;54(8):2550–7. https://doi.org/10.1002/art.21955.
3. Petri M. Infection in systemic lupus erythematosus. Rheum Dis Clin N Am. 1998;24(2):423–56. https://doi.org/10.1016/s0889-857x(05)70016-8.
4. Duffy KN, Duffy CM, Gladman DD. Infection and disease activity in systemic lupus erythematosus: a review of hospitalized patients. J Rheumatol. 1991;18(8):1180–4. 1941820.
5. Zonana-Nacach A, Camargo-Coronel A, Yañez P, Sánchez L, Jimenez-Balderas FJ, Fraga A. Infections in outpatients with systemic lupus erythematosus: a prospective study. Lupus. 2001;10(7):505–10. https://doi.org/10.1191/096120301678416088.
6. Danza A, Ruiz-Irastorza G. Infection risk in systemic lupus erythematosus patients: susceptibility factors and preventive strategies. Lupus. 2013;22(12):1286–94. https://doi.org/10.1177/0961203313493032.
7. Ruiz-Irastorza G, Olivares N, Ruiz-Arruza I, Martinez-Berriotxoa A, Egurbide MV, Aguirre C. Predictors of major infections in systemic lupus erythematosus. Arthritis Res Ther. 2009;11(4):R109. https://doi.org/10.1186/ar2764. Epub 2009 Jul 15.
8. Furer V, Rondaan C, Heijstek MW, Agmon-Levin N, van Assen S, Bijl M, et al. 2019 update of EULAR recommendations for vaccination in adult patients with autoimmune inflammatory rheumatic diseases. Ann Rheum Dis. 2020;79(1):39–52. https://doi.org/10.1136/annrheumdis-2019-215882 Epub 2019 Aug 14.

9. Saad CG, Borba EF, Aikawa NE, et al. Immunogenicity and safety of the 2009 non-adjuvanted influenza a/H1N1 vaccine in a large cohort of autoimmune rheumatic diseases. Ann Rheum Dis. 2011;70(6):1068–73. https://doi.org/10.1136/ard.2011.150250.
10. Pisoni C, Sarano J, Benchetrit G, et al. Antipneumococcal Vaccination in Patient with Systemic Lupus Erythematosus. Medicina (B Aires). 2003;63(5):388–92 PMID: 14628647 (Article in Spanish).
11. Pugès M, Biscay P, Barnetche T, Truchetet MÉ, Richez C, Seneschal J, et al. Immunogenicity and impact on disease activity of influenza and pneumococcal vaccines in systemic lupus erythematosus: a systematic literature review and meta-analysis. Rheumatology (Oxford). 2016;55(9):1664–72. https://doi.org/10.1093/rheumatology/kew211 Epub 2016 May 9.
12. Yazdany J, Tonner C, Trupin L, Panopalis P, Gillis JZ, Hersh AO, et al. Provision of preventive health care in systemic lupus erythematosus: data from a large observational cohort study. Arthritis Res Ther. 2010;12(3):R84. https://doi.org/10.1186/ar3011. Epub 2010 May 12.
13. Vieira de Rezende RP, Mattos GA, De Mello Leal Augusto R, et al. Predictors for Seasonal Influenza Vaccination and Reasons for Inadequate Vaccination Coverage Against a Broad Spectrum of Vaccine-Preventable Diseases: A cross-sectional study among a Brazilian cohort of adult patients with systemic lupus erythematosus. Lupus. 2019;28(6):794–6. https://doi.org/10.1177/0961203319846383 Epub 2019 May 1.
14. Lawson EF, Trupin L, Yelin EH, Yazdany J. Reasons for failure to receive pneumococcal and influenza vaccinations among immunosuppressed patients with systemic lupus erythematosus. Semin Arthritis Rheum. 2015;44(6):666 https://doi.org/10.1016/j.semarthrit.2015.01.002 Epub 2015 Jan 22.
15. Assala M, Groh M, Blanche P, Vinter C, Cohen P, le Guern V, et al. Pneumococcal and influenza vaccination rates in patients treated with corticosteroids and/or immunosuppressive therapies for systemic autoimmune diseases: a cross-sectional study. Joint Bone Spine. 2017;84(3):365–6. https://doi.org/10.1016/j.jbspin.2016.03.013 Epub 2016 Jun 22.
16. Chehab G, Richter JG, Brinks R, Fischer-Betz R, Winkler-Rohlfing B, Schneider M. Vaccination coverage in systemic lupus erythematosus-a cross-sectional analysis of the German long-term study (LuLa cohort). Rheumatology (Oxford). 2018;57(8):1439–47. https://doi.org/10.1093/rheumatology/key120
17. Third National Survey of Risk Factors for Non-communicable Diseases. National Ministry of Health, National Institute of Statistics and Census, Argentina. Available at: https://bancos.salud.gob.ar/sites/default/files/2018-10/0000000544cnt-2015_09_04_encuesta_nacional_factores_riesgo.pdf (article in Spanish).
18. Huerta J M, Tormo M J, Egea-Caparrós J M, et al. Accuracy of self-reported diabetes, hypertension and hyperlipidemia in the adult Spanish population. DINO study findings. Rev Esp Cardiol 2009;62(2):143–152. doi: https://doi.org/10.1016/s1885-5857(09)71532-4. (article in Spanish).
19. Mangtani P, Shah A, Roberts JA. Validation of influenza and pneumococcal vaccine status in adults based on self-report. Epidemiol. Infect. 2007;135(1):139–43. https://doi.org/10.1017/S0950268806006479 Epub 2006 Jun 2.
20. Martin LM, Leff M, Calonge N, Garrett C, Nelson DE. Validation of self-reported chronic conditions and health services in a managed care population. Am J Prev Med. 2000;18(3):215–8. https://doi.org/10.1016/s0749-3797(99)00158-0.
21. Tisnado DM, Adams JL, Liu H, Damberg CL, Chen WP, Hu FA, et al. What is the concordance between the medical record and patient self-report as data sources for ambulatory care? Med Care. 2006;44(2):132–40. https://doi.org/10.1097/01.mlr.0000196952.15921.bf.
22. Grande ED, Fullerton S, Taylor AW. Reliability of self-reported health risk factors and chronic conditions questions collected using the telephone in South Australia, Australia. BMC Med Res Methodol. 2012;12(1):108. https://doi.org/10.1186/1471-2288-12-108.
23. Stolses Bergamo Francisco PM, Azevedo Barros MB, José Segri N, Goi Porto Alves MC, CLG C, Carvalho Malta D. Comparison of estimates for the self-reported chronic conditions among household survey and telephone survey--Campinas (SP), Brazil. Rev Bras Epidemiol. 2011;14(Suppl 1):5–15. https://doi.org/10.1590/s1415-790x2011000500002.
24. Campinas Municipal Health Survey (ISACAMP) 2008, Brazil. Available at: https://www.fcm.unicamp.br/fcm/sites/default/files/questionario_portugues.pdf (article in Portuguese).
25. Surveillance of Risk and Protective Factors for Chronic Diseases by Telephone Survey (VIGITEL) 2007. Available at: http://bvsms.saude.gov.br/bvs/publicacoes/vigilancia_risco_doencas_inquerito_telefonico_2007.pdf (article in Portuguese).
26. Ng E, Vanderloo SE, Geiss L, Johnson JA. Concordance between self-report and a survey-based algorithm for classification of type 1 and type 2 diabetes using the 2011 population-based survey on living with chronic diseases in Canada (SLCDC)-diabetes component. Can J Diabetes. 2013;37(4):249–53. https://doi.org/10.1016/j.jcjd.2013.05.007 Epub 2013 Aug 2.
27. Bienek AS, Gee ME, Nolan RP, et al. Methodology of the 2009 Survey on Living with Chronic Diseases in Canada--hypertension component. Chronic Dis Inj Can. 2013;33(4):267–76 PMID: 23987223. (article in French).
28. Domenicantonio RD, Cappai G, Cascini S, et al. Validation of algorithms for the identification of subjects with chronic disease using health information systems. Epidemiol Prev. 2018;42(5–6):316–25 (article in Italian). https://doi.org/10.19191/EP18.5-6.P316.100.
29. Pons-Estel GJ, Ugarte-Gil MF, Alarcón GS. Epidemiology of systemic lupus erythematosus. Expert Rev Clin Immunol. 2017;13(8):799–814. https://doi.org/10.1080/1744666x.2017.1327352.
30. Population estimates and projections updates for the Latin America and the Caribbean countries. Economic Commission for Latin America and the Caribbean (ECLAC). Available at: https://www.cepal.org/es/notas/actualizacion-estimaciones-proyecciones-poblacion-paises-america-latina-caribe.
31. Pan American Health Organization. 2017 Influenza Vaccine Coverage. Available at: http://ais.paho.org/imm/InfluenzaCoverageMap.asp.
32. Fine MJ, Auble TE, Yealy DM, et al. A prediction rule to identify low-risk patients with community-acquired pneumonia. N Engl J Med. 1997;336(4):243–50. https://doi.org/10.1056/NEJM199701233360402.
33. Squance ML, Reeves G, Attia J, et al. Self-reported Lupus flare: Association with everyday home and personal product exposure. Toxicol Rep. 2015;2:880–8. https://doi.org/10.1016/j.toxrep.2015.05.010. eCollection 2015.
34. Pan American Health Organization. Third dose of diphtheria toxoid, tetanus toxoid and pertussis vaccine. 2018. https://www.paho.org/hq/index.phpoption=com_topics&view=rdmore&cid=7342&item=vacunacion&type=statistics&Itemid=40929&lang=es. Accessed 24 Aug 2020.
35. Guzman-Holst A, DeAntonio R, Prado-Cohrs D. et al. Barriers to vaccination in Latin America: A systematic literature review. Vaccine. 2020;38(3):470–81. https://doi.org/10.1016/j.vaccine.2019.10.088. Epub 2019 Nov 22.
36. McCarthy EM, Azeez MA, Fitzpatrick FM, et al. Knowledge, attitudes, and clinical practice of rheumatologists in vaccination of the at-risk rheumatology patient population. J Clin Rheumatol. 2012;18(5):237–41. https://doi.org/10.1097/RHU.0b013e3182611547.
37. Navarro-Millan I, Cornelius-Schecter A, O'Beirne RJ, et al. Views of primary care physicians and rheumatologists regarding screening and treatment of hyperlipidemia among patients with rheumatoid arthritis. BMC Rheumatol. 2020;4:14. https://doi.org/10.1186/s41927-020-0112-5. eCollection 2020.
38. Bartels CM, Roberts TJ, Hansen KE, et al. Rheumatologist and Primary Care Management of Cardiovascular Disease Risk in Rheumatoid Arthritis: Patient and Provider Perspectives. Arthritis Care Res (Hoboken). 2016;68(4):415–23. https://doi.org/10.1002/acr.22689.
39. Daniels NA, Nguyen TT, Gildengorin G, et al. Adult immunization in university-based primary care and specialty practices. J Am Geriatr Soc. 2004;52:1007Y1012. https://doi.org/10.1111/j.1532-5415.2004.52273.x.
40. Pennant KN, Costa JJ, Fuhlbrigge AL, et al. Improving influenza and pneumococcal vaccination rates in ambulatory specialty practices. Open Forum Infect Dis. 2015;2:ofv119. https://doi.org/10.1093/ofid/ofv119.
41. Skull SA, Andrews RM, Byrnes GB, et al. Validity of self-reported influenza and pneumococcal vaccination status among a cohort of hospitalized elderly inpatients. Vaccine. 2007;25(25):4775–83. https://doi.org/10.1016/j.vaccine.2007.04.015. Epub 2007 Apr 26.
42. Rolstad S, Adler J, Rydén A. Response burden and questionnaire length: is shorter better? A review and meta-analysis. Value Health. 2011;14(8):1101–8. https://doi.org/10.1016/j.jval.2011.06.003. Epub 2011 Aug 2.
43. Yazdany J, Yelin EH, Panopalis P, et al. Validation of the systemic lupus erythematosus activity questionnaire in a large observational cohort. Arthritis Rheum. 2008;59(1):136–43. https://doi.org/10.1002/art.23238.

17

Dualities of the vitamin D in systemic sclerosis

Laiana Schneider[1,2*], Vanessa Hax[2], Odirlei Monticielo[2,3], Tamires Ferri Macedo[3], Roberta Kern Menna Barreto[3], Natália Aydos Marcondes[4] and Rafael Chakr[2,3]

Abstract

Background: Systemic sclerosis (SSc) is a chronic disease characterized by autoimmunity, vasculopathy, and visceral and cutaneous fibrosis. Vitamin D has several functions in the immunological system, and different studies have suggested a potential role in triggering autoimmune diseases. Patients with SSc may present with low serum levels of vitamin D, but the association between hypovitaminosis D and disease onset or any clinical manifestation is still obscure. Our goal was to verify the causal relationship between hypovitaminosis D and SSc onset or any particular clinical manifestation in the literature.

Methods: A systematic literature review was performed through February 24th, 2021 on Pubmed, Lilacs/BIREME, and Cochrane databases. The eligible studies were read in full text, and, in the absence of exclusion criteria, were included in this review after consensus between two reviewers.

Results: Forty articles met the eligibility criteria and the main results of each study are described. In most studies, SSc patients showed a higher prevalence of vitamin D deficiency and insufficiency compared to controls. Additionally, in some reports serum levels of vitamin D were inversely correlated with the severity of SSc. Oral supplementation did not seem to affect serum levels of vitamin D. Four of the included studies were with experimental models.

Conclusion: In conclusion, vitamin D deficiency seems to have a role in susceptibility to SSc, as well as in the clinical manifestations of the disease.

Keywords: Vitamin D, Systemic sclerosis, 25-hydroxyvitamin D, Deficiency

Introduction

Systemic sclerosis (SSc) is a multisystemic autoimmune disease with a complex pathophysiology. SSc is characterized by the presence of autoantibodies and arises from the interrelation between vascular dysfunction, adaptive and innate immunity dysregulation, and excess activation of fibroblasts and similar cells, resulting in the development of progressive tissue fibrosis [1–3]. With a multifactorial etiology, several environmental and genetic factors seem to trigger the onset of SSc and its outcomes [1]. SSc affects predominantly young adults and has an important impact on quality of life and mortality rates [4]. Treatment is multidisciplinary, with a focus on symptoms management and predominant visceral injuries. A better understanding of the pathophysiology behind the disease could help advance research on this area and allow for the development of new therapeutic options [4].

Vitamin D is a steroid hormone known for its function on the regulation of calcium homeostasis and bone metabolism. The active metabolite of vitamin D (calcitriol) is formed by the activation of a precursor on skin exposed to ultraviolet B (UVB) radiation [5]. Serum

* Correspondence: laia_schneider@hotmail.com
[1]Programa de Pós-Graduação em Medicina: Ciências Médicas, Universidade Federal do Rio Grande do Sul, Porto Alegre, Brazil
[2]Serviço de Reumatologia, Hospital de Clínicas de Porto Alegre, Universidade Federal do Rio Grande do Sul, 2350 Ramiro Barcelos St, Room 645, Porto Alegre, RS 90035-903, Brazil

vitamin D levels may vary according to factors such as food intake (although to a lesser extent), bowel absorption, exposure to sunlight, and renal and hepatic metabolisms [5–7]. Vitamin D receptors (VDR) are present in antigen-presenting cells, natural killer cells, and activated B- and T-cell lymphocytes [5], which reinforces the evidence of its multiple immunomodulatory actions on adaptive and innate immune responses [8]. Vitamin D has a predominantly immunosuppressive effect, inhibiting proinflammatory cytokines production (IL6 and IL-17), stimulating anti-inflammatory cytokines production (IL4 and IL-10), and polarizing the Th1 response (IL-1, TNF-α, IFN-γ) into a Th2 response (autoantibodies, TGF-β) [5, 6]. Additionally, vitamin D inhibits the Th17 response and stimulates regulatory T cells. The immunomodulatory and tolerant effects of vitamin D on the adaptive and innate immune systems seem to play a protective role in the development of autoimmunity [6].

Hypovitaminosis D has been reported in several autoimmune diseases. Serum vitamin D levels are significantly lower in patients with SSc compared to healthy individuals [6]. Some studies have reported vitamin D insufficiency (< 30 ng/ml) in over 80% of patients with SSc [9, 10], usually in association with worse quality of life and lower bone mass [10–14]. The role of hypovitaminosis D in SSc pathophysiology and its possible therapeutic impact have been the subject of various studies in different scenarios. Therefore, this systematic review aims to verify the causal relationship between hypovitaminosis D and SSc onset or any particular clinical manifestation of the disease.

Methods

A comprehensive search in PubMed, Lilacs/BIREME, and Cochrane Library databases was performed through February 24th, 2021. The keywords used were "systemic sclerosis" and "vitamin D". No restrictions for language, year or type of publication were added (Supplemental file 1).

After excluding duplicate studies, two reviewers independently reviewed all the articles found in different databases. Initially, titles and summaries were analyzed according to the eligibility criteria and all studies on the association between serum vitamin D levels and the clinical and pathophysiological aspects of SSc or on the role of vitamin D in the pathophysiology of SSc were selected. The selected articles were read in full and, in the absence of exclusion criteria, were included in this review after consensus between two reviewers. If no consensus were reached, a third reviewer would decide on study inclusion. The question that guided studies selection was: "What is the role of vitamin D in the pathophysiology and in the clinical manifestations of SSc?", so all observation or intervention studies assessing vitamin D levels and its correlation with clinical and/or pathophysiological manifestations were eligible for inclusion in this review. We included all clinical and experimental studies published after peer-review, that would address the question guiding paper selection. Articles describing vitamin D levels on SSc patients without evaluation of clinical and/or pathophysiological manifestations were excluded, as well as other review articles and research on SSc therapy or treatment. Preprint studies were not included. In addition, the reference sections of the relevant articles were scanned for additional references that could have been missing from the databases.

Most of the studies included in this review defined vitamin D deficiency as a serum level < 10 ng/ml and insufficiency as a serum level of 10–30 ng/ml.

Results

Overall, 391 publications were identified in the different databases: 162 in PubMed, 211 in Lilacs/BIREME, and 10 in Cochrane Library. Of these, 118 were excluded after summary analysis, 205 were duplicate studies, two were not available online, and one was an erratum. Additionally, 17 publications were excluded after full text review for not meeting the eligibility criteria, and 12 were excluded due to being review articles. Eight additional articles were included after reference review. At the end of the selection process, 40 articles were included in this systematic review. Four included studies were experimental models on the effect of vitamin D or a vitamin D analogue. These data are shown in the flowchart on Fig. 1.

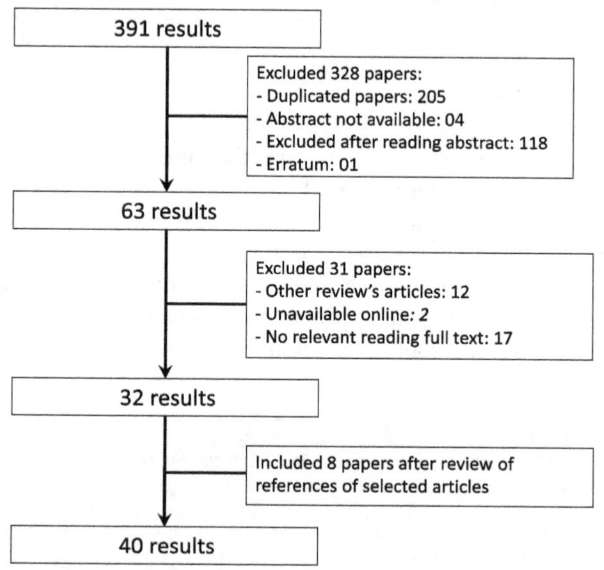

Fig. 1 Flowchart with the selection of articles for the systematic review

Characteristics of the selected articles, number of subjects, serum levels of vitamin D, proportion of patients with vitamin D < 10 and < 30 ng/mL and the main results of each study are presented in Table 1. Most studies showed vitamin D deficiency and insufficiency in SSc patients, regardless of season or oral vitamin D supplementation. Some studies identified association of vitamin D levels with clinical and pathophysiological manifestations, such as an inverse correlation of vitamin D levels with disease severity. Other reports did not identified an association between SSc manifestations and vitamin D.

The methodology and the main results of the experimental studies included in this review are summarized in Table 2.

Discussion

In the last two decades, several authors have reported lower levels of vitamin D in patients with SSc compared to healthy individuals [11–14, 16, 21, 25, 38, 48]. Despite the well-known seasonal variations in serum vitamin D levels, with peak values in summer [41], SSc patients present consistently lower levels throughout all seasons [38, 41]. Initially, we intended to estimate the mean serum vitamin D level among SSc patients across studies, but the great population heterogeneity could lead this estimation to substantial misinterpretation and inaccuracy. Seasonal variation, age, gender, comorbidities, life habits and drug treatment were some of the factors that could falsely impact this measure.

The evidence behind the association between hypovitaminosis D and SSc onset is scarce [15, 29–31, 34, 38]. So far, no published study has properly demonstrated this cause-effect relationship. Future research needs to add more on biologic plausibility, temporality, intensity, consistency and dose-response effect of hypovitaminosis D and SSc onset. An inception cohort study would be a suitable design. However, it may not be feasible due to the very low incidence of SSc in the general population. Longitudinal case-control studies would be the alternative; nonetheless vitamin D levels may not be generally available for comparison between groups.

Recently, An et al. (2017) have performed a meta-analysis to investigate the association between vitamin D and SSc, which included six case-control studies with a total of 554 SSc patients and 321 healthy controls. Meta-analysis results showed that SSc patients suffered from decreased vitamin D levels compared with healthy controls and in diffused SSc patients the vitamin D levels were significantly lower than those in limited SSc. Vitamin D level was not associated with Rodnan score, systolic pulmonary pressure, gastrointestinal ulcer, or pulmonary involvement, so the authors suggested that lower vitamin D levels in SSc patients may not be a factor accelerating disease severity [49].

On the other hand, some studies have shown an association between vitamin D deficiency and severity of SSc [9, 16, 41]. Hypovitaminosis D is common in SSc and patients with vitamin D deficiency have a greater frequency of pulmonary disease, lower diffusion and higher estimated pulmonary hypertension compared to patients with vitamin D insufficiency [8, 22, 37]. Additionally, these patients have higher inflammatory markers [9, 22] and Cruz-Domínguez et al. (2017) have demonstrated lower vitamin D levels in patients with and without calcinosis [24]. Park et al. (2017) demonstrated that vitamin D deficiency is an independent risk factor for digital ulcers in SSc, suggesting an involvement with the microangiopathic manifestations of the disease. However, the study could not demonstrate an association with macrovascular conditions in SSc patients, such as arterial stiffness and atherosclerosis [35], which suggests that vitamin D may act differently on micro- and macrovascular mechanisms in SSc. Caimmi et al. (2019) found in a retrospective cohort study that a decrease in 25-hydroxyvitamin D (25(OH)D) is associated with the risk of developing digital ulcers after 5 years [20]. In spite of this, no consensus has been reached, and further studies are needed to clarify the association between low vitamin D levels and the vascular involvement of the disease [18, 21, 43, 49].

Hypovitaminosis D diagnosis is based on serum 25(OH) D levels, and there is no consensus regarding the ideal values that should be adopted. Several experts agree to define vitamin D deficiency as serum levels below 10 ng/ml [9, 10, 16, 18, 22, 38]. However, this definition is not universal, with some authors suggesting deficiency levels to be lower than 20 ng/ml (50 nmol/l) [39, 41], taking in consideration the regulatory variations of PTH. In turn, vitamin D insufficiency is commonly defined as serum levels between 10 and 30 ng/ml, with levels > 30 ng/ml being considered sufficient [9, 22, 24, 27]. Higher levels of vitamin D do not seem to provide any additional benefits [50]. Nevertheless, the optimal concentration of vitamin D for proper immune system function is not yet well-defined. Studies have demonstrated that genetic polymorphisms in the vitamin D binding protein, in enzymes or even in the VDR could determine variations in 25(OH) D serum levels, further complicating the definition of adequate serum levels [51–53].

Vitamin D deficiency in patients with SSc seems to be multifactorial. In a retrospective cohort comprising 327 SSc patients and 141 controls, Arnson et al. (2011) substantiate an inverse relation between serum vitamin D levels and the extent of cutaneous involvement, they showed that patients with a Rodnan score higher than 10 had a significantly lower serum vitamin D level compared to other patients (17.7 ± 10.4 ng/ml versus 8 ±

Table 1 Characteristics and results of the selected studies

Study	Study design	25(OH) D (ng/ml) levels *		SSc patients with low vitamin D levels		Main results
		SSc patients (n)	Controls (n)	< 10 ng/ml n (%)	< 30 ng/ml n (%)	
Ahmadi et al., 2017 [15]	Cross-sectional	15 ± 4.7 (60)	27.2 ± 8.7 (30)	- -	- -	Serum Klotho and vitamin D lower in SSc patients ($p < 0.001$). Higher intact PTH in SSc patients ($p < 0.001$).
Arnson et al., 2011 [16]	Cross-sectional	13.5 ± 9 (327)	21.6 ± 9.7 (141)	- -	- -	Lower vitamin D levels in SSc patients ($p < 0.001$). Association with lower DLCO ($p < 0.02$). Inverse association with skin extent (mRSS> 10; $p = 0.02$) and RF expression ($p < 0.001$).
Atteritano et al., 2013 [14]	Cross-sectional	18.3 ± 4.1 (54)	39.6 ± 7.5 (54)	- -	- -	Lower vitamin D levels in SSc patients ($p < 0.001$). Association with PTH ($p = 0.001$), osteocalcin ($p < 0.05$), deoxypyridinoline ($p < 0.05$) and BMD on lumbar spine and femur ($p < 0.05$).
Atteritano et al., 2016 [17]	Cross-sectional	25.8 ± 12.8 (40)	35.1 ± 9.1 (40)	0 (0)	20 (50)	Lower vitamin D levels in SSc patients ($p = 0.0003$). Association with skin extent (mRSS> 10; $p = 0.02$) and PASP> 35 mmHg ($p = 0.02$). No association with subtype and autoantibodies.
Belloli et al., 2011 [18]	Cross-sectional	18.1 ± 15.2 (43)	17.3 ± 12 (99 - OA)	15 (34.8)	37 (86)	No significantly difference in insufficiency or deficiency between groups, regardless of disease duration, subtype and autoantibodies.
Braun-Moscovici et al., 2008 [19]	Cross-sectional	- (60)	- -	26[a] (46)	- -	High PTH associated with vitamin D deficiency ($p = 0.01$), calcinosis ($p = 0.009$), and acrosteolysis ($p = 0.015$). No significant correlation between supplementation and vitamin D levels.
Caimmi et al., 2019 [20]	Cohort	(65)	-	-	-	Lower vitamin D levels in patients with incident DU in relation to patients with no incident DU over 5 years (− 17.4 vs 13.0, $p = 0{,}018$).
Calzolari et al., 2009 [21]	Cross-sectional	23(3–92)[b] (18)(60)	39(14–138)[b] (60)	4 (6.7)	38 (63.4)	Lower vitamin D levels in SSc patients ($p < 0.001$). No association with disease subtype, cutaneous ulcers, skin extent, gastrointestinal and joint involvement.
Caramaschi et al., 2010 [22]	Cross-sectional	15.8 ± 9.1 (65)	- -	19 (29.2)	62 (95.4)	Association with lung disease ($p = 0.009$),longer disease duration ($p = 0.026$), lower DLCO ($p = 0.014$), and higher PASP ($p = 0.037$), ESR ($p = 0.001$) and CRP ($p = 0.004$).
Carmel et al., 2015 [23]	Cross-sectional	- (54)	- (41)	- -	39 (82.1)	Anti-25(OH) D IgM antibodies more frequent in SSc patients and in a higher level ($p = 0.002$). No correlation with severity, other autoantibodies and target organ damage.
Corrado et al., 2015 [12]	Cross-sectional	15.7 ± 10.2 (64)	22.9 ± 9.1 (35)	- -	- -	Lower vitamin D levels in patients, especially in diffuse cutaneous SSc ($p < 0.001$). Negative correlation with mRSS ($p < 0.05$). No association with any internal organ involvement.
Cruz-Domínguez et al., 2017 [24]	Cohort	- (109)	- -	- -	- -	Lower vitamin D levels in SSc patients with and without calcinosis (19.1 vs. 13.1; $p = 0.56$).
Di Liberto et al., 2019 [25]	Cross-sectional	22.1 ± 9.7 (45)	-	-	-	Low vitamin D levels in SSc patients. Similar percentage of regulatory T-cells (Tregs) in SSc patients and control group, with higher percentage in SSc patients taking cholecalciferol. Impaired Tregs capability to suppress T cell proliferation in SSc patients. Increase in IL-10 in vitro production of patients Tregs after treatment with (1,25(OH)2D3).
Gambichler et al., 2011 [26]	Cross-sectional	13.1(4–48)[b] (133)	- -	49 (35.8)	123 (89.8)	No association with disease subtype, BMI, lung fibrosis, renal involvement, GERD, digital ulcers, mRSS, autoantibodies and therapy.
Giuggioli et al., 2017 [27]	Cross-sectional	9.8 ± 4.1[d] (140)	- -	40/91[d] (44)	91/91[d] (100)	Lower vitamin D levels in not supplemented patients (9.8 ± 4.1 vs. 26 ± 8.1; $p < 0.0001$), but only 15/49 (31%) supplemented patients reached the normal range of vitamin D.
Groseanu et al., 2016 [8]	Cross-sectional	17.1 ± 9.1 (51)	- -	12 (23.5)	46 (90.2)	Positive correlation with DLCO ($p = 0.019$). Negative correlation of vitamin D with diastolic dysfunction, digital contractures and muscle weakness. No correlation with autoantibodies or skin extent. Higher vitamin D levels in patients with usual supplementation (25.5%), but the difference between groups failed to reach statistical significance ($p = 0.488$).
Gupta et al., 2018 [28]	Cross-sectional	19.5 ± 77.8[c] (38)	100 ± 31.3[c] (38)	13 (34.2)	23 (60.5)	Lower vitamin D levels in SSc patients ($p = 0.001$). Inverse correlationwith mRSS. No correlation with age, disease duration, autoantibodies, digital ulcers, or systemic involvement.
Hajialilo et al., 2017 [29]	Cross-sectional	14.9 ± 4.6 (60)	30.4 ± 7.9 (60)	- -	- -	Serum ET-1 higher in SSc patients ($p = 0.001$). Serum α-Klotho and vitamin D lower in SSc patients ($p = 0.001$). Association of vitamin D with gastrointestinal involvement on Medsger severity scale ($p = 0.003$).
Hax et al., 2020 [30]	Cross-sectional	23.9 ± 8.5 (50)	30.2 ± 6.2 (35)	2 (4%)	36 (72%)	Lower vitamin D levels in SSc patients compared to control group and lower vitamin D levels in SSc patients not taking vitamin D supplementation. No associations between vitamin D and cytokine levels or between vitamind D levels and disease duration.
Ibn-Yacoub et al., 2012 [13]	Cross-sectional	10.9 ± 2.7 (30)	57.4 ± 4.2 (30)	8 (26.7)	30 (100)	Lower vitamin D levels in SSc patients ($p = 0.001$). Association with number of painful ($p = 0.006$) and swollen joints ($p = 0.013$) and anti-Scl70 ($p = 0.027$). Association of vitamin D with BMD

Table 1 Characteristics and results of the selected studies *(Continued)*

Study	Study design	25(OH) D (ng/ml) levels *		SSc patients with low vitamin D levels		Main results
		SSc patients (n)	Controls (n)	< 10 ng/ml n (%)	< 30 ng/ml n (%)	
						on lumbar spine ($p = 0.002$) and femoral neck ($p = 0.032$).
Kamal et al., 2016 [31]	Cross-sectional	- (30)	- (60)	- -	- -	No association between VDR polymorphisms (ApaI and TaqI) and SSc susceptibility. Significant association between ApaI and diffuse cutaneous SSc.
Matsuoka et al., 1991 [32]	Cross-sectional	28 ± 3 (19)	29 ± 3 (19)	- -	- -	Hypovitaminosis D common in SSc patients and healthy controls. No correlation with skin extent.
Montabone et al., 2016 [33]	Cross-sectional	18.5(7.5–37)[b] (35)	- -	4 (11)	30 (85)	Association with a worse physical component on SF-36 and physical function ($p < 0.04$). No association with gastrointestinal, kidney and cardiopulmonary involvement.
Orbach et al., 2007 [34]	Cross-sectional	11 ± 5.8 (229)	- -	- -	- -	Lower vitamin D levels in different autoimmune diseases (SSc, SLE, PM, DM, APS, and RA).
Park et al., 2017 [35]	Cross-sectional	43.7(25–68)[b] (40)	57.5(40–81)[b] (80)	2 (5)	12 (30)	Association with digital ulcers ($p = 0.012$). No association with arterial stiffness, atherosclerosis, autoantibodies, mRSS, lung disease, PASP, ESR and CRP.
Rios Fernández et al., 2010 [36]	Cross-sectional	- (48)	- -	5 (9.5)	39 (81)	No significant vitamin D correlation with PASP or lung fibrosis. Hypovitaminosis D was common, despite 60.4% of patients were taking usual supplementation.
Rios Fernández et al., 2012 [37]	Cross-sectional	- (90)	- -	10 (11)	69 (76.7)	Association of vitamin D with calcinosis ($p < 0.034$), heart involvement ($p < 0.012$), DLCO ($p < 0.006$) and positive ANA ($p < 0.017$). Hypovitaminosis D was common, despite 58.9% of patients were taking usual supplementation. Vitamin D deficiency was not different between groups (52% vs. 66.7%).
Sampaio-Barros et al., 2016 [10]	Cross-sectional	20.7 ± 8.2 (38)	- -	4 (11)	33 (87)	Vitamin D positive correlation with anti-Scl70 ($p = 0.039$) and some SF-36 domains (vitality, social function, emotional role and mental health). Negative correlation with HAQ-reach and HAQ-grip strength. Positive correlation of vitamin D with BMI ($p = 0.038$) and femur BMD ($p = 0.037$).
Seriolo et al., 2011 [38]	Cross-sectional	21.7 ± 13.4 (53)	39.4 ± 15.4 (35)	13 (24)	47 (88)	Seasonal variation in patients and controls (highest values in summer, $p < 0.01$). Significantly lower levels in SSc patients in all seasons.
Shinjo et al., 2011 [39]	Cross-sectional	18.1 ± 6.4 (10)	25.1 ± 6.6 (10)	- -	- -	Lower vitamin D levels in juvenile SSc patients ($p = 0.04$). Positive correlation with femur BMD ($p = 0.02$).
Taylan et al., 2019 [40]	Cross-sectional	8.7(4.5–18)[b] (46)	16.5(9–21)[b] (30)			Lower serum vitamin D levels in SSc patients ($p = 0.02$). No correlation with mRSS.
Trombetta et al., 2017 [41]	Cross-sectional	18.7 ± 9 (154)	- -	- -	124 (80.5)	Association of vitamin D with pulmonary fibrotic changes ($p = 0.04$). Correlation with some domains of Medsger severity scale (peripheral vascular, renal and gastrointestinal involvement). Vitamin D levels not influenced by usual supplementation ($p = 0.81$).
Ursini et al., 2017 [42]	Cohort	15.4(8–25)[b] (124)	- -	- -	13 (89.5)	Inverse correlation with mRSS ($p = 0.03$) and subclinical liver fibrosis (evaluated using the aspartate aminotransferase-to-platelet ratio index; $p = 0.02$). No correlation with age and disease duration.
Vacca et al., 2009 [9]	Cross-sectional	19 ± 11 (156)	- -	44 (28)	131 (84)	Association of vitamin D with higher PASP ($p = 0.004$), lung fibrosis ($p = 0.04$), anticentromere ($p = 0.04$) and ESR ($p = 0.008$). No association with calcinosis, HAQ, or Medsger severity score. Negative correlation with EDAS ($p = 0.04$). Vitamin D levels not influenced by usual supplementation ($p = 0.1$).
Zhang et al., 2017 [43]	Cross-sectional	26.5 ± 6.3 (60)	36.3 ± 14.2 (60)	- -	45 (75)	Lower vitamin D levels in SSc patients ($p < 0.001$). More frequent lung involvement, but without significance ($p = 0.08$). No difference in joint involvement, autoantibodies, ESR and CRP.

Abbreviations: *ANA* antinuclear antibodies, *APS* antiphospholipid syndrome, *BMD* bone mineral density, *BMI* body mass index, *CRP* C-reactive protein, *DLCO* diffusion capacity of carbon monoxide, *DM* dermatomyositis, *DU* digital ulcers, *EDAS* European Disease Activity Score, *ESR* erythrocyte sedimentation rate, *ET-1* Endotelina 1, *GERD* gastroesophageal reflux disease, *HAQ* Health Assessment Questionnaire, *mRSS* modified Rodnan skin score, *OA* osteoarthritis, *PASP* pulmonary arterial systolic pressure on Doppler echocardiography, *PM* polymyositis, *RA* rheumatoid arthritis, *RF* rheumatoid factor, *SF-36* Short-Form-36 Questionnaire, *SLE* systemic lupus erythematosus, *SSc* systemic sclerosis, *TGF-β* transforming growth factor β, *VDR* vitamin D receptor

* Data are presented as mean ± standard deviation, except when indicated otherwise

[a]These author presented only the proportion of patients with 25(OH) D < 12 ng/ml

[b]Median (25–75th percentile)

[c]Median ± IQR

[d]Vitamin D levels only in non-supplemented patients (91/140)

10.1 ng/ml; $p = 0.02$) [16], a result recently replicated in another study [17]. Since then, other authors also demonstrated an inverse correlation between serum vitamin D levels and the extent of cutaneous involvement [11, 12, 28, 42]. On the other hand, some studies did not evidence the same correlation between cutaneous involvement and vitamin D levels [8, 26, 32, 35, 40, 49]. These authors suggest that the epidermal synthesis could

Table 2 Characteristics and results of the selected experimental models of systemic sclerosis

Author	Year	Research Design	Main results
Slominski et al. [44]	2013	Culture of skin fibroblasts from patients and controls	Efficacy of vitamin D in inhibiting TGF-induced collagen synthesis and inhibiting cell proliferation in fibroblasts from patients and controls; vitamin D suppressed fibrogenesis in a bleomycin-induced sclerosis model.
Terao et al. [45]	2015	Experimental model	Effect of vitamin D analogue on periostin expression in fibroblasts and bleomycin-induced sclerosis model; maxacalcitol reduces the expression of periostin and TGF-β and suppresses the Th2 response.
Usategui et al. [46]	2014	Cutaneous fibrosis in animal model	Effect of the topical analogue of vitamin D (calcipotriol) on cytokines and the development of fibrosis in rats with bleomycin-induced sclerosis; calcipotriol overexpressed Th2 axis expression, with antifibrotic effect.
Zerr et al. [47]	2014	Culture of skin fibroblasts from patients and controls	Expression of VDR in experimental model and fibroblasts; effect of paricalcitol on bleomycin-induced fibrosis model and overexpression of TGF-β receptor (TBRICA); VDR characterization as a negative regulator of TGF-β / Smad pathway signaling.

Abbreviations: *TGF-β* transforming growth factor β, *VDR* Vitamin D receptor

remain virtually normal, and that the hepatic and renal hydroxylation mechanisms of vitamin D could also work normally in this disease. Gastrointestinal involvement in SSc seems to contribute to vitamin D malabsorption, although these data are still controversial [19, 22]. Furthermore, it is possible that some medications used by SSc patients, such as corticosteroids or anticonvulsants for neuropathic pain control, could interfere with vitamin absorption [16]. In spite of this, not all authors were able to evidence differences in vitamin D levels between patients on and off these medications [41]. In addition to the cutaneous and gastrointestinal involvement, reduced sun exposure due to physical incapacity, self-image disorders, depression, and social and psychological limitations could compound the deficit [9, 34]. As one might expect, serum vitamin D levels could simply reflect a better health in general due to better life habits, such as exercise, outdoor activities and a healthier diet. This hypothesis is corroborated by previous research showing an association between low levels of 25(OH) D and a worse quality of life and physical function in SSc patients [10, 33].

Many authors have explored the association between lower vitamin D levels and SSc phenotype. Sampaio-Barros et al. (2016) demonstrated an association between lower serum vitamin D levels, underlying vascular involvement and the production of anti-Scl70 autoantibodies [10]. In addition, lower levels of vitamin D were described in patients with diffuse cutaneous SSc when compared with limited cutaneous disease [12, 49]. On the other hand, Vacca et al. (2009) showed an association between lower serum vitamin D levels and the presence of anti-centromere autoantibodies [9]. Other authors, however, have failed to demonstrate any association between serum vitamin D levels and disease subtype or specific autoantibodies [18, 43]. Therefore, the role of vitamin D in the clinical and serological phenotypes of SSc is not yet well known. Further studies should seek to clarify the possible associations between hypovitaminosis D and disease subtype, also considering the prognostic impact of these findings.

Considering the pathogenesis of SSc, several studies have suggested that vitamin D is related to the regulation of cellular immunity mechanisms [6–8]. The synthesis of 1,25 dihydroxyvitamin D (1,25(OH)2D) and presence of VDR in activated immune cells have attracted the attention of several researchers. Vitamin D acts as a regulator of innate and adaptive immune responses, promoting monocyte differentiation into macrophages, modulating macrophage response and inhibiting production of chemokines and inflammatory cytokines [54]. Polymorphisms in the VDR gene also seem to be associated with vitamin D deficiency, as suggested by Kamal et al. (2016). The authors found no association between VDR polymorphisms (ApaI and TaqI) and susceptibility to SSc, but reported an association between the ApaI polymorphism and disease subtype [31]. In a recent study, an association between some VDR single nucleotide polymorphisms and SSc susceptibility was stablished [55].

Interestingly, Carmel et al. (2015) reported a higher frequency and an increased level of anti-25(OH) D IgM antibodies in SSc patients when compared to controls, similarly to what has been described in patients with systemic lupus erythematosus (SLE). However, the same study reported lower levels of anti-25(OH) D IgG antibodies in SSc patients than in controls [23]. The pathophysiological significance and clinical relevance of these autoantibodies in SSc remains controversial.

Vitamin D also seems to have an important role in modulating TGF-β activity, an essential factor in collagen production by fibroblasts. Zerr et al. (2015) analyzed VDR expression in fibroblasts of SSc patients and in a murine model of bleomycin-induced fibrosis. The authors characterized the VDR as a negative regulator of TGF-β signaling. Furthermore, they demonstrated that treatment with a vitamin D analogue (paricalcitol) was able to restore VDR signaling and reduce the pro-fibrotic effects of TGF-β on fibroblasts [47]. Similar findings were described in a study on skin fibroblast cultures from SSc patients and controls, which demonstrated the inhibitory effects of vitamin D in collagen and hyaluronate production induced by TGF [44]. The research of Boelsma et al. (1995) supports these findings by demonstrating evidence of cutaneous fibrosis in humans, which was also correlated with lower serum levels of vitamin D [56]. However, this finding could also result from reduced vitamin D production due to cutaneous fibrosis [57]. When assessing the therapeutic use of topical vitamin D analogues on SSc patients with hypovitaminosis D, a reduction in cutaneous fibrosis was observed. These results may be due to the role of vitamin D in reducing pro-fibrotic signaling by TGF-β and in inducing a polarization of the local immune response by producing potentially pro-fibrotic Th2 cytokines [45, 46]. A study by Ahmadi et al. (2017) analyzed the serum levels of fibroblast growth factor 23 (FGF-23), which has an essential role in the kidney-bone axis, and its membrane co-receptor Klotho. Klotho is a protein predominantly expressed in the renal tubules and possibly involved in calcium and phosphate homeostasis, prevents hyperphosphatemia, fibrosis, arteriosclerosis and inflammation [15]. A deficiency in α-Klotho expression has been studied for its potential involvement in endothelial dysfunction, microangiopathy, calcinosis and fibrosis, which are common features of scleroderma. Serum levels of soluble Klotho tend to decrease with age, and a defect in its gene increases the risk for age-related diseases. Significantly lower serum levels of Klotho in SSc patients were identified [29]. It is believe that an increase in inflammatory markers could reduce the renal expression of this protein [15].

In two independent European cohorts, Vacca et al. (2011) assessed the frequency of vitamin D insufficiency and deficiency in SSc patients. These studies found no difference in serum levels between SSc patients under the standard dose of vitamin D supplementation (800 IU/day) or under placebo [58]. In a Spanish retrospective cohort, Rios-Fernández et al. (2010) also described a high prevalence of vitamin D deficiency in SSc patients and corroborated the finding that supplementation with the usual dose of vitamin D was insufficient (60.4% of patients with low vitamin D levels were taking supplements) [36]. Therefore, conventional vitamin D supplementation (800 IU/day) does not seem to correct deficiency in SSc patients. Higher doses could be needed, especially in patients with severe disease or high inflammatory activity.

In a cross-sectional study with 140 SSc patients, 91 patients did not receive vitamin D supplementation, while 49 received 8000 to 12,500 IU of 25(OH) D weekly for a minimum period of 6 months. Non-supplemented patients had lower serum levels of vitamin D (9.8 ± 4.1 vs. 26 ± 8.1 ng/ml, $p < 0.0001$), although less than one-third of supplemented patients had reached normal levels by the end of the study [27]. In contrast, a retrospective cohort by Trombetta et al. (2017) was not able to demonstrate any changes on serum vitamin D levels in SSc patients supplemented with 1000 IU/day of cholecalciferol for 6 to 12 months [41]. The authors raised several hypotheses to justify these findings, with the strongest ones pointing to an interference in vitamin D activation caused by cutaneous fibrosis and to cholecalciferol malabsorption [27]. In spite of the variation in results for studies on vitamin D supplementation and the need for further research, most experts still recommend correcting vitamin D deficiency. The dose required to achieve and maintain adequate 25(OH) D levels depends on several factors. Some authors have suggested that a raise of 1 ng/ml of 25(OH) D in serum levels would require about 100 IU/day of vitamin D intake for approximately 3 months to reach a steady state once supplementation is initiated [59, 60]. In spite of this estimate, individual responses can vary, and the known risk factors for vitamin D deficiency should be considered for a personalized therapeutic approach.

Our study has some limitations. The major one is the lack of prospective cohort studies or randomized controlled trials assessing the role of vitamin D in the pathophysiology and in the clinical manifestations of SSc, so no definitive conclusions could be drawn regarding cause-effect relationship between hypovitaminosis D and SSc onset or any clinical manifestation. Besides, literature on Medline/EMBASE was not included in this systematic literature review due to access restrictions, however, considering the great number of overlaps between Medline/EMBASE and Medline/PubMed, it is not likely that any major study was left out of this review. Also, we have chosen to include as many peer-reviewed articles as possible, in this regard, a quality assessment of included articles was not performed and methodologically distinct studies were included. Our article selection strategy was based on the fact that systematic reviews evaluate areas where evidence may be too heterogeneous for comparison and a meta-analysis study is not possible [61, 62].

Conclusion

In conclusion, vitamin D deficiency is frequent in SSc patients and seems to be associated with some clinical and serological features of the disease. However, to date, there is no evidence that the usual supplementation interferes with vitamin D deficiency, and its clinical impact remains uncertain. Further randomized trials on the clinical effects of vitamin D supplementation are necessary to verify the effects of vitamin D on the clinical characteristics of SSc, as well as to identify the potential role of vitamin D on immunomodulation and treatment of the disease. Thus, the optimal dosage of vitamin D supplementation and the need for monitoring of 25(OH) D serum levels in SSc patients are still open fields for research. Further studies are also needed to clarify the relationship between serum vitamin D levels and the pathophysiology of SSc. It remains unclear if vitamin D deficiency is an epiphenomenon or if it actually determines an increase in susceptibility and a worse prognosis for this complex disease.

Abbreviations

1,25(OH)2D: 1,25 dihydroxyvitamin D; 25(OH)D: 25-hydroxyvitamin D; ANA: Antinuclear antibodies; APS: Antiphospholipid syndrome; BMD: Bone mineral density; BMI: Body mass index; CRP: C-reactive protein; DLCO: Diffusion capacity of carbon monoxide; DM: Dermatomyositis; DU: Digital ulcers; EDAS: European Disease Activity Score; ESR: Erythrocyte sedimentation rate; ET-1: Endotelina 1; FGF-23: Fibroblast growth factor 23; GERD: Gastroesophageal reflux disease; HAQ: Health Assessment Questionnaire; mRSS: Modified Rodnan skin score; OA: Osteoarthritis; PASP: Pulmonary arterial systolic pressure on Doppler echocardiography; PM: Polymyositis; RA: Rheumatoid arthritis; RF: Rheumatoid factor; SF-36: Short-Form-36 Questionnaire; SLE: Systemic lupus erythematosus; SSc: Systemic sclerosis; TGF-β: Transforming growth factor β; Tregs: Regulatory T-cells; UVB: Ultraviolet B; VDR: Vitamin D receptor

Supplementary Information

Additional file 1. search strategy and paper selection.

Acknowledgements

We would like to thank Fernanda Igansi, biologist and clinical research coordinator at the Department of Cardiology of the Hospital de Clínicas de Porto Alegre, for her assistance in reviewing and selecting the articles. We are grateful to the Fundo de Incentivo à Pesquisa e Eventos do Hospital de Clínicas de Porto Alegre (FIPE/HCPA) for the financial support.

Authors' contributions

LS, VH, TFM and RKMB acquired the data, conceived and designed the research, and drafted the manuscript. OM, RC and NAM made a critical revision of the manuscript. All authors read and approved the final manuscript.

Author details

[1]Programa de Pós-Graduação em Medicina: Ciências Médicas, Universidade Federal do Rio Grande do Sul, Porto Alegre, Brazil. [2]Serviço de Reumatologia, Hospital de Clínicas de Porto Alegre, Universidade Federal do Rio Grande do Sul, 2350 Ramiro Barcelos St, Room 645, Porto Alegre, RS 90035-903, Brazil. [3]Faculdade de Medicina, Universidade Federal do Rio Grande do Sul, Porto Alegre, Brazil. [4]Laboratório Zanol, Porto Alegre, Brazil.

References

1. Murdaca G, Contatore M, Gulli R, Mandich P, Puppo F. Genetic factors and systemic sclerosis. Autoimmun Rev. 2016;15(5):427–32. https://doi.org/10.1016/j.autrev.2016.01.016.
2. Denton CP, Black CM, Abraham DJ. Mechanisms and consequences of fibrosis in systemic sclerosis. Nat Clin Pract Rheumatol. 2006;2(3):134–44. https://doi.org/10.1038/ncprheum0115.
3. Zimmermann AF, Pizzichini MM. Update on etiopathogenesis of systemic sclerosis. Rev Bras Reumatol. 2013;53(6):516–24. https://doi.org/10.1016/j.rbr.2013.01.001.
4. Desbois AC, Cacoub P. Systemic sclerosis: An update in 2016. Autoimmun Rev. 2016;15(5):417–26. https://doi.org/10.1016/j.autrev.2016.01.007.
5. Bivona G, Agnello L, Pivetti A, Milano S, Scazzone C, Sasso BL, et al. Association between hypovitaminosis D and systemic sclerosis: true or fake? Clin Chim Acta. 2016;458:115–9. https://doi.org/10.1016/j.cca.2016.04.026.
6. Rosen Y, Daich J, Soliman I, Brathwaite E, Shoenfeld Y. Vitamin D and autoimmunity. Scand J Rheumatol. 2016;45(6):439–47. https://doi.org/10.3109/03009742.2016.1151072.
7. Pelajo CF, Lopez-Benitez JM, Miller LC. Vitamin D and autoimmune rheumatologic disorders. Autoimmun Rev. 2010;9(7):507–10. https://doi.org/10.1016/j.autrev.2010.02.011.
8. Groseanu L, Bojinca V, Gudu T, Saulescu I, Predeteanu D, Balanescu A, et al. Low vitamin D status in systemic sclerosis and the impact on disease phenotype. Eur J Rheumatol. 2016;3(2):50–5. https://doi.org/10.5152/eurjrheum.2015.0065.
9. Vacca A, Cormier C, Piras M, Mathieu A, Kahan A, Allanore Y. Vitamin D deficiency and insufficiency in 2 independent cohorts of patients with systemic sclerosis. J Rheumatol. 2009;36(9):1924–9. https://doi.org/10.3899/jrheum.081287.
10. Sampaio-Barros MM, Takayama L, Sampaio-Barros PD, Bonfa E, Pereira RM. Low vitamin D serum levels in diffuse systemic sclerosis: a correlation with worst quality of life and severe capillaroscopic findings. Rev Bras Reumatol Engl Ed. 2016;56(4):337–44. https://doi.org/10.1016/j.rbre.2016.05.006.
11. Corrado A, Colia R, Mele A, Di Bello V, Trotta A, Neve A, et al. Correction: relationship between body mass composition, bone mineral density, skin fibrosis and 25(OH) vitamin D serum levels in systemic sclerosis. PLoS One. 2015;10(11):e0142748. https://doi.org/10.1371/journal.pone.0142748.
12. Corrado A, Colia R, Mele A, Di Bello V, Trotta A, Neve A, et al. Relationship between body mass composition, bone mineral density, skin fibrosis and 25(OH) vitamin D serum levels in systemic sclerosis. PLoS One. 2015;10(9):e0137912. https://doi.org/10.1371/journal.pone.0137912.
13. Ibn Yacoub Y, Amine B, Laatiris A, Wafki F, Znat F, Hajjaj-Hassouni N. Bone density in Moroccan women with systemic scleroderma and its relationships with disease-related parameters and vitamin D status. Rheumatol Int. 2012;32(10):3143–8. https://doi.org/10.1007/s00296-011-2150-1.
14. Atteritano M, Lasco A, Mazzaferro S, Macri I, Catalano A, Santangelo A, et al. Bone mineral density, quantitative ultrasound parameters and bone metabolism in postmenopausal women with depression. Intern Emerg Med. 2013;8(6):485–91. https://doi.org/10.1007/s11739-011-0628-1.
15. Ahmadi R, Hajialilo M, Ghorbanihaghjo A, Mota A, Raeisi S, Bargahi N, et al. FGF-23, Klotho and vitamin D levels in scleroderma. Iran J Public Health. 2017;46(4):530–6.
16. Arnson Y, Amital H, Agmon-Levin N, Alon D, Sanchez-Castanon M, Lopez-Hoyos M, et al. Serum 25-OH vitamin D concentrations are linked with various clinical aspects in patients with systemic sclerosis: a retrospective cohort study and review of the literature. Autoimmun Rev. 2011;10(8):490–4. https://doi.org/10.1016/j.autrev.2011.02.002.
17. Atteritano M, Santoro D, Corallo G, Visalli E, Buemi M, Catalano A, et al. Skin involvement and pulmonary hypertension are associated with vitamin D insufficiency in scleroderma. Int J Mol Sci. 2016;17(12).
18. Belloli L, Ughi N, Marasini B. Vitamin D in systemic sclerosis. Clin Rheumatol. 2011;30(1):145–6. https://doi.org/10.1007/s10067-010-1564-6.
19. Braun-Moscovici Y, Furst DE, Markovits D, Rozin A, Clements PJ, Nahir AM, et al. Vitamin D, parathyroid hormone, and acroosteolysis in systemic sclerosis. J Rheumatol. 2008;35(11):2201–5. https://doi.org/10.3899/jrheum.071171.
20. Caimmi C, Bertoldo E, Pozza A, Caramaschi P, Orsolini G, Gatti D, et al. Vitamin D serum levels and the risk of digital ulcers in systemic sclerosis: a longitudinal study. Int J Rheum Dis. 2019;22(6):1041–5. https://doi.org/10.1111/1756-185X.13554.
21. Calzolari G, Data V, Carignola R, Angeli A. Hypovitaminosis D in systemic sclerosis. J Rheumatol. 2009;36(12):2844 author reply 5.
22. Caramaschi P, Dalla Gassa A, Ruzzenente O, Volpe A, Ravagnani V, Tinazzi I, et al. Very low levels of vitamin D in systemic sclerosis patients. Clin Rheumatol. 2010;29(12):1419–25. https://doi.org/10.1007/s10067-010-1478-3
23. Carmel NN, Rotman-Pikielny P, Lavrov A, Levy Y. Vitamin D antibodies in systemic sclerosis patients: findings and clinical correlations. Isr Med Assoc J. 2015;17(2):80–4.

24. Cruz-Dominguez MP, Garcia-Collinot G, Saavedra MA, Medina G, Carranza-Muleiro RA, Vera-Lastra OL, et al. Clinical, biochemical, and radiological characterization of the calcinosis in a cohort of Mexican patients with systemic sclerosis. Clin Rheumatol. 2017;36(1):111–7. https://doi.org/10.1007/s10067-016-3412-9.
25. Di Liberto D, Scazzone C, La Rocca G, Cipriani P, Lo Pizzo M, Ruscitti P, et al. Vitamin D increases the production of IL-10 by regulatory T cells in patients with systemic sclerosis. Clin Exp Rheumatol. 2019;37(Suppl 119(4)):76–81.
26. Gambichler T, Chrobok I, Hoxtermann S, Kreuter A. Significantly decreased serum 25-hydroxyvitamin d levels in a large german systemic sclerosis cohort. J Rheumatol. 2011;38(11):2492–3 author reply 4.
27. Giuggioli D, Colaci M, Cassone G, Fallahi P, Lumetti F, Spinella A, et al. Serum 25-OH vitamin D levels in systemic sclerosis: analysis of 140 patients and review of the literature. Clin Rheumatol. 2017;36(3):583–90. https://doi.org/10.1007/s10067-016-3535-z.
28. Gupta S, Mahajan VK, Yadav RS, Mehta KS, Bhushan S, Chauhan PS, et al. Evaluation of serum vitamin D levels in patients with systemic sclerosis and healthy controls: results of a pilot study. Indian Dermatol Online J. 2018;9(4):250–5. https://doi.org/10.4103/idoj.IDOJ_328_17.
29. Hajialilo M, Noorabadi P, Tahsini Tekantapeh S, Malek MA. Endothelin-1, alpha-Klotho, 25(OH) Vit D levels and severity of disease in scleroderma patients. Rheumatol Int. 2017;37(10):1651–7. https://doi.org/10.1007/s00296-017-3797-z.
30. Hax V, Gasparin AA, Schneider L, Monticielo OA, Soares HMF, Streit MDA, et al. Vitamin D and cytokine profiles in patients with systemic sclerosis. J Clin Rheumatol. 2020;26(7):289–94. https://doi.org/10.1097/RHU.0000000000001112.
31. Kamal A, Gamal SM, Elgengehy FT, Alkemary AK, Siam I. Association of VDR ApaI and TaqI gene polymorphisms with the risk of scleroderma and Behcet's disease. Immunol Investig. 2016;45(6):531–42. https://doi.org/10.1080/08820139.2016.1180302.
32. Matsuoka LY, Dannenberg MJ, Wortsman J, Hollis BW, Jimenez SA, Varga J. Cutaneous vitamin D3 formation in progressive systemic sclerosis. J Rheumatol. 1991;18(8):1196–8.
33. Montabone E, Data V, Carignola R. Vitamin D status and quality of life in systemic sclerosis patients. J Clin Rheumatol. 2016;22(4):229–30. https://doi.org/10.1097/RHU.0000000000000406.
34. Orbach H, Zandman-Goddard G, Amital H, Barak V, Szekanecz Z, Szucs G, et al. Novel biomarkers in autoimmune diseases: prolactin, ferritin, vitamin D, and TPA levels in autoimmune diseases. Ann N Y Acad Sci. 2007;1109(1):385–400. https://doi.org/10.1196/annals.1398.044.
35. Park EK, Park JH, Kweon SM, Kim GT, Lee SG. Vitamin D deficiency is associated with digital ulcer but not with atherosclerosis or arterial stiffness in patients with systemic sclerosis: a pilot study. Clin Rheumatol. 2017;36(6):1325–33. https://doi.org/10.1007/s10067-017-3622-9.
36. Rios Fernandez R, Fernandez Roldan C, Callejas Rubio JL, Ortego CN. Vitamin D deficiency in a cohort of patients with systemic scleroderma from the south of Spain. J Rheumatol. 2010;37(6):1355; author reply 6. https://doi.org/10.3899/jrheum.091143.
37. Rios-Fernandez R, Callejas-Rubio JL, Fernandez-Roldan C, Simeon-Aznar CP, Garcia-Hernandez F, Castillo-Garcia MJ, et al. Bone mass and vitamin D in patients with systemic sclerosis from two Spanish regions. Clin Exp Rheumatol. 2012;30(6):905–11.
38. Seriolo B, Molfetta L, Cutolo M. Seasonal variations in serum levels of 25-hydroxyvitamin D in patients with systemic sclerosis. Clin Rheumatol. 2011;30(3):445–6. https://doi.org/10.1007/s10067-011-1684-7.
39. Shinjo SK, Bonfa E, de Falco CV, Pereira RM. Low bone mass in juvenile onset sclerosis systemic: the possible role for 25-hydroxyvitamin D insufficiency. Rheumatol Int. 2011;31(8):1075–80. https://doi.org/10.1007/s00296-010-1421-6.
40. Taylan A, Birlik M, Kenar G, Toprak B, Gundogdu B, Gurler O, et al. Osteoprotegrin interacts with biomarkers and cytokines that have roles in osteoporosis, skin fibrosis, and vasculopathy in systemic sclerosis: a potential multifaceted relationship between OPG/RANKL/TRAIL and Wnt inhibitors. Mod Rheumatol. 2019;29(4):619–24. https://doi.org/10.1080/14397595.2018.1500736.
41. Trombetta AC, Smith V, Gotelli E, Ghio M, Paolino S, Pizzorni C, et al. Vitamin D deficiency and clinical correlations in systemic sclerosis patients: a retrospective analysis for possible future developments. PLoS One. 2017;12(6):e0179062. https://doi.org/10.1371/journal.pone.0179062.
42. Ursini F, D'Angelo S, Padula A, Leccese P, Abignano G, Mennillo GA, et al. Vitamin D deficiency in systemic sclerosis: a possible role of subclinical liver fibrosis? Retrospective analysis from an Italian cohort. Clin Rheumatol. 2017;36(12):2871–2. https://doi.org/10.1007/s10067-017-3709-3.
43. Zhang L, Duan Y, Zhang TP, Huang XL, Li BZ, Ye DQ, et al. Association between the serum level of vitamin D and systemic sclerosis in a Chinese population: a case control study. Int J Rheum Dis. 2017;20(8):1002–8. https://doi.org/10.1111/1756-185X.12794.
44. Slominski A, Janjetovic Z, Tuckey RC, Nguyen MN, Bhattacharya KG, Wang J, et al. 20S-hydroxyvitamin D3, noncalcemic product of CYP11A1 action on vitamin D3, exhibits potent antifibrogenic activity in vivo. J Clin Endocrinol Metab. 2013;98(2):E298–303. https://doi.org/10.1210/jc.2012-3074.
45. Terao M, Yang L, Matsumura S, Yutani M, Murota H, Katayama I. A vitamin D analog inhibits Th2 cytokine- and TGFbeta -induced periostin production in fibroblasts: a potential role for vitamin D in skin sclerosis. Dermatoendocrinol. 2015;7(1):e1010983. https://doi.org/10.1080/19381980.2015.1010983.
46. Usategui A, Criado G, Del Rey MJ, Fare R, Pablos JL. Topical vitamin D analogue calcipotriol reduces skin fibrosis in experimental scleroderma. Arch Dermatol Res. 2014 Oct;306(8):757–61. https://doi.org/10.1007/s00403-014-1466-6.
47. Zerr P, Vollath S, Palumbo-Zerr K, Tomcik M, Huang J, Distler A, et al. Vitamin D receptor regulates TGF-beta signalling in systemic sclerosis. Ann Rheum Dis. 2015;74(3):e20. https://doi.org/10.1136/annrheumdis-2013-204378.
48. Antico A, Tampoia M, Tozzoli R, Bizzaro N. Can supplementation with vitamin D reduce the risk or modify the course of autoimmune diseases? A systematic review of the literature. Autoimmun Rev. 2012;12(2):127–36. https://doi.org/10.1016/j.autrev.2012.07.007.
49. An L, Sun MH, Chen F, Li JR. Vitamin D levels in systemic sclerosis patients: a meta-analysis. Drug Des Devel Ther. 2017;11:3119–25. https://doi.org/10.2147/DDDT.S144860.
50. Ross AC, Manson JE, Abrams SA, Aloia JF, Brannon PM, Clinton SK, et al. The 2011 report on dietary reference intakes for calcium and vitamin D from the Institute of Medicine: what clinicians need to know. J Clin Endocrinol Metab. 2011;96(1):53–8. https://doi.org/10.1210/jc.2010-2704.
51. Cantorna MT, Mahon BD. Mounting evidence for vitamin D as an environmental factor affecting autoimmune disease prevalence. Exp Biol Med (Maywood). 2004;229(11):1136–42. https://doi.org/10.1177/153537020422901108.
52. McGrath JJ, Saha S, Burne TH, Eyles DW. A systematic review of the association between common single nucleotide polymorphisms and 25-hydroxyvitamin D concentrations. J Steroid Biochem Mol Biol. 2010;121(1–2):471–7. https://doi.org/10.1016/j.jsbmb.2010.03.073.
53. Hewison M. An update on vitamin D and human immunity. Clin Endocrinol. 2012;76(3):315–25. https://doi.org/10.1111/j.1365-2265.2011.04261.x.
54. Helming L, Bose J, Ehrchen J, Schiebe S, Frahm T, Geffers R, et al. 1alpha,25-Dihydroxyvitamin D3 is a potent suppressor of interferon gamma-mediated macrophage activation. Blood. 2005;106(13):4351–8. https://doi.org/10.1182/blood-2005-03-1029.
55. Li J, Chen SY, Liu HH, Yin XD, Cao LT, Xu JH, et al. Associations of vitamin D receptor single nucleotide polymorphisms with susceptibility to systemic sclerosis. Arch Med Res. 2019;50(6):368–76. https://doi.org/10.1016/j.arcmed.2019.09.006.
56. Boelsma E, Pavel S, Ponec M. Effects of calcitriol on fibroblasts derived from skin of scleroderma patients. Dermatology. 1995;191(3):226–33. https://doi.org/10.1159/000246550.
57. Pattanaik D, Brown M, Postlethwaite BC, Postlethwaite AE. Pathogenesis of systemic sclerosis. Front Immunol. 2015;6:272.
58. Vacca A, Cormier C, Mathieu A, Kahan A, Allanore Y. Vitamin D levels and potential impact in systemic sclerosis. Clin Exp Rheumatol. 2011;29(6):1024–31.
59. Hollis BW. Editorial: the determination of circulating 25-hydroxyvitamin D: no easy task. J Clin Endocrinol Metab. 2004;89(7):3149–51. https://doi.org/10.1210/jc.2004-0682.
60. Schneider L, Dos Santos AS, Santos M, da Silva Chakr RM, Monticielo OA. Vitamin D and systemic lupus erythematosus: state of the art. Clin Rheumatol. 2014;33(8):1033–8.
61. Gurevitch J, Koricheva J, Nakagawa S. S Gavin. Meta-analysis and the science of research synthesis. Nature. 2018;555(7695):175–82. https://doi.org/10.1038/nature25753.
62. Lee YH. An overview of meta-analysis for clinicians. Korean J Intern Med. 2018;33(2):277–83. https://doi.org/10.3904/kjim.2016.195.

18

Rheumatologist perspective of the Brazilian consensus for detection of auto antibodies in HEp-2 CELLS

Isadora Carvalho Medeiros Francescantonio[1], Leandro Augusto Rodrigues dos Santos[1], Paulo Luiz Carvalho Francescantonio[1], Luiz Eduardo Coelho Andrade[2] and Wilson de Melo Cruvinel[1*]

Abstract

Objective: To evaluate the perception of rheumatologists regarding the recommendations of the Brazilian Consensus for detection of Autoantibodies (BCA) on HEp-2 Cells by Indirect Immunofluorescence assay (IFA) and how BCA recommendations help in clinical practice.

Methodology: A structured questionnaire regarding the BCA recommendations for detection and interpretations of autoantibodies in HEp-2 cells was applied to randomly selected rheumatologists. The results were tabulated using the Microsoft® Excel program, expressed as a simple percentage and the dichotomous data were analyzed using the Chi-square test and the Epi Info® program.

Results: Four hundred fuorteen rheumatologists participated in the study: 70% of them considered their knowledge of the HEp-2 IFA test satisfactory or excellent, and 43% said they knew the BCA recommendations in general, without distinguishing the edition of the BCA to which they refer. The Revista Brasileira de Rheumatologia/ Advances in Rheumatology was the means of dissemination most consulted by specialists (50%). According to the rheumatologists' opinion, the most relevant pattern was the homogeneous nuclear (78%) and 65% stated they were satisfied with the BCA recommendations at a level of satisfaction greater than or equal to 80%. There was no significant difference in the perception of rheumatologists from the several Brazilian geographic regions.

Conclusion: Brazilian rheumatologists are aware of the BCA guidelines and most are satisfied with the content published, considering that the BCA recommendations assist positively in the clinical practice. Most rheumatologists recognize the patterns associated with rheumatic autoimmune diseases and have used BCA recommendations to interpret the results of the HEp-2 IFA test.

Keywords: Anti-nuclear antibodies, ANA, HEp-2, Autoimmunity

Introduction

The evaluation of autoantibodies by indirect immunofluorescence in HEp-2 cells (IFA HEp-2) represents, in the current context, a relevant tool for the diagnostic investigation of systemic autoimmune diseases in the scope of rheumatology, hepatology, pulmonology, dermatology, hematology, and other medical specialties [1]. In recent years, the test methodology has undergone an intense improvement and standardization process, especially regarding diagnostic performance and interpretation [2–6]. Such standardization procedures began in Brazil in 2000, in Goiania, with the first Brazilian Consensus for antinuclear antibodies detection on HEp-2 cells (BCA), serving as a reference for other international standardization initiatives, with emphasis for the International Consensus on ANA Patterns - ICAP [7–11].

* Correspondence: melocruvinel@gmail.com
[1] Pontifícia Universidade Católica de Goiás (PUC Goiás), Escola de Ciências Médicas, Farmacêuticas e Biomédicas, Avenida Universitária 1.440, Setor Universitário, Goiânia, GO, Brazil

Five editions of the BCA and four international Workshops were published on the matter [2–11].

The first BCA was motivated by three main aspects: 1) heterogeneous nomenclature of the immunofluorescence patterns in Brazil since the same pattern had different denominations; 2) absence of parametric guidelines for reading the slides; and 3) lack of an algorithm for pattern organization into coherent classification groups [2].

The BCA organized the various patterns into coherent groups and stratified them in a classification tree [2]. The recognition, denomination, and classification of the patterns followed morphological criteria, i.e., the nomenclature and classification obeyed and reflected the distinctive morphological characteristics of each pattern. Besides, the first edition of the BCA encompassed the initial sample dilution approach for assay screening and indicated a systematic protocol for reading the slides [2].

Standardization recommendations were improved along successive BCA editions, encompassing new recommendations based on the doubts that arose by using the recommendations and classifications established in previous versions [3–6].

In 2014, during the 12th Workshop on Autoantibodies and Autoimmunity in São Paulo - Brazil, the First International Consensus on ANA Patterns (ICAP) was held [7]. With participation of European, North American, South American, and Asian specialists, this initiative adopted the Brazilian Consensus basic guidelines and defined a classification tree with three groups: nuclear, cytoplasmic, and mitotic [7]. In their first edition, the patterns received alphanumeric codes from AC-1 to AC-28 [7]. Some patterns discussed were not incorporated into the classification tree, reserved for subsequent discussions [7]. The first ICAP has already highlighted some clinical correlations of the patterns presented [7]. The international ICAP group produced four additional publications that, like BCA, have progressively improved the initial recommendations based on the practical application of the proposed algorithm, community feedback, and the acquisition of new scientific information [8–11].

In 2018, the fourth ICAP workshop, held in Germany during the 13th Dresden Autoantibody Symposium, recognized and incorporated the AC-0 pattern into the classification tree, defined as the pattern for a negative reaction; the AC-XX pattern, used to report patterns not included in the tree; and the AC-29 pattern, corresponding to the characteristic compound pattern caused by anti-topoisomerase I antibodies [9, 11].

The V BCA, held in 2016 during the XXXIII Brazilian Congress of Rheumatology, had as main objective the harmonization between the algorithms of the Brazilian and International Consensus [6]. Thus, the V BCA incorporated the ICAP alphanumeric code system for the classification of BCA patterns. However, in some specific points, the original arrangement of BCA was maintained: 1) the recognition of 33 patterns was kept while ICAP recognizes 30 patterns; 2) nucleolar patterns were maintained as a distinct group; 3) the dichotomous classification of the speckled nuclear pattern was preserved in two subgroups, with positive metaphase plate and negative metaphase plate, respectively; 4) the centromere pattern linked to the group of speckled nuclear patterns was maintained; 5) the speckled pattern with isolated dots was maintained in the subgroup of the negative metaphase plate patterns; 6) the Mitotic chromosomal pattern (AC-28) was not incorporated; 7) the concept of compound patterns was maintained, encompassing the CENP-F and Topo I patterns, among the rest of the group of compound patterns [6]. Finally, the V BCA recommends the designation (ANA - anti-cell antibody test) for the assay, in Portuguese *"FAN - Pesquisa de Anticorpos Anticélula"* [6]. With respect to the name of the test, it is worth noting that the following VI BCA Workshop, during the 36th Brazilian Congress of Rheumatology, held in Fortaleza in 2019, decided to adhere to the ICAP recommendation, stating that the name of the test should emphasize the method (indirect immunofluorescence assay on HEp-2 cells - HEp-2 IFA). The designation HEp-2 IFA contemplates reactivity against the various cellular domains and not only to the nucleus, as is the case for antinuclear antibody test.

Based on the BCA pioneering spirit and the development of ICAP in recent years, there has been a continuous wide-ranging international discussion that has led to significant evolution and implementation of methodological and interpretative criteria. It included the recognition of more than 30 simple patterns, the inclusion of new patterns, several possibilities of compound patterns, as well as progressive encouragement to the implementation of standardized parameters of reading, interpretation, and quality control of the HEp-2 IFA test [2–5]. Faced with this continually changing reality, physicians who deal with the interpretation of HEp-2 IFA reports daily must be updated and able to interpret the results in all their magnitude and carry out a relevant clinical correlation for patients' benefit.

As a screening test for the presence of autoantibodies, there is no perfect association between the pattern and the specific autoantibody in the sample. For this reason, isolated HEp-2 IFA results do not allow definitive clinical conclusions. Concerning immunological associations, various patterns suggest certain autoantibodies; however, specific immunoassays must confirm these in any given sample. Thus, the potential benefit of HEp-2 IFA in the clinical practice depends on the attending physician's knowledge about its limitations, the significance of each immunofluorescence pattern, and the impact of the titer [12]. Its use in the clinical practice comes up against some obstacles, such as the historical paradigm that a positive HEp-2 IFA test necessarily implies autoimmune disease as well as the contrasts in the previous literature and BCA/ICAP recommendations regarding pattern designation and correlations with autoantibodies and diseases [12].

Systemic Lupus Erythematosus (SLE), characterized by an extremely high frequency of positive HEp-2 IFA results, can elicit different patterns according to the type of underlying autoantibody [12]. However, a positive HEp-2 IFA result happens in several other diseases, up to 35% at the 1/40 dilution [13] including asymptomatic individuals that show a positivity rate between 12 and 20% positivity at the 1/80 dilution [14]. This positivity rate in apparently healthy individuals reflects possibly a certain degree of physiological autoimmunity. This tendency seems exacerbated in patients with non-autoimmune diseases, which present a higher frequency and titer of HEp-2 IFA than healthy individuals [13–15].

The unawareness of the limitation that a positive HEp-2 IFA test may occur in non-autoimmune individuals could lead to an incorrect diagnosis of autoimmunity, generating exposure to unnecessary and potentially harmful treatment [12]. This scenario can be exacerbated because of the significant heterogeneity of methodological protocols and criteria for the exam interpretation. Therefore, to support the assistant physician's clinical reasoning, consistent standardization in the test methodology, interpretation, and reporting is essential [7, 16].

Regarding the clinical laboratory and the direct patient care, the consensus in HEp-2 IFA aim to offer such standardization guidelines to health professionals, aiming to ensure the best results for patients' treatment. It is up to the professional involved in dealing with this test to know the methodological and interpretation guidelines and to contribute to its improvement. Considering that BCA is completing two decades of existence, it is essential to investigate its penetration among the specialist most frequently interested in its use, that is, the rheumatologist. This study intended to evaluate rheumatologists' knowledge about BCA guidelines and how BCA recommendations help their clinical practice.

Methodology

This is a cross-sectional quantitative study, carried out using a structured questionnaire drawn up together with the Laboratory Committee of the Brazilian Society of Rheumatology (SBR). The work was approved by the research ethics committee of the Pontifícia Universidade Católica de Goiás (PUC Goiás), under the number 2872574.

The virtual questionnaire development used HTML5, CSS3, JQuery, and PHP 5, in a MySQL database hosted on a server with Linux Operating System and Apache 2.2 web server. The structured questionnaire form was applied using a virtual platform at the official electronic address of the Brazilian Consensus as well as using a physical form during the 36th Brazilian Congress of Rheumatology in Fortaleza, Ceará (detailed below).

The SBR Laboratory Committee sent an e-mail to all rheumatologists enrolled in the SBR with an invitation to participate in the survey, with the respective link to access the form. The invitation link directed the participant to the official page of the Brazilian Consensus (http://www.hep-2.com.br), where the physician first accessed the informed consent form. After voluntary agreement, the participant was directed to the survey form. To avoid double responses by the same physician, participants provided their e-mail, and the platform restricted one response to each e-mail address. The questionnaire was available online to participants for the entire survey period, which was from January to December 2019, so that during the entire survey period the participants could edit their responses. After confirming responses, the participant no longer had access to edit the submitted form. Participants that did not complete the form as well as non-rheumatologists were excluded from the survey.

In addition to the virtual platform, face-to-face data collection took place during the 36th Brazilian Congress of Rheumatology. With authorization from SBR, the congress participants were approached and invited to fill in the survey form, either online, as detailed in the previous paragraph, or using a physical questionnaire form to be posted on the digital platform. From these two platforms, we obtained responses from 521 participants. Participants that did not complete the form and those that did not refer to themselves as rheumatologists had their records dismissed and therefore 414 participants were eligible to compose the sample.

The data analysis used a simple percentage method from the Microsoft® Excel 2016 program and the Chi-square test was used to dichotomous comparisons by geographic regions, after excluding the non-responders and non-rheumatologists, using the Epi Info™ program. A threshold of 0.05 was defined for the establishment of statistical significance.

Results

The SBR database registers 2359 rheumatologists as members. Of these, 3.7% (87) are in the North region, 15.4% (363) in the Northeast, 7.8% (185) in the Midwest, 57.6% (1559) in the Southeast, and 15.8% (365) in the South region of the country. The sample consisted of 414 participants, representing 17.5% of the SBR member-rheumatologists. This amount was considered satisfactory since a representative sample would correspond to 331 participants, with a 95% confidence interval, calculated by the software BioEstat 5.3.

As shown in Table 1, there were participants from all Brazilian regions, covering the 26 Brazilian states and the Federal District, with the largest number of participants from the Southeast followed by Northeast, South, Midwest, and North regions. Five participants (1.2%) did not answer question regarding the Brazilian region.

Regarding the nature of the institutions where the rheumatologists worked (public and private), the group proved quite heterogeneous. Among the 414 participants, 44% (184) work in institutions of the Brazilian Unified Health System, 7% (29) in state public universities and 17% (70) in federal public universities, 72% (298) in private institutions, and 10% (42) in private universities. One hundred and sixty-one (39.0%) participants stated that they work simultaneously in public and private institutions. Of the total, 25 (6%) participants did not answer this question.

One of the aspects evaluated was the self-perception of rheumatologists' knowledge about BCA guidelines. As detailed in Table 2, we observed a considerable variation in this parameter: 70% of the participants said they had satisfactory or excellent knowledge, 19% average knowledge, and 8% scarce or insufficient knowledge. Only 3% of respondents did not answer this query. When we grouped the degree of knowledge attributed to the BCA into two categories, we verified no statistically significant difference between the country's five regions (Table 2).

Table 1 Distribution of rheumatologists and participants according to the state of the federation

Region	State	Number of rheumatologists	Number of study participants
North 18 (4%)	Acre	5 (0.2%)[a]	1 (20%)[b]
	Amazonas	17 (1%)	5 (29%)
	Amapá	5 (0.2%)	1 (20%)
	Pará	30 (1%)	6 (20%)
	Rondônia	11 (1%)	2 (18%)
	Roraima	2 (0.1%)	1 (50%)
	Tocantins	13 (1%)	2 (15%)
Northeast 72 (17%)	Alagoas	27 (3%)	4 (15%)
	Bahia	65 (3%)	10 (15%)
	Ceará	75 (3%)	16 (21%)
	Maranhão	13 (1%)	6 (46%)
	Paraíba	38 (2%)	3 (8%)
	Pernambuco	47 (2%)	16 (34)
	Piauí	24 (1%)	6 (25%)
	Rio Grande do Norte	34 (2%)	8 (24%)
	Sergipe	18 (1%)	3 (17%)
Midwest 37 (9%)	Federal District	105 (5%)	13 (12%)
	Goiás	56 (3%)	16 (29%)
	Mato Grosso	26 (1%)	2 (8%)
	Mato Grosso do Sul	45 (2%)	6 (13%)
Southeast 230 (56%)	Espírito Santo	71 (3%)	7 (10%)
	Minas Gerais	260 (12%)	50 (19%)
	Rio de Janeiro	163 (8%)	42 (26%)
	São Paulo	563 (26%)	131 (23%)
South 52 (13%)	Paraná	179 (8%)	29 (16%)
	Rio Grande do Sul	167 (8%)	8 (5%)
	Santa Catarina	91 (4%)	15 (16%)
	BRAZIL	2150 (100%)[c]	409 (19%)

[a] Percentage concerning the total number of rheumatologists in the country; [b] Percentage concerning the total number of rheumatologists in the respective State; [c] Total rheumatologists in Brazil, data obtained from the federal council of medicine

Table 2 Rheumatologists' self-assessment regarding knowledge about the Brazilian Consensus on antinuclear antibodies

Region	N	NE	CO	S	SE	SR	Total
Total Participants	**18 (4%)[a]**	**72 (17%)**	**37 (9%)**	**52 (13%)**	**230 (56%)**	**5 (1%)**	**414 (100%)**
Knowledge about the Brazilian Consensus in IFA-HEp 2:							
Satisfactory	14 (78%)[b]	38 (53%)	20 (54%)	29 (56%)	138 (60%)	2 (40%)	241 (58%)
Limited	2 (11%)	4 (6%)	2 (5%)	3 (6%)	9 (4%)	1 (20%)	21 (5%)
Reasonable	1 (5,5%)	19 (26%)	8 (22%)	14 (27%)	37 (16%)	1 (20%)	80 (19%)
Excellent	1 (5,5%)	10 (14%)	3 (8%)	4 (8%)	30 (13%)	1 (20%)	49 (12%)
Insufficient	0 (0%)	0 (0%)	1 (3%)	2 (4%)	8 (3%)	0 (0%)	11 (3%)
I don't know yet	0 (0%)	0 (0%)	0 (0%)	0 (0%)	1 (0%)	0 (0%)	1 (0%)
Did not answer	0 (0%)	1 (1%)	3 (8%)	0 (0%)	7 (3%)	0 (0%)	11 (3%)
Satisfactory/Excellent	15 (83%)	48 (68%)	23 (68%)	33 (63%)	168 (75%)	3 (60%)	290 (72%)[c]
Medium/Little/Insufficient	3 (17%)	23 (32%)	11 (30%)	19 (58%)	54 (23%)	2 (40%)	113 (27%)[c]

[a] Percentage in relation to the total number of participants; [b] Percentage of total participants in the region; [c] Percentage in relation to the total of respondents in each region. Chi-square test: $p = 0.237$

The knowledge of each edition of the BCA by the participants showed an increase over the successive editions: 16% (65) of the participants said they knew the first BCA, 14% (60) the second BCA, 28% (114) the third BCA, 36% (151) the fourth BCA and 37% (155) the fifth BCA, with 43% (180) saying that they know the recommendations in general without distinguishing the edition of the BCA which they refer to. Only 2% (10) said they were unaware of the Brazilian Consensus and 3% (13) of the participants did not answer this query.

Concerning the first access to the BCA material, 50% (205) of the participants were introduced to the BCA by the Brazilian Journal of Rheumatology, currently Advances in Rheumatology, 1% (6) by the Brazilian Journal of Clinical Pathology and Laboratory Medicine, 28% (114) in conferences at congresses, 30% (125) by Internet search, 5% (17) by communications from scientific societies and 14% (60) by the official BCA website (www.hep-2.com.br). A total of 4% (18) did not inform the source of information for BCA access, and 5% (19) did not answer this query. It is worth noting that the form allowed indicating more than one possibility; therefore, several participants informed more than one source for learning about BCA.

The frequency of HEp-2 IFA tests requested by the participants averaged 10.7 tests per week, with little significant variation among the five regions of the country (Table 3).

When asked about the use of BCA recommendations to support clinical correlations, 86% (354) of the participants stated that they use the recommendations daily, while 10% (44) said they do not use them at all, and 4% (16) of the participants did not answer this query (Table 4). The analysis using the 5 × 2 chi-square test, comparing the country's macro-regions, did not show any statistically significant difference for this parameter.

Regarding BCA's contributions to the HEp-2 IFA report, 76% (315) of the participants consider that the process of nomenclature standardization has made their understanding clearer, while 7% (29) think otherwise. In this assessment, 17% (70) did not answer this query (Table 4). The analysis using the chi-square test showed that there was no statistically significant difference among the five macro-regions of the country.

Assessing the influence of BCA on clinical correlations, 78% of participants (321) believe that BCA has made clinical correlations clearer, while 5% (17) think otherwise and 17% (72) of participants have not responded to this question (Table 4). Again, the analysis using the chi-square test showed that no statistically significant difference among the five macro-regions of the country.

Table 3 Frequency of HEp-2 IFA tests requested per week by rheumatologists in the five Brazilian macro-regions

Geographic region	N	NE	CO	S	SE	NS	Total
Number of rheumatologists	18 (4%)	72 (17%)	37 (9%)	52 (13%)	230 (56%)	5 (1%)	414 (100%)
Average (standard deviation) IFA-HEp2 exams ordered per week							
Average	**9.5 ± 8.96**	**11.8 ± 14.83**	**12.5 ± 11.04**	**8.3 ± 6.45**	**11.0 ± 9.85**	**10.7 ± 10.69**	
No answer	2	2	7	3	20	1	35

N North, *NE* Northeast; *CO* Midwest; *S* South; *SE* Southeast, *NS* Not specified

Table 4 Rheumatologist's perception of the role of the Brazilian Consensus in clinical practice

Geographic Macro-Region	N	NE	CO	S	SE	SR	Total
Number of rheumatologists	18 (4%)	72 (17%)	37 (9%)	52 (13%)	230 (56%)	5 (1%)	414 (100%)
Do you rely on BCA recommendations to support clinical correlations? *							
Yes	13 (72%)	64 (89%)	33 (89%)	46 (88%)	193 (84%)	5 (100%)	354 (86%)
No	3 (17%)	6 (8%)	1 (3%)	5 (10%)	29 (13%)	0 (0%)	44 (10%)
Did not answer	2 (11%)	2 (3%)	3 (8%)	1 (2%)	8 (3%)	0 (0%)	16 (4%)
Did BCA make the understanding of the report clearer? **							
Yes	15 (83%)	60 (83%)	29 (78%)	40 (77%)	168 (73%)	3 (60%)	315 (76%)
No	1 (6%)	2 (3%)	1 (3%)	4 (8%)	19 (8%)	2 (40%)	29 (7%)
Did not answer	2 (11%)	10 (14%)	7 (19%)	8 (15%)	43 (19%)	0 (0%)	70 (17%)
Has the Consensus made clinical correlations clearer? ***							
Yes	14 (78%)	61 (85%)	28 (76%)	43 (83%)	172 (75%)	3 (60%)	321 (78%)
No	1 (5%)	2 (3%)	2 (5%)	0 (0%)	14 (6%)	2 (40%)	21 (5%)
Did not answer	3 (17%)	9 (12%)	7 (19%)	9 (17%)	44 (19%)	0 (0%)	72 (17%)

N North, *NO* Northeast; *CO* Midwest; *S* South; *SE* Southeast, *SR* No region.
Chi-square test: *$p = 0.329$, **$p = 0.386$, ***$p = 0.59$

When asked about the information that should be present in the HEp-2 IFA report, 76% (316) indicated the identification of the pattern name, 25% (103) supported the inclusion of the international alphanumeric code of the pattern (AC code from ICAP), 63% (261) the final title, 47% (194) the cell compartment that appears fluorescent, 32% (134) the information about the chromosomal metaphase plate, 38% (158) the note with the pattern clinical relevance, and 35% (144) the HEp-2 IFA patterns in previous exams, with 19% (79) of the participants not answering this query. It is worth noting that the form allowed indicating more than one possibility; therefore, several participants informed more than one item to be included in the report.

Table 5 details the participants' perception of the importance of different nuclear patterns. Most rheumatologists demonstrated intimacy with the various nuclear patterns, and the perceived relevance varied among patterns. The most recognized nuclear patterns were the homogeneous (AC-1), coarse speckled (AC-5), and centromere (AC-3). The fine speckled nuclear pattern (AC-4) was considered relevant by just over half of the participants, while the dense fine speckled (AC-2) and reticular coarse speckled (BAC-4) patterns were considered pertinent by about 1/3 of the participants. The other nuclear patterns were considered relevant by only a small portion of the participants. One percent said they were unfamiliar with these patterns, and 0.5% did not consider these types of pattern to be necessary.

Regarding the nucleolar group, still in Table 5, these patterns were also recognized by most of the participants. The most acknowledged patterns were the homogeneous (AC-8) and the punctate (AC-10). Only 9% of participants did not confirm familiarity with this group of patterns, and 1% did not consider them essential.

When asked about the importance of the cytoplasmic pattern group, the most acknowledged was the fine speckled (AC-20) and the reticular speckled (AC-21). In general, the interviewees were less familiar with the cytoplasmic group of patterns, but only 16% said they did not know any the of the cytoplasmic patterns (Table 5).

Regarding the mitotic group patterns, the most acknowledged were the mitotic spindle fibers and the Spindle fibers NuMA-2 (AC-25). Also the mitotic group of patterns was unknown for many of the participants, with 26% saying they did not know them at all. In the histograms presented in Fig. 1, it is possible to verify in global terms the percentage of relevance attributed by rheumatologists to each group of patterns: nuclear, nucleolar, cytoplasmic, and mitotic.

Figure 2 shows the degree of satisfaction of the participants regarding the contributions of the Consensus (Brazilian and International) to clinical practice, graded on a scale from 0 to 10. The BCA was rated as ≥7.0 by 74% of the participants, as ≥8.0 by 65%, and as ≥9.0 by 41% of the participants.

When asked about the awareness on the International Consensus (ICAP), 50% (208) of the participants said they know it, and 30% (123) said they do not know it, and 20% (83) of the participants did not answer this query. In relation to the assessment of ICAP's contribution to the clinical practice, on a scale of 0 to 10 regarding the participant's satisfaction with the contributions of ICAP to clinical practice, 50% assigned a score ≥ 7.0, and 22.5% a score ≤ 6.0.

Table 5 Distribution of nuclear, nucleolar, cytoplasmic and mitotic apparatus patterns according to the relevance perceived by rheumatologists in different Brazilian macro-regions

Macro-region	N	NE	CO	S	SE	SR	Total
Total	18 (4%)	72 (17%)	37 (9%)	52 (13%)	230 (56%)	5 (1%)	414 (100%)
Nuclear patterns							
Reticular coarse	28%[a]	28%	24%	40%	34%	20%	32%
Quasi-homogeneous	17%	29%	35%	33%	17%	20%	23%
Homogenous	78%	83%	78%	71%	79%	40%	78%
Dense fine speckled	39%	33%	35%	23%	30%	60%	31%
Centromere	44%	63%	59%	75%	67%	20%	65%
Fine speckled	56%	56%	49%	58%	56%	40%	55%
Large/coarse speckled	83%	82%	62%	75%	71%	40%	73%
Multiple nuclear dots	6%	8%	14%	10%	5%	0%	7%
Smooth/Punctate nuclear envelope	11%	8%	8%	13%	11%	0%	10%
Pleomorfic/PCNA	6%	14%	11%	13%	16%	0%	14%
Not familiar with the patterns	0%	0%	0%	0%	1%	0%	1%
Considers the patterns unimportant	0,5%	1%	0%	0%	0%	0%	0%
Did not answer	11%	7%	19%	13%	14%	40%	13%
Nucleolar patterns							
Homogeneous nucleolar	67%	58%	70%	67%	61%	40%	62%
Clumpy nucleolar	11%	13%	24%	19%	22%	40%	20%
Punctate nucleolar	44%	43%	49%	40%	43%	60%	44%
Not familiar	6%	8%	5%	8%	10%	0%	9%
Unimportant	0%	4%	0%	0%	0%	0%	1%
Did not answer	17%	11%	19%	15%	15%	40%	15%
Cytoplasmic patterns							
Fibrillar linear	17%	14%	8%	21%	14%	0%	14%
Fibrillar filamentous	6%	11%	14%	19%	9%	0%	11%
Fibrillar segmental	6%	8%	5%	13%	10%	0%	9%
Discrete dots	17%	14%	19%	19%	18%	0%	17%
Dense fine speckled	22%	32%	30%	21%	29%	20%	28%
Fine speckled	17%	33%	35%	27%	42%	20%	36%
Reticular/AMA	22%	33%	35%	40%	30%	60%	33%
Polar speckled	6%	14%	14%	17%	9%	20%	11%
Rods and rings	6%	28%	22%	19%	13%	0%	17%
Not familiar with the patterns	6%	13%	11%	17%	18%	0%	16%
Considers unimportant the patterns	11%	57%	0%	2%	0%	0%	2%
Did not answer	17%	13%	19%	15%	17%	40%	17%
Mitotic patterns							
Spindle fibers	0%	24%	32%	19%	38%	40%	31%
Centrosome	11%	19%	24%	25%	18%	20%	19%
Spidle fibers NuMA II	28%	32%	27%	40%	31%	0%	32%
Intercellular bridge	6%	21%	8%	17%	11%	20%	13%
Not familiar with the patterns	33%	31%	14%	29%	26%	20%	26%
Considers unimportant the patterns	6%	13%	0%	2%	0%	0%	3%
Did not answer	22%	14%	22%	17%	19%	40%	18%

[a] Frequency of participants who consider the pattern relevant (in brackets the percentage relative to the total number of participants who answered this question in the respective region of the country)
N North, *NE* Northeast; *CO* Midwest; *S* South; *SE* Southeast, *SR* No region

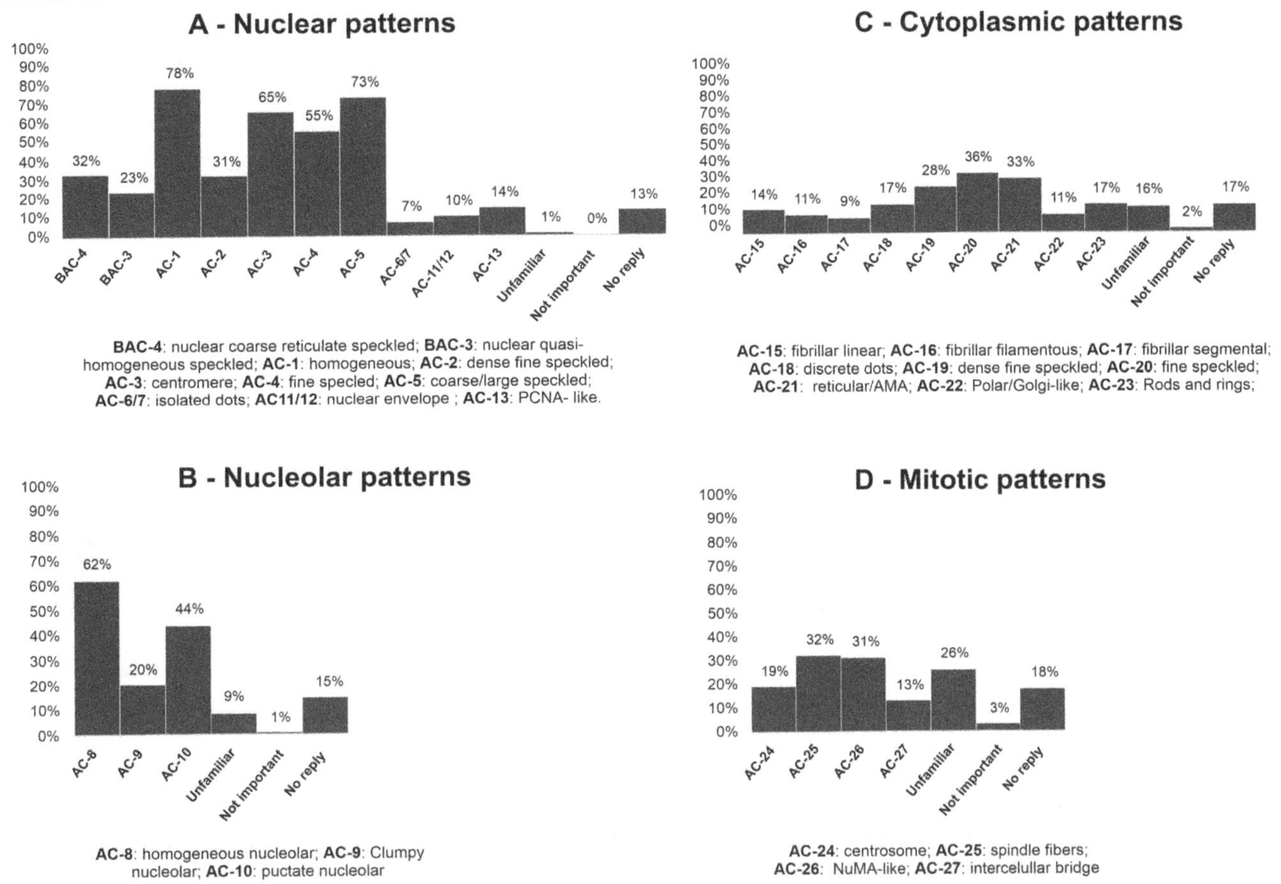

Fig. 1 Relevance attribute by rheumatologist to the four groups of autoantibody patterns in HEp-2 cells: nuclear, nucleolar, cytoplasmic and mitotic. Histograms depict the frequency of participants that classify the patterns as relevant. Unfamiliar and Not important refer to the group of patterns in each cell compartment.

Discussion

The present study analyzed Brazilian rheumatologists' opinions about BCA's recommendations, the first evaluation of medical opinion 20 years after the first BCA Workshop [2]. Of the 414 participants included in the study, all are self-reported rheumatologists. The group contained representatives from the 26 Brazilian States and the Federal District, and these specialists operate in 127 Brazilian cities.

Systemic Autoimmune Rheumatic Diseases (SARD), a major object of study by the rheumatologist, consist of a group of diseases whose investigation may include the identification of autoantibodies, which function as diagnostic markers [12, 17]. These autoantibodies can be screened by the indirect immunofluorescence assay in HEp-2 cells, being expressed as immunofluorescence patterns [12]. Autoantibodies are part of the classification criteria of several SARD. In SLE, for example, the HEp-2 IFA test is positive in 95 to 100% of patients; in Systemic Sclerosis, in 60–80%; in Sjögren's Syndrome, in 40–70%; in Dermatomyositis, in 30–80% [18]. When a 1: 80 serum dilution is considered in healthy individuals, there is a 10–13% positivity of the test [14, 18]. Thus, the test alone does not determine any diagnosis [18]. It is just one of the classification criteria that can also be used in the list of diagnostic elements [19].

Among the limitations of the test are the fact that healthy individuals may have a positive test; diseases can be associated with different HEp-2 IFA patterns; variation between patterns may depend on variations in the test substrate [12, 14]. Thus, the clinical relevance depends on the close correlation between the clinical context and the HEp-2 IFA pattern, both of which will to guide the next step, i.e., for the determination of disease-associated autoantibodies [12, 18].

Most of the participants in this study, 70% (290), considered their knowledge regarding the HEp-2 IFA test to be satisfactory or excellent. In comparison, 27% (112) considered it unsatisfactory. This percentage of 27% is considered high since the test is a diagnostic tool for frequent diseases in this specialist's clinical practice. Therefore, it is necessary to reinforce BCA's educational actions through continuing education projects in partnership with the Brazilian Society of Rheumatology. The

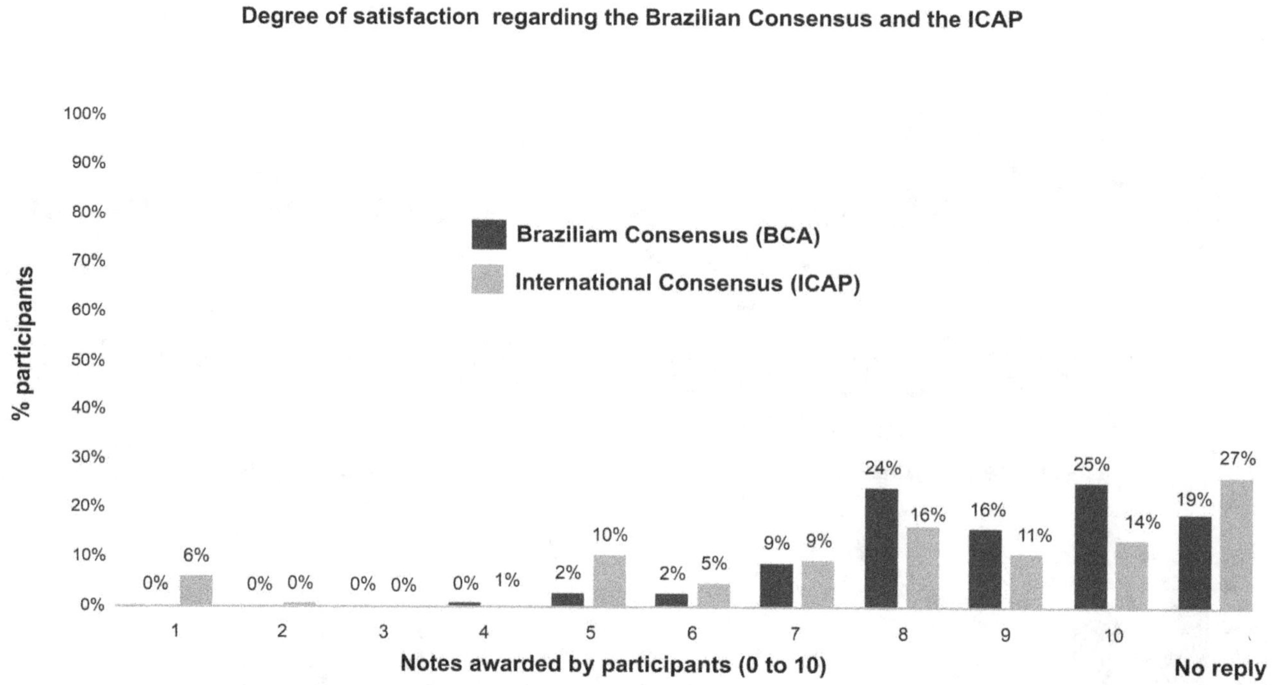

Fig. 2 Degree of satisfaction attribute of rheumatologist regarding the contributions of the Brazilian Consensus and the ICAP to clinical practice,

use of the HEp-2 IFA test in clinical practice is an important diagnostic tool and can only reach its full potential if there is complete knowledge of the specialists on how to interpret the test report. When this does not occur, the chance of misdiagnosis increases, and healthy individuals may be considered sick and vice versa. In addition, the correct ordering of reflex disease-specific antibodies is strongly helped by the knowledge of the relevance of HEp-2 IFA patterns [18].

The BCA was created to help the access to information about the HEp-2 IFA test and to systematize the interpretation of patterns regarding applicability in clinical practice. In addition, the standardized BCA nomenclature allows the reports to be reliable, reproducible, and suitable for long-term comparison [6–10]. The BCA information has been disseminated for about 20 years, and, in a way, it has been helping and guiding the rheumatologists' clinical practice when it comes to the HEp-2 IFA test interpretation. This action has been successful since only 2% of the study participants reported not knowing BCA.

About the use of BCA recommendations in clinical practice, 86% (354) of the participants stated that they use these guidelines to facilitate clinical correlations, 76% (315) consider that the proposed nomenclature standardization process made the understanding of the reports clearer, and 78% (321) believe that BCA has made the clinical correlations as explicit as possible. Also, 65% of the participants said that their satisfaction with the BCA information is greater than or equal to 80%. Therefore, we conclude that the BCA information has been useful for those who use such information in their routine operation.

Regarding the ways of getting to know the BCA material, 50% of the participants had access to the BCA by the journal *Advances in Rheumatology*, previously Brazilian Journal of Rheumatology, while only 14% actively sought an update through the BCA web page (http://www.hep-2.com.br/). Such data reinforces the need for joint work among the BCA team, rheumatologists, the SBR Laboratory Commission, and the Brazilian Society of Rheumatology, aiming to disseminate information and expand access.

When asked about the importance of several patterns, the participants considered the homogeneous nuclear pattern (AC-1) as the most important (78%). Such information is consistent because this pattern is present almost exclusively in individuals with autoimmune diseases, especially in SLE [12, 20]. This pattern is related to anti-native DNA antibodies, which occur in 50–80% of individuals with SLE and is used to monitor disease activity. It is also related to the anti-nucleosome antibody, also a specific marker for SLE. Finally, the AC-1 pattern is associated with the anti-histone antibody, which is also frequently related to SLE and in drug-induced SLE [4, 12, 15].

Another pattern also pointed out as relevant was the nuclear centromere/AC-3 (65%), strongly associated to systemic sclerosis and, as such, included in the classification criteria for this disease [12]. Its positivity in individuals with this diagnosis is around 70% [18].

The coarse speckled nuclear pattern (AC-5) was also considered relevant by 73% of the participants. It can be found in individuals with SLE, systemic sclerosis, undifferentiated connective tissue disease, systemic sclerosis overlap syndrome - autoimmune myopathy, and mixed connective tissue disease [12, 20]. Its frequency varies among these autoimmune diseases, being virtually 100% in mixed connective tissue disease [20].

The fine speckled nuclear pattern (AC-4) was deemed essential by 55% of the participants and it is associated with the presence of anti-SS-B/La and anti-SS-A/Ro autoantibodies, found in Sjögren's syndrome, SLE, cutaneous lupus erythematosus, neonatal lupus, rheumatoid arthritis, myositis associated with systemic sclerosis, and polymyositis [12, 20]. Its frequency in individuals with these disease varies from 15 to 65% [20].

Among the participants, 62% of them find the homogeneous nucleolar pattern (AC-8) important. It is associated with anti-PM/Scl antibody when it is accompanied by a nuclear fine speckled pattern, being observed mainly in the association of systemic sclerosis and inflammatory myopathy [12, 20]. Other thant that, the AC-8 pattern may indicate the rare anti-To/Th antibodies. Interestingly, a low number of rheumatologists attributed importance to the clumpy nucleolar pattern (AC-9). However, this pattern is associated with the anti-fibrillarin antibody, a specific marker of systemic sclerosis. Considering the high number of rheumatologists who attributed importance to homogeneous nucleolar patterns (62%) and nucleolar speckled patterns (40 to 60%), many can speculate that several rheumatologists were mistaken when answering the questionnaire, taking the nucleolar patterns by nuclear patterns. This possible mistake could explain the high degree of importance given to the homogeneous nucleolar pattern, since the homogeneous nuclear pattern (AC-1) has justified importance. However, this is a speculative possibility that would need further investigation.

In general, the patterns best known by rheumatologists are related to recurrent diseases in the clinical practice and the same disease can be associated with different patterns [10, 20]. With this perspective, the relevance attributed by rheumatologists to the four groups of autoantibody patterns was greater for the nuclear and nucleolar patterns, followed by cytoplasmic and mitotic.

It is noteworthy that some patterns with no established clinical correlation were also considered important by a large number of specialists. As examples, we have the *quasi*-homogeneous speckled nuclear pattern (BAC-3) that was considered necessary by 23% of the participants; and the nuclear reticular coarse speckled (BAC-4), which was deemed important by 32% of the participants. In contrast, the dense fine speckled cytoplasmic pattern (AC-19), associated with the presence of anti-P-ribosomal protein antibody in SLE, was considered relevant. Other clinically relevant patterns that were not highly rated by the participants were the fine speckled cytoplasmic pattern (AC-20) (36%), associated with anti-Jo1 antibody in polymyositis, and the reticular cytoplasmic pattern (AC-21) (33%), associated with the presence of anti-mitochondria antibody in Primary Biliary Cholangitis [12].

Due to the design of the questionnaire, the study does not allow us to conclude on the reasons why rheumatologists attributed importance to some patterns. Possible criteria would include the clinical correlation of the pattern and its frequency on the clinical practice.

Concerning the type of information that should be included in the HEp-2 IFA report, 76% (316) of the participants indicated the identification of the pattern and 63% (261) the final titer. It should be emphasized that the dilution of 1:80 is used for SARD screening, but this screening dilution results in 13.3% positivity in healthy individuals, a fact that the physician must be aware of [21]. Healthy individuals tend to present lower HEp-2 IFA titers, due to the lower serum concentration of natural autoantibodies [12, 21]. Still on the aspects that the rheumatologist considers important in the HEp-2 IFA report, 35% (144) referred that the history of previous patterns is an important information in the report. SARD are associated with a varied range of autoantibodies, which may fluctuate over time depending on the period of the disease in which the individual is tested [22–25]. Between periods of disease activity and remission, there may be a predominance of one antibody over the other, thus changing the titer and the pattern found [22–26]. Therefore, recording the history of patterns may be relevant for this monitoring. In addition, occasional changes in the pattern may herald a transformation in the clinical scenario. The typical example is a person with ill-defined symptoms that presents the dense fine nuclear pattern (AC-2) for years and comes to the clinical visit bringing a HEp-2 IFA report with the homogeneous nuclear pattern (AC-1). This change in the HEp-2 IFA indicates the appearance of novel autoantibodies that may shed light into the clinical investigation of such a patient. The standardization of the information in the report and the way in which it is presented to the attending physician facilitates the monitoring of the data provided by the screening exam over time and allows a temporal and comprehensive analysis of the patient's condition.

Conclusion

The Brazilian Consensus on HEp-2 IFA has been used by the Brazilian community of rheumatologists for two decades and has played an important role in the clinical practice. The data presented here indicate that the guidelines regarding standardization contribute to the uniformity in the presentation of results and in the scope of clinical interpretation.

However, as usually occurs in voluntary response sample studies, responders are differentiated in terms of motivation on the subject of the research. In addition, the sampling represents one fifth of SBR members. These limitations should be taken into consideration and the findings and conclusions should not be freely generalized.

Brazilian rheumatologists are knowledgeable about the BCA literature and most evaluate positively the content available, considering that the recommendations help in clinical practice. Experts also recognize the patterns most commonly associated with rheumatic autoimmune diseases and have used BCA recommendations to interpret the related laboratory findings.

On the other hand, the study pointed out that there is an opportunity to expand the knowledge of rheumatologists on the content of BCA by means of continuous education, contributing to the update and dissemination of BCA concepts and nomenclature. In parallel, it is equally important to communicate the harmonization of international recommendations to those of the BCA. These initiatives should allow rheumatologists to take the best of the HEp-2 IFA test, contributing to an accurate diagnosis, optimal therapy and greater chances of treatment success.

Abbreviations

AC: Anti-cell; ANA: Antinuclear antibody; BCA: Brazilian consensus for detection of autoantibodies; HEp-2: Human epithelial type 2 cells; ICAP: International consensus on ANA patterns; IFA: Indirect immunofluorescent Assay; SARD: Systemic autoimmune rheumatic diseases; SBR: Brazilian rheumatology society; SLE: Systemic lupus erythematosus

Acknowledgements

Sociedade Brasileira de Reumatologia (SBR) (in English, Brazilian Rheumatology Society) and the SBR's Laboratory Commission.

Authors' contributions

WMC, LEA, PLCF are design of the questionnaire. ICMF and LARS applied the questionnaire with the support of the SBR laboratory commission. ICMF and LARS elaborate of the first paper draft. WMC, LEA, PLCF are review of the manuscript. All authors read and approved the final manuscript.

Author details

Pontifícia Universidade Católica de Goiás (PUC Goiás), Escola de Ciências Médicas, Farmacêuticas e Biomédicas, Avenida Universitária 1.440, Setor Universitário, Goiânia, GO, Brazil. [2]Disciplina de Reumatologia, Escola Paulista de Medicina, Universidade Federal de São Paulo (UNIFESP), Divisão de Imunologia, Fleury Medicina e Saúde, São Paulo, SP, Brazil.

References

1. Tan EM. Antinuclear antibodies: diagnostic markers for autoimmune diseases and probes for cell biology. Adv Immunol. 1989;44:93–151. https://doi.org/10.1016/S0065-2776(08)60641-0.
2. Dellavance A, Júnior AG, Cintra AF, Ximenes AC, Nuccitelli B, Mühlen CA, et al. I consenso nacional para padronização dos laudos de FAN HEp-2 the first Brazilian consensus for standardization of ANA in HEp-2 Cells. J Bras Patol Med Lab. 2002;38(3):201–16.
3. Dellavance A, Junior AG, Cintra AFU, Ximenes AC, Nuccitelli B, Taliberti BH. II Brazilian consensus on antinuclear factor in HEp-2 cells (*) II Brazilian consensus on antinuclear antibodies in HEp-2 cells nucleolus, cytoplasm and mitotic apparatus, as wel as its clinical associations. Rev Bras Reumatol. 2003;43(3):129–40. https://doi.org/10.1590/S0482-50042003000300002.
4. Francescantonio PLC, Andrade LEC, de Melo Cruvinel, W, Nuccitelli B, Taliberti BH, et al. III Consenso Brasileiro para Pesquisa de Autoanticorpos em Células HEp-2 : perspectiva histórica, controle de qualidade e associações clínicas. Jornal Brasileiro de Patologia Clínica Vol. 2009;45:185–99.
5. Francescantonio PLC, de Melo Cruvinel, W, Dellavance A, Andrade LEC, Taliberti BH, von Mühlen CA, et al. IV Consenso Brasileiro para pesquisa de autoanticorpos em células HEp-2. Rev Bras Reumatol. 2014;54(1):44–50. https://doi.org/10.1016/j.rbr.2013.10.001.
6. de Melo Cruvinel, W, Andrade LEC, von Mühlen CA, Dellavance A, Ximenes AC, Bichara CD, et al. V Brazilian consensus guidelines for detection of anti-cell autoantibodies on HEp-2 cells. Adv Rheumatol. 2019;59(1):28.
7. Chan EKL, Damoiseaux J, Carballo OG, Conrad K, de Melo Cruvinel, W, Francescantonio PLC, et al. Report of the first international consensus on standardized nomenclature of antinuclear antibody HEp-2 cell patterns 2014–2015. Front Immunol. 2015;6. https://doi.org/10.3389/fimmu.2015.00412.
8. Chan EKL, Damoiseaux J, de Melo Cruvinel, W, Carballo OG, Conrad K, Francescantonio PLC, et al. Report on the second international consensus on ANA pattern (ICAP) workshop in Dresden 2015. Lupus. 2016;25(8):797–804. https://doi.org/10.1177/0961203316640920.
9. Andrade LEC, Klotz W, Herold M, Conrad K, Rönnelid J, Fritzler MJ, et al. International consensus on antinuclear antibody patterns: definition of the AC-29 pattern associated with antibodies to DNA topoisomerase i. Clin Chem Lab Med. 2018;56(10):1783–8. https://doi.org/10.1515/cclm-2018-0188.
10. Damoiseaux J, von Mühlen CA, Garcia-De La Torre I, Carballo OG, de Melo Cruvinel W, PLC F, et al. International consensus on ANA patterns (ICAP): the bumpy road towards a consensus on reporting ANA results. Autoimmun Highlights. 2016;7(1):1–8. https://doi.org/10.1007/s13317-016-0075-0.
11. Herold M, Klotz W, Andrade LEC, Conrad K, de Melo Cruvinel, W, Damoiseaux J, et al. International consensus on antinuclear antibody patterns: defining negative results and reporting unidentified patterns. Clin Chem Lab Med. 2018;56(10):1799–802. https://doi.org/10.1515/cclm-2018-0052.
12. Damoiseaux J, Andrade LEC, Carballo OG, Conrad K, Francescantonio PLC, Fritzler MJ, et al. Clinical relevance of HEp-2 indirect immunofluorescent patterns: the international consensus on ANA patterns (ICAP) perspective. Ann Rheum Dis. 2019;78(7):879–89. https://doi.org/10.1136/annrheumdis-2018-214436.
13. Tan EM, Feltkamp TEW, Smolen JS, Butcher B, Dawkins R, Fritzler MJ, et al. Range of antinuclear antibodies in "healthy" individuals. Arthritis Rheum. 1997 Sep;40(9):1601–11. https://doi.org/10.1002/art.1780400909.
14. Satoh M, Chan EKL, Ho LA, Rose KM, Parks CG, Cohn RD, et al. Prevalence and sociodemographic correlates of antinuclear antibodies in the United States. Arthritis Rheum. 2012;64(7):2319–27. https://doi.org/10.1002/art.34380.
15. Agustinelli RA, Rodrigues SH, Mariz HA, Prado MS, Andrade LEC. Distinctive features of positive anti-cell antibody tests (indirect immunofluorescence on HEp-2 cells) in patients with non-autoimmune diseases. Lupus. 2019;28:629–34.
16. Dellavance A, Andrade LEC. Detection of autoantibodies by indirect immunofluorescence Cytochemistry on Hep-2 cells. Methods Mol Biol. 2019; 1901:19–46.
17. Satoh M, Vázquez-Del Mercado M, Chan EKL. Clinical interpretation of antinuclear antibody tests in systemic rheumatic diseases. Mod Rheumatol. 2009;19(3):219–28. https://doi.org/10.3109/s10165-009-0155-3.
18. Kavanaugh A, Tomar R, Reveille J, Solomon DH, Homburger HA. Guidelines for clinical use of the antinuclear antibody test and tests for specific

autoantibodies to nuclear antigens. Arch Pathol Lab Med. 2000;124(1):71–81. https://doi.org/10.5858/2000-124-0071-GFCUOT.
19. Petri M, Orbai AM, Alarcõn GS, Gordon C, Merrill JT, Fortin PR, et al. Derivation and validation of the systemic lupus international collaborating clinics classification criteria for systemic lupus erythematosus. Arthritis Rheum. 2012;64(8):2677–86. https://doi.org/10.1002/art.34473.
20. Alessandra D, Coelho ALE. Como interpretar e valorizar adequadamente o teste de anticorpos antinúcleo. J Bras Patol Med Lab. 2007;43(3):157–68.
21. Mariz HA, Sato EI, Barbosa SH, Rodrigues SH, Dellavance A, Andrade LEC. Pattern on the antinuclear antibody-HEp-2 test is a critical parameter for discriminating antinuclear antibody-positive healthy individuals and patients with autoimmune rheumatic diseases. Arthritis Rheum. 2011;63(1):191–200. https://doi.org/10.1002/art.30084.
22. Hargraves MM. Discovery of the LE cell and its morphology. Mayo Clin Proc. 1969;44(9):579–99.
23. Fritzler MJ. Antinuclear antibodies in the investigation of rheumatic diseases. Bull Rheum Dis. 1985;35(6):1–10 PMID: 3879803.
24. von Mühlen CA, Tan EJM. Autoantibody in the diagnosis of systemic rheumatic diseases. Semin Arthritis Rheum. 1995;24(5):323–58. https://doi.org/10.1016/S0049-0172(95)80004-2.
25. Evans J. Antinuclear antibody testing in systemic autoimmune disease. Clin Chest Med. 1998;19(4):613–25. https://doi.org/10.1016/S0272-5231(05)70106-4.
26. Prado MS, Dellavance A, Rodrigues SH, Marvulle V, Andrade LEC. Changes in the result of antinuclear antibody immunofluorescence assay on HEp-2 cells reflect disease activity status in systemic lupus erythematosus. Clin Chem Lab Med. 2020;58(8):1271–81.

19

Pain and fatigue are predictors of quality of life in primary Sjögren's syndrome

Laiza Hombre Dias[1,2], Samira Tatiyama Miyamoto[3], Raquel Altoé Giovelli[2,4], Caerê Iamonde Maciel de Magalhães[5] and Valeria Valim[1,2,6*]

Abstract

Background: Few studies have evaluated the relation of quality of life (QoL) with symptoms and disease activity in primary Sjögren's syndrome (pSS). There is also scant information on the predictors of QoL in this population. The aim of this study was to assess QoL in patients with pSS and to investigate their possible predictors.

Methods: In a cross-sectional study, 77 patients with pSS were evaluated using the following questionnaires: Functional Assessment of Chronic Illness Therapy Fatigue Subscale (FACIT-Fatigue), EULAR Sjögren's Syndrome Patient Reported Index (ESSPRI), EULAR Sjögren's Syndrome Disease Activity Index (ESSDAI), Short Form-36 Health Survey (SF-36) and World Health Organization Quality of Life Assessment (WHOQOL-BREF). Seventy-seven healthy controls responded to the SF-36 and WHOQOL-BREF. The Mann-Whitney test, t-test, Pearson and Spearman correlation, and multiple regression analysis were used in the statistical analysis.

Results: Patients with pSS and healthy controls were matched by gender and age. The mean scores for the ESSDAI, ESSPRI and FACIT-Fatigue were 3.34 ± 4.61, 6.58 ± 2.29 and 26.17 ± 11.02, respectively. Patients had a lower employment rate (36.4% versus 62.3%, $p < 0.01$) and higher work disability (10.4% versus 1.3%, $p < 0.01$). SF-36 and WHOQOL-BREF values were lower in patients with pSS ($p < 0.001$), except in the WHOQOL-BREF environment domain. Pain (ESSPRI), fatigue (FACIT-Fatigue), antinuclear antibody (ANA), anti-Ro-SSA and economic class (Brazilian Economic Classification Criteria - CCEB) were independent predictors of QoL.

Conclusions: The main predictors of poor QoL in patients with pSS were pain and fatigue, and these symptoms had an impact regardless of disease activity, age, schooling, marital status, work disability and fibromyalgia.

Keywords: Sjögren's syndrome, Quality of life, Pain, Fatigue

Introduction

Primary Sjögren syndrome (pSS) is an autoimmune, chronic and systemic disease that causes an inflammatory lymphocyte infiltrate with dysfunction of the salivary and lacrimal glands, leading to xerostomia and xerophthalmia. Epigenetic mechanisms such as DNA demethylation in epithelial cells and altered expression of microRNAs in salivary glands act on genetically susceptible patients, leading to the production of pathogenic autoantibodies [1]. Primary Sjögren syndrome affects mainly Caucasian women in the 4th to 5th decade of life and presents a broad clinical spectrum, with extraglandular manifestations occurring in more than two-thirds of cases, the most common being arthralgia or arthritis, Raynaud's phenomenon, skin vasculitis, interstitial pneumonitis and pulmonary fibrosis, peripheral neuropathy, and tubulointerstitial and glomerular nephritis [2–4].

Fatigue, a physical or mental feeling of tiredness, also affects approximately 70% of these patients and is strongly associated with psychosocial factors, occupational dysfunction and a greater number of medical visits but not with sicca severity or laboratory features [5, 6].

* Correspondence: val.valim@gmail.com
[1]Department of Clinical Medicine, Cassiano Antonio Moraes University Hospital / EBSERH, Federal University of Espírito Santo (Ufes), Av. Marechal Campos, 1468, Maruípe, Vitória, ES CEP: 29075-910, Brazil
[2]Brazilian Society of Rheumatology, São Paulo, Brazil

In pSS, pain can be explained by different reasons, such as arthritis, pain amplification, and neuropathy. Arthritis is usually symmetrical, predominantly in peripheral and small joints, and may precede or appear simultaneously with sicca symptoms. Small-fiber neuropathy is the most common cause of neuropathic pain and is characterized by distal paraesthesias, allodynia, and burning and itching sensations. Half of the pSS patients present widespread pain, and combined with fatigue and sleep disorders, the diagnosis of associated fibromyalgia may be considered [7].

PSS patients have low quality of life (QoL) in the physical, emotional and social dimensions evaluated by different instruments, such as the Short Form-36 Health Survey (SF-36), the *World Health Organization Quality of Life – BREF* (WHOQOL-BREF) and the EuroQol 5-dimensions (EQ-5D) [8–20]. There is also an increase in health expenditures, both individual and social, and a higher frequency of work withdrawal in this population. QoL can be influenced by several factors, such as age, schooling and socioeconomic level [6, 9, 11, 12, 21].

Considering the aspects related to the disease itself, pain, fatigue and dryness are associated with worse QoL [11–13, 16, 17, 19, 22]. Comorbidities such as depression, anxiety, and fibromyalgia are also negatively correlated [11, 18]. The association with immunological and biological variables is controversial or weak. Hypergammaglobulinemia, the presence of anti-SSA/Ro, anti-SSB/La antibodies, antinuclear antibody (ANA) or rheumatoid factor (RF), cytopenias, high cytokine levels or salivary gland biopsy do not correlate with worse QoL, while extraglandular manifestations, mainly articular and pulmonary, are poorly correlated [13]. Few studies have evaluated the relationship of QoL with symptoms and disease activity as measured by EULAR Sjögren's Syndrome Patient Reported Index (ESSPRI) and EULAR Sjögren's Syndrome Disease Activity Index (ESSDAI) [17, 19]. There is also little information on the predictors of QoL in this population [11, 17, 19].

The objective of this study was to evaluate whether disease activity or symptoms such as pain, dryness, and fatigue are predictors of QoL regardless of other clinical-epidemiological features in patients with pSS.

Methods

A cross-sectional study was conducted from January to July 2013 at the University Hospital of Federal University of Espírito Santo (HUCAM), in Vitória, Brazil.

PSS patients who met the American – European classification criteria (AECG) [23] and signed the informed consent form (ICF) were included. Secondary Sjögren syndrome patients were excluded.

The control group consisted of healthy individuals matched by gender and age who were in external circulation areas of the hospital, as well as donors from the blood bank. The exclusion criteria were having autoimmune rheumatic disease at < 18 years of age and any other comorbidity. All patients signed the ICF. The Research Ethics Committee (REC) of HUCAM, protocol number 178.520, approved the project on January 30, 2013.

Demographic data such as age, gender, self-reported color, level of schooling, income by the Brazilian Economic Classification Criteria (CCEB) [24], labor status, work disability (sick leave or early retirement), as well as clinical data such as diagnosis of fibromyalgia (American College of Rheumatology - ACR 1990 or ACR 2010) [25, 26], salivary gland biopsy, presence of antinuclear antibodies (ANA), rheumatoid factor (RF), anti-SSA/Ro and anti-SSB/La were collected from medical records and physician interview.

Minor salivary gland biopsies were performed and analyzed by rheumatologists and pathologists with experience in pSS and were considered positive when the histopathology showed one or more lymphocytic infiltrates with more than 50 mononuclear cells in an area of 4 mm^2 [24]. The anti-SSA/Ro and anti-SSB/La laboratory tests were performed by the hemagglutination technique, while ANA was performed by indirect immunofluorescence and RF by the latex test.

To evaluate the activity of the disease, two physicians experienced in pSS applied the ESSDAI. It has 12 domains of systemic evaluation (constitutional, lymphadenopathy, glandular, articular, cutaneous, respiratory, renal, muscular, peripheral and central nervous system, hematological and biological). The domains have different weights in the final score, 0 to 123, according to the level of activity [27, 28]. Values lower than 5 are considered to indicate low disease activity; values from 5 to 13, moderate activity; and values greater than or equal to 14, high activity [29].

Symptoms and QoL were assessed using self-administered questionnaires, and a trained professional was available to assist participants when needed. PSS patients answered the ESSPRI, which measures three symptoms related to the disease: dryness, pain and fatigue. Each domain ranges from 0 to 10, and the result is the average of the three domains [30]. Values less than 5 are considered acceptable [29].

Fatigue in pSS patients was evaluated through the Functional Assessment of Chronic Illness Therapy - fatigue (FACIT-fatigue). The FACIT system originally developed to evaluate QoL in cancer patients has been widely used in several chronic diseases. Its score ranges from 0 to 52, and its value is inversely proportional to the degree of fatigue [31].

The SF-36 and WHOQOL-BREF questionnaires were used to assess QoL in pSS patients and healthy controls. The SF-36 is an easy-to-administer instrument consisting of 36 items divided into 8 domains: physical functioning, physical role functioning, bodily pain, general health, vitality, social functioning, emotional role functioning and mental health. These can be grouped into two components that summarize the dimensions: physical (PCS) and mental (MCS) component summaries. Its final score ranges from 0 to 100, and the higher the score, the better the overall health condition [32]. Developed by the World Health Organization (WHO), the WHOQOL-BREF is an abbreviated version of the WHOQOL-100. It is composed of 26 questions. The first two questions are general QoL issues, and the remaining 24 facets will form four domains: physical, psychological, social relations and environment. The total score ranges from zero to 100, and the higher its value, the better the QoL [33, 34].

The chi-square, Fisher and likelihood ratio association tests were used for qualitative variables among patients with pSS and healthy controls. The Kolmogorov-Smirnov test was used to evaluate the normal distribution of the data. For quantitative variables, the Mann-Whitney test was used when there was a breakdown of normality, and with normal data, the t test was used. Pearson or Spearman tests were used in the correlations. To identify independent predictors for quality of life, stepwise linear regression analysis was performed. The variables considered in the analysis were age, weight, body mass index (BMI), smoking, alcoholism, marital status, schooling, fibromyalgia, CCEB, work disability (sick leave or early retirement), ESSDAI, ESSPRI, FACIT-Fatigue, salivary gland biopsy, ANA, anti-SSA/Ro, anti-SSB/La and RF. Variables with a statistical significance level of 10% were included in the multiple regression analysis. Statistical significance was set at a p value of ≤0.05. The Statistical Package for the Social Sciences (SPSS), version 20.0, Armonk, New York (NY), 2011 software was used.

Results

Of 127 pSS outpatients, 27 were excluded because they did not meet the AECG, and 33 were not willing to participate.

Seventy-seven pSS patients and 77 healthy women were included, aged 27 to 67 years. Groups were similar in age, ethnicity, schooling, marital status and economic classification. Patients had a lower employment rate (36.4% versus 62.3%, $p < 0.01$) and higher work disability (10.4% versus 1.3%, $p < 0.01$). Moreover, the patients had a low disease activity (ESSDAI 3.34 ± 4.61) and a low frequency of autoantibodies, characterizing a sample with mild disease. Biological and articular domains were the most frequently affected. In contrast, the patients presented a high level of symptoms (ESSPRI 6.58 ± 2.29). Among patients with pSS, the percentage of fibromyalgia was 42.9% (Table 1).

Table 1 Demographic and clinical data in pSS patients and healthy controls

	pSS ($n = 77$)	Controls ($n = 77$)
Age, mean, years	52.34 (9.03)	52.27 (8.91)
Ethnicity		
Black (%)	11.7	13
Brown (%)	59.7	49.4
White (%)	24.7	37.7
Indigenous (%)	2.6	0
Education		
< 8 years (%)	50.7	57.2
≥ 8 years (%)	48.1	40.3
Never studied (%)	1.2	2.5
Marital status		
Married (%)	66.2	63.6
Not married (%)	14.3	13
Divorced/widow (%)	19.5	23.4
CCEB		
A (%)	1.3	0
B (%)	23.4	26.6
C (%)	52	49.3
D (%)	18.2	24
E (%)	0	0
*Employment rate (%)	36.4	62.3
Work disability (%)*	10.4	1.3
Positive salivary biopsy (focus score ≥ 1) (%)	90.5	
Anti-SSA/Ro (%)	33.3	
Anti-SSB/La (%)	24	
Antinuclear antibody (%)	68.9	
Rheumatoid factor (%)	29.2	
Fibromyalgia (%)	42.9	
FACIT-*Fatigue*, mean, SD	26.17 (11.02)	
ESSPRI, mean, SD	6.58 (2.29)	
Fatigue, mean, SD	6.38 (2.57)	
Dryness, mean, SD	6.53 (2.78)	
Pain, mean, SD	6.84 (3.12)	
Extra glandular manifestations (%)	49.4	
ESSDAI, mean SD	3.34 (4.61)	

pSS Primary Sjögren Syndrome, *CCEB* Brazilian Economic Classification Criteria, *FACIT* Fatigue – Functional Assessment of Chronic Illness Therapy-Fatigue, *SD* standard deviation, *ESSPRI* EULAR Sjögren's syndrome patient reported index
*$p < 0.01$

The QoL measured by SF-36 and WHOQOL-BREF was worse in patients with pSS than in healthy controls, except for the environment domain tested by WHOQOL-BREF, which was similar for both groups (Table 2).

Table 2 Comparison of quality of life between pSS patients and healthy controls

SF-36	pSS (n = 77)	Controls (n = 77)
*Physical functioning	37.3 ± 24.2	80.5 ± 20.8
*Physical role functioning	27.6 ± 35.9	73.4 ± 37.2
*Bodily pain	36.7 ± 22.2	69.5 ± 21.4
*General health	43.2 ± 17.9	69.5 ± 20.0
*Vitality	37.2 ± 20.6	64.8 ± 20.9
*Social functioning	48.3 ± 26.9	74.8 ± 23.1
*Emotional role functioning	31.1 ± 38.6	69.3 ± 40.0
*Mental health	46.2 ± 22.3	67.8 ± 23.0
*PCS	33.1 ± 9.1	48.9 ± 8.5
*MCS	37.2 ± 11.4	46.8 ± 12.3
WHOQOL-BREF		
*Physical health	41.6 ± 16.8	67.7 ± 16.8
*Psychological health	53.4 ± 18.8	63.9 ± 15.9
*Social relations	55.5 ± 22.0	65.4 ± 18.2
Environment	49.1 ± 12.7	53.0 ± 16.5

SF-36 Short Form 36 Health Survey, *pSS* primary Sjögren's Syndrome, *PSC* Physical Component Summary, *MCS* Mental Component Summary, *WHOQOL-BREF* World Health Organization Quality of Life Assessment
*$p < 0.01$

Table 3 Comparison of quality of life between patients with acceptable and non-acceptable ESSPRI

	ESSPRI	
	Acceptable	Non-acceptable
SF36		
*Physical functioning	63.44 ± 29.08	30.83 ± 17.54
Physical role functioning	35.94 ± 43.75	25.00 ± 33.19
*Bodily pain	55.06 ± 25.69	31.80 ± 18.56
*General health	53.75 ± 19.21	40.57 ± 16.66
Vitality	47.19 ± 34.92	34.92 ± 18.31
Social functioning	54.66 ± 47.02	47.02 ± 27.27
**Emotional role functioning	52.08 ± 25.00	25.00 ± 34.51
**Mental health	56.00 ± 24.57	43.87 ± 21.05
*PCS	40.21 ± 10.88	31.28 ± 7.62
MCS	40.83 ± 13.14	36.31 ± 10.84
WHOQOL-BREF		
*Physical health	56.70 ± 19.25	37.54 ± 13.76
**Psychological health	63.02 ± 16.66	50.90 ± 18.75
*Social relations	71.35 ± 14.58	51.11 ± 21.94
**Environment	54.88 ± 9.20	47.53 ± 13.23

ESSPRI EULAR Sjögren's syndrome patient reported index, *SF-36* Short Form-36 Health Survey, *PCS* Physical Component Summary, *MCS* Mental Component Summary, *WHOQOL-BREF* World Health Organization quality of life – BREF
*$p < 0.01$; **$p < 0.05$

In the pSS group, patients with a nonacceptable ESSPRI (≥ 5) had all WHOQOL-BREF and most SF-36 domains worse than patients with an acceptable ESSPRI (Table 3). Patients with pSS and fibromyalgia had worse QoL values in bodily pain (SF-36) and physical health (WHOQOL-BREF) (Table 4).

There was a moderate-to-strong correlation of FACIT-Fatigue with all domains of QoL questionnaires. The ESSPRI also correlated with all QoL domains. The ESSDAI showed only a weak correlation with the emotional role functioning domain of the SF-36 and did not correlate with fatigue indexes (FACIT-Fatigue) and ESSPRI (Table 5).

In the regression analysis, pain (ESSPRI), fatigue (FACIT-Fatigue), antinuclear antibody (ANA), anti-Ro-SSA and economic class (Brazilian Economic Classification Criteria - CCEB) were independent predictors of QoL. The symptoms measured by FACIT-Fatigue and ESSPRI pain were the main predictors of poor QoL, regardless of age, marital status, schooling, work disability, disease activity and fibromyalgia. In the PCS of the SF-36, the predictors for the worst values were pain, fatigue, and the presence of ANA and anti-SSA/Ro autoantibodies. Fatigue was the only predictor in the MCS of the SF-36 and psychological health domain of the WHOQOL-BREF. Pain interfered with the PCS of the SF-36, physical health, social relations and environmental domains of the WHOQOL-BREF (Table 6).

Table 4 Comparison of QoL between pSS patients with fibromyalgia

		Fibromyalgia	
		Yes	No
SF-36	Physical functioning	30.9 ± 18.9	42.6 ± 26.5
	Physical role functioning	22.0 ± 30.5	32.4 ± 39.1
	*Bodily pain	25 ± 15.3	45.6 ± 22.4
	General health	37.9 ± 17.2	47.4 ± 17.4
	Vitality	30.9 ± 17.4	42.2 ± 21.4
	Social functioning	42.3 ± 25.2	53.7 ± 27.7
	Emotional role functionig	28.3 ± 38.3	34.1 ± 39.0
	Mental health	41.7 ± 22.7	49.6 ± 21.4
	PCS	29.7 ± 6.5	35.8 ± 9.8
	MCS	35.7 ± 11.6	38.6 ± 11.1
WHOQOL-BREF	*Physical health	35.5 ± 15.3	46.2 ± 16.5
	Social relations	51.0 ± 23.0	58.9 ± 20.9
	Environment	45.6 ± 11.4	51.8 ± 13.1
	Psychological health	48.7 ± 19.3	56.8 ± 17.8

QoL Quality of Life, *pSS* primary Sjögren's Syndrome, *SF-36* Short Form 36 Health Survey, *PSC* Physical Component Summary, *MCS* Mental Component Summary, *WHOQOL-BREF* World Health Organization Quality of Life Assessment
*$p < 0.01$

Table 5 Correlation of quality of life, disease activity, symptoms and fatigue

	ESSDAI	ESSPRI dryness	ESSPRI fatigue	ESSPRI pain	ESSPRI Total	FACIT-Fatigue
SF36						
Physical functioning	0.04	−0.44**	−0.29*	− 0.55**	− 0.56**	0.53**
Physical role functioning	0.01	−0.17	−0.08	− 0.23*	−0.24*	0.35**
Bodily pain	0.03	−0.33**	−0.23*	− 0.59**	−0.53**	0.56**
General health	−0.08	−0.27*	− 0.17	−0.34**	− 0.34**	0.56**
Vitality	−0.04	−0.23*	− 0.26*	−0.36**	− 0.39**	0.56**
Social functioning	−0.01	−0.33**	− 0.18	−0.21	− 0.29*	0.45**
Emotional role functioning	−0.24**	−0.31**	− 0.11	−0.23	− 0.29*	0.48**
Mental health	0.04	−0.21	−0.23*	− 0.31**	−0.28*	0.46**
PCS	0.06	−0.35**	−0.21	− 0.53**	−0.5**	0.46**
MCS	−0.14	−0.2	− 0.17	−0.12	− 0.24*	0.48**
Whoqol Bref						
Physical health	−0.09	−0.34**	− 0.19	−0.43**	− 0.50**	0.68**
Psychological health	−0.08	−0.32**	− 0.19	−0.36**	− 0.38**	0.56**
Social relations	−0.03	−0.17	− 0.2	−0.34**	− 0.33**	0.37**
Environment	−0.01	−0.19	− 0.18	−0.49**	− 0.34**	0.32**
ESSDAI		−0.11	−0.01	− 0.04	−0.08	− 0.06

ESSDAI EULAR Sjögren's syndrome disease activity index, *ESSPRI* EULAR Sjögren's syndrome patient reported index, *FACIT* Fatigue - Functional Assessment of Chronic Illness Therapy-Fatigue, *SF-36* Short Form-36 Health Survey, *PCS* Physical Component Summary, *MCS* Mental Component Summary, *WHOQOL-BREF* World Health Organization quality of life - BREF

*$p < 0.01$; '**$p < 0.05$

Discussion

Here, PSS patients were found to have lower QoL scores than healthy controls, corroborating previous studies in other countries [11–13, 15–19, 22]. The relevance of the present data was to demonstrate that symptoms, but not disease activity, were the main predictors of low QoL.

Few studies have performed multivariate analyses to identify predictors of QoL in pSS. Cornec et al. corroborated the results of our study, showing that disease activity is not associated with greater QoL impairments in 120 French patients with moderate-to-high levels of systemic activity, despite the low level of disease activity in our patients [35]. Disease activity (ESSDAI) was also not a predictor of QoL in 639 pSS patients from United Kingdom (UK) [18] and in 104 Korean patients [17]. In contrast, Omma et al. found that the ESSDAI was an independent determinant of all SF-36 domains, with the exception of the vitality domain, in 105 patients from Turkey, most of whom had low to moderate levels of disease activity [36]. As in Liu et al.'s study [37], our results showed that pain and fatigue were independently associated with a low physical component summary (PCS) of the SF-36 and that fatigue was associated with a low mental component summary (MCS) of the SF-36. In the Cornec et al. study, only pain was associated [35]. Omma et al. demonstrated that the ESSPRI was an independent determinant of bodily pain, general health, mental health and PCS of the SF-36, while fatigue was

Table 6 Predictors of quality of life

	SF-36		WHOQOL-BREF									
	PCS R^2: 0.56		MCS R^2: 0.22		Physical health R^2: 0.52		Psychological health R^2: 0.36		Social relations R^2: 0.23		Environment R^2: 0.30	
	ß	*p*-value	ß	*p*-value	ß	*p*-value	ß	*p*-value	ß	*p*-value	ß	*p*-value
ESSPRI-pain	−1.16	0.00			−1.48	0.00			−1.53	0.06	−1.63	0.00
FACIT-Fatigue	0.31	0.00	0.51	0.00	0.88	0.00	1.00	0.00	0.48	0.04		
ANA	−4.64	0.01										
Anti-SSA/Ro	−4.09	0.01										
CCEB									− 4.91	0.05	−3.9	0.01

SF-36 Short Form-36 Health Survey, *WHOQOL-BREF* World Health Organization quality of life - BREF, *PCS* Physical Component Summary, *MCS* Mental Component Summary, *ANA* Antinuclear Antibody, *CCEB* Brazilian Economic Classification Criteria

significantly correlated with four or more domains of the SF-36 [36].

Results showed a correlation between the ESSDAI only and the emotional aspects domain of the SF-36, and yet this correlation was weak, not being confirmed as a predictor of QoL in patients with pSS. Sharing a similar result, a cohort in the UK using the EQ-5D to assess QoL demonstrated a weak correlation with the ESSDAI [19]. Yacoub et al. used the degree of activity in salivary gland biopsy, immunological status and severity of systemic involvement as a way of assessing disease activity, and they found no correlation with QoL or fatigue [13]. It is not clear why there is a weak association between disease activity (ESSDAI) and QoL. One possible answer could be the wide range of ESSDAI scores (0–123) in samples with low mean activity. In addition, ESSDAI is an index that does not assess established damage, only current activity; thus, perhaps the patient's perception about the QoL is not modified at that moment, but when there is an established organic dysfunction. Other studies correlating injury rates with disease activity and QoL could better elucidate the issue.

QoL was worse in patients with higher nonacceptable ESSPRI, and it was not associated with ESSDAI, corroborating that symptoms (fatigue, pain and dryness) impact QoL more than disease activity.

In pSS, QoL has been found to be associated with fatigue, pain/articular involvement, ocular and oral involvement, pruritus, sexual dysfunction, impaired sleep, pulmonary manifestations, psychological dysfunction and impaired physical function [20]. On the other hand, delayed diagnosis, protracted course of the disease, and the lack of social support are also causes of the decline in the quality of life in these patients [37].

Fatigue is considered a hallmark of pSS [5]. In the present study, fatigue (FACIT-fatigue) was strongly associated with all dimensions of QoL and was an independent risk factor for the physical and mental aspects of QoL in both instruments, SF-36 and WHOQOL-BREF. In contrast, there was no association between fatigue and disease activity measured by the ESSDAI. Taken together, the results suggest that fatigue is itself associated with pSS but may not be explained by disease activity.

Recent evidence has shown weak or no association with inflammatory biomarkers such as interleukin (IL)-1b, IL-2, IL-6, IL-10 and tumor necrosis factor alpha (TNF-α). In the same direction, immunosuppressors and biological therapy failed to treat fatigue in pSS [38]. However, Howard et al. showed that lower levels of the pro-inflammatory cytokines inducible protein (IP)-10 and interferon-gamma (IFN-γ), together with pain and depression, were the most important predictors of fatigue [39], and Davies et al. demonstrated that TNF-α and LT-α have an inverse relationship with fatigue severity in pSS [40]. A proteomic study of cerebrospinal fluid showed that some proteins that are increased in pSS have a role in the downregulation of inflammation and in the cellular stress defense (hemopexin, pigment epithelium-derived factor, clusterin, osteopontin, and selenium-binding protein 1). These results suggest that some fatigue signaling pathways are associated with "cellular protection and defense" and are not directly related to proinflammatory factors [41]. Nonetheless, the evidence for an association between fatigue and disease activity – or any other inflammatory markers – remains controversial.

In fact, the pathogenesis of fatigue in pSS is unknown but seems to be associated with a lower aerobic capacity and lower physical activity levels, sleep disturbances, autonomic dysfunction, depression, psychological profiles, and fibromyalgia [38]. It is noteworthy that, in the multiple regression models, fatigue measured by FACIT-Fatigue was the only predictor of the MCS of SF-36 and the psychological component of WHOQOL-BREF. These data indicate that this symptom impacts not only the physical aspects but also the mental health of these individuals. Other studies have pointed to depression as an important determinant of poor QoL along with fatigue in these patients [11, 17, 18], which could partially explain the low values of the determination coefficients in the mental domain of the SF-36, as well as in the psychological, social relations and environmental domains of the WHOQOL-BREF. However, we did not evaluate psychiatric disorders, such as depression or anxiety, which is a limitation of this study. Interestingly, aerobic exercise has been found to improve fatigue, but not QoL and depression [42], and resistance exercise has been found to improve QoL [43]. Clearly, many efforts still need to be made to elucidate the pathogenesis of fatigue, as well as to identify pharmacological and nonpharmacological therapies to treat fatigue and improve the QoL in pSS.

Pain was a determinant for lower QoL in the physical, social relations and environmental domains but not for mental aspects. A large proportion of patients with pSS have noninflammatory musculoskeletal pain without the laboratory or clinical abnormalities of arthritis. Among patients with pSS, cases of pain amplification syndrome are associated with a benign pole of the disease, with a low frequency of autoantibodies and extraglandular manifestations [44].

The prevalence of fibromyalgia in pSS varies from 12 to 55% [7]. In our study, the prevalence was 42.9%. This large range can certainly be explained by the various criteria to diagnose fibromyalgia as well as pSS that have been applied over time. Indeed, pain and fatigue are common symptoms in both fibromyalgia and pSS, and the association of the two can be a misleading factor.

However, in the present study, fatigue and pain were the main predictors of poor QoL, regardless of the diagnosis of fibromyalgia, indicating that pSS itself was associated with poor QoL. Lendrem et al. found no difference in QoL between those with fibromyalgic symptoms and those without [18]. Notwithstanding, our study did not investigate other factors, such as subclinical autonomic dysfunction and sleep disorders, that could contribute to pain and fatigue in these patients with pSS without fibromyalgia [45].

The present study demonstrated a contribution of ANA and Anti-Ro/SSA, even if discrete, to worse values in the SF-36 physical domain. This information differs from the findings of other studies in which no correlation was found between antibodies and QoL [9, 13, 18]. However, it is well established in the literature that patients with positive autoantibodies evolve to greater glandular dysfunction and systemic manifestations [46, 47].

Although dryness is the main symptom and causes great discomfort in pSS patients, it was not a predictor of QoL, as demonstrated in previous studies [11, 35]. A review on QoL in pSS mentioned that it is possible this may reflect an inadequacy of single VAS scales, as is often used in such studies, to capture the breadth and impact of oral and ocular involvement. That review also showed that non-SS sicca syndrome patients have an impairment of QoL similar to that observed in pSS and other chronic diseases such as rheumatoid arthritis, systemic lupus erythematosus and fibromyalgia [20].

In the comparison between patients and healthy controls, SF-36 and WHOQOL-BREF domains were worse in patients with pSS, showing that the disease had a negative influence on the different aspects of QoL. Interestingly, the environmental domain, which is associated with transportation-related and residential conditions, in pSS was similar to that in healthy controls, probably because both groups showed similar socioeconomic levels.

Other relevant information included the lower number of employed individuals and the greater amount of sick leave among pSS patients compared to healthy controls. Patients with pSS also generate a higher cost to the health system, since they use more medical services, have higher hospitalization rates and use more medications [11, 20]. These data demonstrate how much the disease interferes not only emotionally and physically but also socially and individually, affecting employers and the government, increasing social security costs and reducing the life expectancy of the worker.

The study has limitations. Medications used by patients and other comorbidities were not collected. These data could have enriched the analysis, as some medications can yield adverse effects and other diseases may have symptoms with negative impacts on QoL. Questionnaires about emotional aspects such as depression and anxiety were also not applied, and these data could have improved the values of the mental domain determination coefficients.

Conclusion

This study demonstrated that the main predictors of poor QoL in patients with pSS were pain and fatigue, independent of disease activity, age, schooling, work disability, marital status and fibromyalgia.

Abbreviations

ANA: Antinuclear antibody; BMI: Body mass index; CCEB: Brazilian Economic Classification Criteria; ESSDAI: EULAR Sjögren's Syndrome Disease Activity Index; ESSPRI: EULAR Sjögren's Syndrome Patient Reported Index; FACIT-Fatigue: Functional Assessment of Chronic Illness Therapy Fatigue Subscale; pSS: Primary Sjögren's syndrome; QoL: Quality of life; RF: Rheumatoid factor; SF-36: Short Form-36 Health Survey; WHOQOL-BREF: World Health Organization Quality of Life Assessment

Acknowledgements

Not applicable.

Authors' contributions

All authors contributed to the conception and design of the study, analysis and interpretation of the data. In addition, all authors performed a critical review and read and approved the final version of this manuscript.

Author details

[1]Department of Clinical Medicine, Cassiano Antonio Moraes University Hospital / EBSERH, Federal University of Espírito Santo (Ufes), Av. Marechal Campos, 1468, Maruípe, Vitória, ES CEP: 29075-910, Brazil. [2]Brazilian Society of Rheumatology, São Paulo, Brazil. [3]Department of Integrated Health Education, Federal University of Espírito Santo (Ufes), Av. Marechal Campos, 1468, Maruípe, Vitória, ES CEP: 29075-910, Brazil. [4]Department of Clinical Medicine, School of Sciences of Santa Casa de Misericórdia de Vitória (Emescam), Av. Nossa Senhora da Penha 2190, Vitória, ES 29045-925, Brazil. [5]Federal University of Espírito Santo (Ufes), Av. Marechal Campos, 1468, Maruípe, Vitória, ES CEP: 29075-910, Brazil. [6]Brazilian Sjögren Syndrome Commission, São Paulo, Brazil.

References

1. Cafaro G, et al. One year in review 2019: Sjögren's syndrome. Clin Exp Rheumatol. 2019;37 Suppl 118(3):3–15.
2. Patel R, Shahane A. The epidemiology of Sjögren's syndrome. Clin Epidemiol. 2014;6:247–55.
3. Ramos-Casals M, Solans R, Rosas J, Camps MT, Gil A, del Pino-Montes J, et al. Primary Sjögren syndrome in Spain: clinical and immunologic expression in 1010 patients. Medicine (Baltimore). 2008;87(4):210–9. https://doi.org/10.1097/MD.0b013e318181e6af.
4. Kassan SS, Moutsopoulos HM. Clinical manifestations and early diagnosis of Sjögren syndrome. Arch Intern Med. 2004;164(12):1275–84. https://doi.org/10.1001/archinte.164.12.1275.
5. Segal B, Thomas W, Rogers T, Leon JM, Hughes P, Patel D, et al. Prevalence, severity, and predictors of fatigue in subjects with primary Sjögren's syndrome. Arthritis Rheum. 2008;59(12):1780–7. https://doi.org/10.1002/art.24311.
6. Westhoff G, Dorner T, Zink A. Fatigue and depression predict physician visits and work disability in women with primary Sjögren's syndrome: results from a cohort study. Rheumatology (Oxford). 2012;51(2):262–9. https://doi.org/10.1093/rheumatology/ker208.
7. Vitali C, Del Papa N. Pain in primary Sjögren's syndrome. Best Pract Res Clin Rheumatol. 2015;29(1):63–70. https://doi.org/10.1016/j.berh.2015.05.002.

8. Strömbeck B, Ekdahl C, Manthorpe R, Wikström I, Jacobsson L. Health-related quality of life in primary Sjögren's syndrome, rheumatoid arthritis and fibromyalgia compared to normal population data using SF-36. Scand J Rheumatol. 2000;29(1):20–8. https://doi.org/10.1080/030097400750001761.
9. Belenguer R, Ramos-Casals M, Brito-Zerón P, del Pino J, Sentís J, Aguiló S, et al. Influence of clinical and immunological parameters on the health-related quality of life of patients with primary Sjögren's syndrome. Clin Exp Rheumatol. 2005;23(3):351–6.
10. Lopez-Jornet P, Camacho-Alonso F. Quality of life in patients with Sjögren's syndrome and sicca complex. J Oral Rehabil. 2008;35(12):875–81. https://doi.org/10.1111/j.1365-2842.2008.01919.x.
11. Segal B, Bowman SJ, Fox PC, Vivino FB, Murukutla N, Brodscholl J, et al. Primary Sjögren's syndrome: health experiences and predictors of health quality among patients in the United States. Health Qual Life Outcomes. 2009;7(1):46. https://doi.org/10.1186/1477-7525-7-46.
12. Meijer JM, Meiners PM, Huddleston Slater JJR, Spijkervet FKL, Kallenberg CGM, Vissink A, et al. Health-related quality of life, employment and disability in patients with Sjögren's syndrome. Rheumatology (Oxford). 2009; 48(9):1077–82. https://doi.org/10.1093/rheumatology/kep141.
13. Ibn Yacoub Y, et al. Primary Sjögren's syndrome in Moroccan patients: characteristics, fatigue and quality of life. Rheumatol Int. 2012;32(9):2637–43. https://doi.org/10.1007/s00296-011-2009-5.
14. Baturone R, Soto MJ, Márquez M, Macías I, Montes de Oca M, Medina F, et al. Health-related quality of life in patients with primary Sjögren's syndrome: relationship with serum levels of proinflammatory cytokines. Scand J Rheumatol. 2009;38(5):386–9. https://doi.org/10.1080/03009740902973821.
15. Inal V, Kitapcioglu G, Karabulut G, Keser G, Kabasakal Y. Evaluation of quality of life in relation to anxiety and depression in primary Sjögren's syndrome. Mod Rheumatol. 2010;20(6):588–97. https://doi.org/10.3109/s10165-010-0329-z.
16. Enger TB, Palm Ø, Garen T, Sandvik L, Jensen JL. Oral distress in primary Sjögren's syndrome: implications for health-related quality of life. Eur J Oral Sci. 2011;119(6):474–80. https://doi.org/10.1111/j.1600-0722.2011.00891.x.
17. Cho HJ, Yoo JJ, Yun CY, Kang EH, Lee HJ, Hyon JY, et al. The EULAR Sjögren's syndrome patient reported index as an independent determinant of health-related quality of life in primary Sjögren's syndrome patients: in comparison with non-Sjögren's sicca patients. Rheumatology (Oxford). 2013; 52(12):2208–17. https://doi.org/10.1093/rheumatology/ket270.
18. Lendrem D, Mitchell S, McMeekin P, Bowman S, Price E, Pease CT, et al. Health-related utility values of patients with primary Sjögren's syndrome and its predictors. Ann Rheum Dis. 2014;73(7):1362–8. https://doi.org/10.1136/annrheumdis-2012-202863.
19. Lendrem D, Mitchell S, McMeekin P, Gompels L, Hackett K, Bowman S, et al. Do the EULAR Sjögren's syndrome outcome measures correlate with health status in primary Sjögren's syndrome? Rheumatology (Oxford). 2015;54(4): 655–9. https://doi.org/10.1093/rheumatology/keu361.
20. Miyamoto ST, Valim V, Fisher BA. Health-related quality of life and costs in Sjögren's syndrome. Rheumatology. 2019. https://doi.org/10.1093/rheumatology/key370.
21. Callaghan R, Prabu A, Allan RB, Clarke AE, Sutcliffe N, Pierre YS, et al. Direct healthcare costs and predictors of costs in patients with primary Sjögren's syndrome. Rheumatology (Oxford). 2007;46(1):105–11. https://doi.org/10.1093/rheumatology/kel155.
22. Kamel UF, Maddison BA, Whitaker R. Impact of primary Sjögren's syndrome on smell and taste: effect on quality of life. Rheumatology (Oxford). 2009; 48(12):1512–4. https://doi.org/10.1093/rheumatology/kep249.
23. Vitali C, Bombardieri S, Jonsson R, Moutsopoulos HM, Alexander EL, Carsons SE, et al. Classification criteria for Sjögren's syndrome: a revised version of the European criteria proposed by the American-European Consensus Group. Ann Rheum Dis. 2002;61(6):554–8. https://doi.org/10.1136/ard.61.6.554.
24. Associação Brasileira de Empresas de Pesquisa. Critério de Classificação econômica Brasil. São Paulo: Associação Brasileira de Empresas de Pesquisa; 2012. p. 4.
25. Wolfe F, et al. The American College of Rheumatology 1990 Criteria for the classification of fibromyalgia. Report of the Multicenter Criteria Committee. Arthritis Rheum. 1990;33(2):160–72.
26. Wolfe F, Clauw DJ, Fitzcharles MA, Goldenberg DL, Katz RS, Mease P, et al. The American College of Rheumatology preliminary diagnostic criteria for fibromyalgia and measurement of symptom severity. Arthritis Care Res. 2010;62(5):600–10. https://doi.org/10.1002/acr.20140.
27. Seror R, Ravaud P, Bowman SJ, Baron G, Tzioufas A, Theander E, et al. EULAR Sjögren's syndrome disease activity index: development of a consensus systemic disease activity index for primary Sjögren's syndrome. Ann Rheum Dis. 2010;69(6):1103–9. https://doi.org/10.1136/ard.2009.110619.
28. Serrano EV, Valim V, Miyamoto ST, Giovelli RA, Paganotti MA, Cadê NV. Transcultural adaptation of the "EULAR Sjögren's syndrome disease activity index (ESSDAI)" into Brazilian Portuguese. Rev Bras Reumatol. 2013;53(6): 483–93. https://doi.org/10.1016/j.rbr.2013.04.003.
29. Seror R, Bootsma H, Saraux A, Bowman SJ, Theander E, Brun JG, et al. Defining disease activity states and clinically meaningful improvement in primary Sjögren's syndrome with EULAR primary Sjögren's syndrome disease activity (ESSDAI) and patient-reported indexes (ESSPRI). Ann Rheum Dis. 2016;75(2):382–9. https://doi.org/10.1136/annrheumdis-2014-206008.
30. Seror R, Ravaud P, Mariette X, Bootsma H, Theander E, Hansen A, et al. EULAR Sjögren's syndrome patient reported index (ESSPRI): development of a consensus patient index for primary Sjögren's syndrome. Ann Rheum Dis. 2011;70(6):968–72. https://doi.org/10.1136/ard.2010.143743.
31. Cella D, Yount S, Sorensen M, Chartash E, Sengupta N, Grober J. Validation of the functional assessment of chronic illness therapy fatigue scale relative to other instrumentation in patients with rheumatoid arthritis. J Rheumatol. 2005;32(5):811–9.
32. Ciconelli RM, et al. Brazilian-Portuguese version of the SF-36. A reliable and valid quality of life outcome measure. Rev Bras Reumatol. 1999;39(3):143–50.
33. World Health Organization (WHO). WHOQOL-BREF: Introduction, administration, scoring and generic version of the assessment. Geneva: Whoqol Group; 1996.
34. Fleck MP, Louzada S, Xavier M, Chachamovich E, Vieira G, Santos L, et al. Application of the Portuguese version of the abbreviated instrument of quality life WHOQOL-bref. Rev Saude Publica. 2000;34(2):178–83. https://doi.org/10.1590/S0034-89102000000200012.
35. Cornec D, Devauchelle-Pensec V, Mariette X, Jousse-Joulin S, Berthelot JM, Perdriger A, et al. Severe health-related quality of life impairment in active primary Sjögren's syndrome and patient-reported outcomes: data from a large therapeutic trial. Arthritis Care Res. 2017;69(4):528–35. https://doi.org/10.1002/acr.22974.
36. Omma A, Tecer D, Kucuksahin O, Sandikci SC, Yildiz F, Erten S. Do the European league against rheumatism (EULAR) Sjögren's syndrome outcome measures correlate with impaired quality of life, fatigue, anxiety and depression in primary Sjogren's syndrome? Arch Med Sci. 2018;14(4):830–7. https://doi.org/10.5114/aoms.2017.70300.
37. Liu Z, Dong Z, Liang X, Liu J, Xuan L, Wang J, et al. Health-related quality of life and psychological status of women with primary Sjögren's syndrome: a cross-sectional study of 304 Chinese patients. Medicine (Baltimore). 2017; 96(50):e9208. https://doi.org/10.1097/MD.0000000000009208.
38. Miyamoto ST, Lendrem DW, Ng WF, Hackett KL, Valim V. Managing fatigue in patients with primary Sjögren's syndrome: challenges and solutions. Open Access Rheumatol. 2019;11:77–88. https://doi.org/10.2147/OARRR.S167990.
39. Howard Tripp N, Tarn J, Natasari A, Gillespie C, Mitchell S, Hackett KL, et al. Fatigue in primary Sjögren's syndrome is associated with lower levels of proinflammatory cytokines. RMD Open. 2016;2(2):e000282. https://doi.org/10.1136/rmdopen-2016-000282.
40. Davies K, et al. Fatigue in primary Sjögren's syndrome (pSS) is associated with lower levels of proinflammatory cytokines: a validation study. Rheumatol Int. 2019;39(11):1867–73. https://doi.org/10.1007/s00296-019-04354-0.
41. Larssen E, et al. Fatigue in primary Sjögren's syndrome: a proteomic pilot study of cerebrospinal fluid. SAGE Open Med. 2019;7:2050312119850390.
42. Miyamoto ST, Valim V, Carletti L, Ng WF, Perez AJ, Lendrem DW, et al. Supervised walking improves cardiorespiratory fitness, exercise tolerance, and fatigue in women with primary Sjögren's syndrome: a randomized-controlled trial. Rheumatol Int. 2019;39(2):227–38. https://doi.org/10.1007/s00296-018-4213-z.
43. Minali PA, Pimentel CFMG, de Mello MT, Lima GHO, Dardin LP, Garcia ABA, et al. Effectiveness of resistance exercise in functional fitness in women with primary Sjögren's syndrome: randomized clinical trial. Scand J Rheumatol. 2020;49(1):47–56. https://doi.org/10.1080/03009742.2019.1602880.
44. ter Borg EJ, Kelder JC. Lower prevalence of extra-glandular manifestations and anti-SSB antibodies in patients with primary Sjögren's syndrome and widespread pain: evidence for a relatively benign subset. Clin Exp Rheumatol. 2014;32(3):349–53.
45. Giles I, Isenberg D. Fatigue in primary Sjögren's syndrome: is there a link

with the fibromyalgia syndrome? Ann Rheum Dis. 2000;59(11):875–8. https://doi.org/10.1136/ard.59.11.875.

46. Maslinska M, et al. Sjögren's syndrome: still not fully understood disease. Rheumatol Int. 2015;35(2):233–41. https://doi.org/10.1007/s00296-014-3072-5.
47. Theander E, Andersson SI, Manthorpe R, Jacobsson LT. Proposed core set of outcome measures in patients with primary Sjögren's syndrome: 5 year follow up. J Rheumatol. 2005;32(8):1495–502.

20

Hematopoietic stem cell transplantation for systemic sclerosis: Brazilian experience

Álvaro Henrique-Neto[1], Marianna Yumi Kawashima Vasconcelos[1,2], Juliana Bernardes Elias Dias[3], Daniela Aparecida de Moraes[3], Maynara Santana Gonçalves[2,4], Djúlio César Zanin-Silva[2,5], Talita Graminha Zucoloto[1,2,3], Marília de Fátima Cirioli de Oliveira[3,6], Giuliana Martinelli Dotoli[1,2], Luiz Fernando Weffort[3], Vanessa Cristina Leopoldo[3,6] and Maria Carolina Oliveira[2,7*]

Abstract

Background: In the past 20 years, hematopoietic stem cell transplantation (HSCT) has been investigated as treatment for systemic sclerosis (SSc). The goal of HSCT is to eradicate the autoreactive immune system, which is replaced by a new immune repertoire with long-lasting regulation and tolerance to autoantigens. Here, we describe the clinical outcomes of severe and refractory SSc patients that underwent HSCT at a single Brazilian center.

Patients and methods: This is a longitudinal and retrospective study, including 70 adult SSc patients, with an established diagnosis of SSc, and who underwent autologous HSCT from 2009 to 2016. The procedure included harvesting and cryopreservation of autologous hematopoietic progenitor cells, followed by administration of an immunoablative regimen and subsequent infusion of the previously collected cells. Patients were evaluated immediately before transplantation, at 6 months and then yearly until at least 5-years of post-transplantation follow-up. At each evaluation time point, patients underwent clinical examination, including modified Rodnan's skin score (mRSS) assessment, echocardiography, high-resolution computed tomography of the lungs and pulmonary function.

Results: Median (range) age was 35.9 (19–59), with 57 (81.4%) female and median (range) non-Raynaud's disease duration of 2 (1–7) years. Before transplantation, 96% of the patients had diffuse skin involvement, 84.2%, interstitial lung disease and 67%, positive anti-topoisomerase I antibodies. Skin involvement significantly improved, with a decline in mRSS at all post-transplantation time points until at least 5-years of follow-up. When patients with pre-HSCT interstitial lung disease were analyzed, there was an improvement in pulmonary function (forced vital capacity and diffusing capacity of lung for carbon monoxide) over the 5-year follow-up. Overall survival was 81% and progression-free survival was 70.5% at 8-years after HSCT. Three patients died due to transplant-related toxicity, 9 patients died over follow-up due to disease reactivation and one patient died due to thrombotic thrombocytopenic purpura.

(Continued on next page)

* Correspondence: mcarolor@usp.br
[2]Center for Cell-Based Therapy, Ribeirão Preto Medical School, University of São Paulo, Ribeirão Preto, Brazil
[7]Department of Internal Medicine, Ribeirão Preto Medical School, University of São Paulo, Avenida dos Bandeirantes 3900, Ribeirão Preto, SP 14048-900, Brazil

(Continued from previous page)

Conclusions: Autologous hematopoietic progenitor cell transplantation improves skin and interstitial lung involvement. These results are in line with the international experience and support HSCT as a viable therapeutic alternative for patients with severe and progressive systemic sclerosis.

Keywords: Systemic sclerosis, Hematopoietic stem cell transplantation, Stem cells, Progenitor cells, Transplantation

Background

Autologous hematopoietic stem cell transplantation (HSCT) has been investigated as treatment for systemic sclerosis (SSc) for more than two decades, with progress both in choosing the most suitable candidates and in reducing the morbidity and mortality associated with the procedure [1–3]. Patients with severe and rapidly progressive SSc have been enrolled for HCST, and according to data from international transplant registries, the number of transplanted patients per year has progressively increased, reflecting the good outcomes of this therapeutic approach [4].

The initial phase I/II studies were important to establish recommendations and to guide currently adopted transplant procedures [5–12]. Over time, details about patient selection, drugs included in the procedure, patient management and follow-up were discussed and improved around multiple transplantation centers. These studies also evidenced the importance of a proper heart assessment as a strategy to decrease transplant-related mortality. Cardiac dysfunctions that occur during transplantation accounted for many of the transplant-related deaths described in the initial studies [13]. Currently, recommendations for pre-transplantation cardiac assessment are available in the literature [14]. Multivariate analyses have also shown that the experience of the center in transplanting autoimmune diseases has also a significant impact on patient outcomes. Centers with more than 26-transplanted autoimmune disease patients and those with more than 6 years of experience have better disease outcomes over time than less experienced centers [4].

The goal of transplantation is to non-selectively eliminate autoreactive T and B-lymphocytes through high-dose immunosuppression and to reconstitute a new immunological system by infusion of autologous hematopoietic progenitor cells, previously collected and cryopreserved [15]. The strategy promotes an immunological resetting, in which the existing immune system is eradicated, and replaced by a new immune repertoire with adequate long-lasting regulation and tolerance to autoantigens [16, 17]. Studies have described thymic reactivation, increased frequencies of cells with regulatory function, improvement of T-cell receptor diversity and normalization of molecular signatures as post-transplantation mechanisms associated with clinical outcomes [18, 19].

Autologous HSCT has a striking impact on skin involvement, as mRSS significantly declines, starting in the first months after the procedure [2, 5, 20]. Pulmonary function also benefits from transplantation, in most cases stabilizing or, less frequently, improving after HSCT [2, 5, 20]. To date, three prospective and randomized studies have shown that autologous HSCT is superior to conventional therapy with monthly cyclophosphamide infusions in patients with severe and progressive SSc [21–23]. These studies report higher overall survival and progression-free survival rates, as well as better disease control and quality of life in transplanted versus non-transplanted patients. A recent meta-analysis shows that autologous HSCT is superior to conventional therapies in SSc patients, especially in the analyses of risk of death from any cause, skin and lung involvement, and quality of life [24]. Recently, the European League Against Rheumatism (EULAR), the American Society for Transplantation and Cell Therapy (ASCTC) and the Brazilian Society of Bone Marrow Transplantation (SBTMO) have recommended autologous HSCT as treatment for patients with progressive SSc at risk of organ failure [3, 25, 26].

The present study aims to evaluate the outcomes of severe and progressive SSc patients treated with autologous HSCT at a single Brazilian center, and to compare them with the international experience.

Patients and methods

Study design and patient enrolment

This retrospective study included 70 SSc patients older than 18 years of age, diagnosed according to the ACR criteria of 1980 [27] and ACR/EULAR of 2013 [28], who underwent autologous HSCT from November 2009 to May 2016. The institutional ethics committee approved the study (CAAE: 71204717.6.0000.5440) and consent forms were waved due to the retrospective nature of data collection. At enrolment for transplantation, every patient had signed informed consent forms agreeing to participate in HSCT as an experimental protocol, with collection of clinical data and biological samples for the purpose of research.

Patients were eligible for transplantation if up to 60 years of age, and with evidence of skin and/or interstitial lung disease worsening in the past 6 months, despite immunosuppressive therapy. Specifically, transplant indications included diffuse skin involvement with increases in the mRSS [29] by more than 25% (if initial mRSS greater than 14) and/or interstitial lung disease with worsening of pulmonary function detected by reduction in forced vital capacity (FVC) and/or diffusing capacity of lung for carbon monoxide (DLCO) predicted values greater than 10%. Exclusion criteria for the procedure were: left ventricular ejection fraction below 40%, constrictive pericarditis, moderate or severe diastolic dysfunction (evidenced by echocardiography, cardiac MRI or right side catheterism) or ventricular arrhythmias, FVC below 45%, DLCO lower than 40%, systolic pulmonary artery pressure above 40 mmHg by echocardiography or mean pulmonary artery pressure higher than 27 mmHg by right side catheterism, serum creatinine levels higher than 2 mg/dl, aspartate aminotransferase/ alanine transaminase (AST/ALT) serum levels above 3 times the normal limit, total bilirubin serum levels greater than 2 mg/dl (excluding Gilbert's disease), positive serology for HIV or HTLV 1 and 2, previous malignancy, positive pregnancy test, psychiatric disorder and cognitive impairment that compromises treatment adherence or understanding of the consent form. Overlapping autoimmune diseases did not contraindicate enrolment for the procedure.

Experimental procedure and data collection

Immediately before transplantation, all patients underwent a thorough clinical and laboratorial assessment, aiming to evaluate the disease status, as well as possible exclusion conditions. Rodnan's skin score was measured by an experienced rheumatologist. Patients collected blood and urine samples for complete blood counts, biochemical profile, infectious serologies, pregnancy tests (female patients), urine analysis, creatinine clearance, proteinuria, and autoantibody assays. Patients underwent pulmonary function tests, high resolution computed tomography of the lungs, esophageal manometry, 24 h-electrocardiography (Holter) and echocardiography. Patients transplanted after the year 2014 also completed cardiac magnetic resonance and right-side cardiac catheterism with fluid challenge (infusion of 500 ml of saline over 10–15 min) as part of the pre-transplantation screening.

Autologous HSCT comprised a first phase, consisting of mobilization of hematopoietic progenitor cells from the bone marrow into the peripheral blood through infusion of cyclophosphamide at a dose of 2 g/m^2 and granulocyte colony stimulating factor (G-CSF), followed by apheresis and cryopreservation of unmanipulated hematopoietic progenitor cells (aiming for more than 2×10^6 CD34+ cells/kg of patient body weight). After a minimum interval of 2 weeks, patients started the second phase, comprising intense immunoablation, followed by infusion of the previously collected cells (Fig. 1). The standard immunoablative regimen consisted of 200 mg/kg cyclophosphamide plus 4.5 mg/kg anti-thymocyte globulin (ATG). When patients were overweight, cyclophosphamide doses were adjusted for ideal body weight (calculated considering ideal body mass index of 25 kg/m^2). For patients with evidence of heart involvement, but not fulfilling exclusion criteria for transplantation, the regimen consisted of fludarabine 120 mg/m^2 and melphalan 120 mg/m^2 of body surface plus 4.5 mg/kg ATG. Autologous progenitor cells infusions were followed by approximately 7 days of aplasia (destruction of the previous immuno-hematological system), and subsequent recovery of red blood cells, leukocytes and platelets. Neutrophil and platelet engraftment was considered when the patients reached at least 500 neutrophils/µL and at least 20.000 platelets/µL for three consecutive days, respectively, not supported by transfusion.

Patients were evaluated immediately before transplant (pre-HSCT), at 6 months and then yearly, until at least 60 months of follow-up after transplantation, after which patients returned to their original rheumatologist. At each evaluation, patients underwent clinical examination, including mRSS, complete blood counts, biochemical tests, high-resolution computed tomography of the chest and pulmonary function with DLCO. Clinical data were obtained from medical records. Disease progression/reactivation was considered when there was worsening of mRSS values above 25% of baseline (pre-transplant) levels, decline in FVC or DLCO predicted percentages above 10%, scleroderma renal crisis or initiation of immunosuppressive therapy. A HSCT failure would be established if the patient fulfilled the progression criteria at the first (6 months) evaluation after transplant. None of the patients had a HSCT failure. Beyond the fifth year of post-HSCT follow-up, monitoring for survival and late disease reactivation was done by telephone calls, whenever possible.

Statistical analysis

An exploratory data analysis was performed using measures of central position, dispersion and box-plot graphs for quantitative variables. Qualitative variables are presented considering absolute and relative frequencies. Linear regression models of mixed effects were performed to verify the effect of time in relation to the variables where the repeated measures of each patient were considered as a random effect and time as a fixed effect. Comparisons between evaluation periods were performed using orthogonal contrasts. The fit of the model was verified through the analysis of residues. Statistical analyses used SAS software (SAS Institute Inc., NC, USA) version 9.4. Graphs were created with GraphPad Prism (*GraphPad Software*, Inc., CA, EUA) version 9. Significance was set at 0.05.

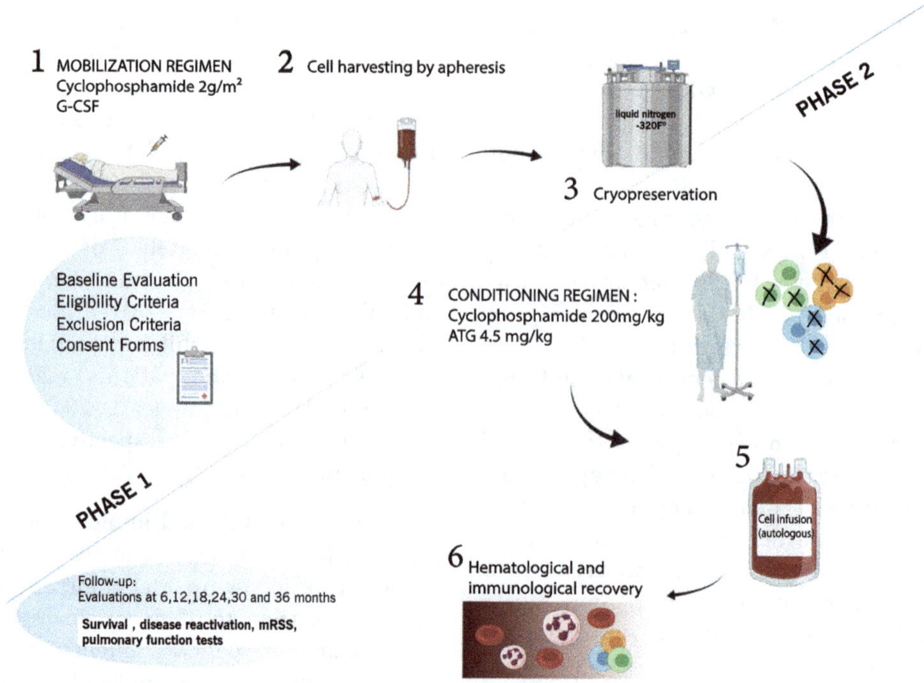

Fig. 1 Study design. Hematopoietic stem cell transplantation comprises two phases. In phase I, patients that fulfill the inclusion criteria for transplantation are thoroughly evaluated for organ involvement, eligibility and exclusion criteria (baseline evaluation). Then, progenitor hematopoietic cells (CD34+) are mobilized from the bone marrow to the peripheral blood by a regimen of cyclophosphamide plus granulocyte-colony stimulating factor (G-CSF). Circulating CD34+ cells are harvested from the peripheral blood through apheresis and cryopreserved, without further manipulation. In phase 2, which begins at least 2 weeks after phase 1, patients are treated with a conditioning regimen consisting of combined high-dose chemotherapy and immunotherapy agents, usually cyclophosphamide 200 mg/kg plus anti-thymocyte globulin (ATG). Subsequently, the previously harvested autologous progenitor cells are thawed at bedside and administered to the patient, intravenously. A period of bone marrow aplasia follows, lasting approximately 7 days, ended by hematological and immunological recovery. Patients are followed-up periodically for hematological and immunological reconstitution and clinical outcomes, until 5-years of follow-up

Results

Seventy transplanted adult SSc patients were initially included in the study, and 66 patients had available data for analysis on long-term follow-up (Fig. 2). Table 1 shows baseline (pre-HSCT) characteristics of all adult transplanted patients. Most subjects presented diffuse SSc, had interstitial lung disease and gastrointestinal involvement. Approximately two thirds of the patients had positive anti-topoisomerase I (anti-SCl70) antibodies and all had been treated with at least one line of immunosuppressive therapy. Fifty-one (73%) patients had progressing interstitial lung disease as indication for HSCT, out of which 46 (90%) had been previously treated with intravenous cyclophosphamide, 11 (21%) with mycophenolate mofetil and 4 (8%) with rituximab.

Immediate transplant outcomes

Sixty-nine patients underwent mobilization with cyclophosphamide and G-CSF, as determined by institutional protocol. One patient was mobilized with G-CSF only, due to a previous episode of acute cardiac insufficiency after a standard cyclophosphamide pulse. Mean (standard deviation, SD) CD34+ cell count was 5.63 (3.21) × 10^6 cells per kilogram of body weight and there were no progenitor harvesting failures. Sixty-five (92.8%) patients received immunoablative conditioning regimen with cyclophosphamide and ATG. The five remaining patients were treated with the fludarabine plus melphalan and ATG regimen, due to cardiac involvement by SSc evidenced by the pre-transplantation screening. All patients presented neutrophil and platelet engraftment at median (range) time of 9 (8–11) and 10 (9–14) days after HSCT, respectively. For the subset of patients transplanted with fludarabine and melphalan, median (range) time for neutrophil engraftment was of 11 (10–13) days, therefore slightly delayed in comparison to the whole group of patients. Platelet engraftment was not different.

Gastrointestinal manifestations, mostly nausea and vomiting, as well as alopecia, are expected side effects of cyclophosphamide and occurred in all patients (Table 2). Acute myocardial toxicity, verified by echocardiography as a decrease in left ventricle ejection fraction of more than 10% and increase in serum troponin levels, was detected in four of the patients treated with high-dose cyclophosphamide. Most patients presented fever while

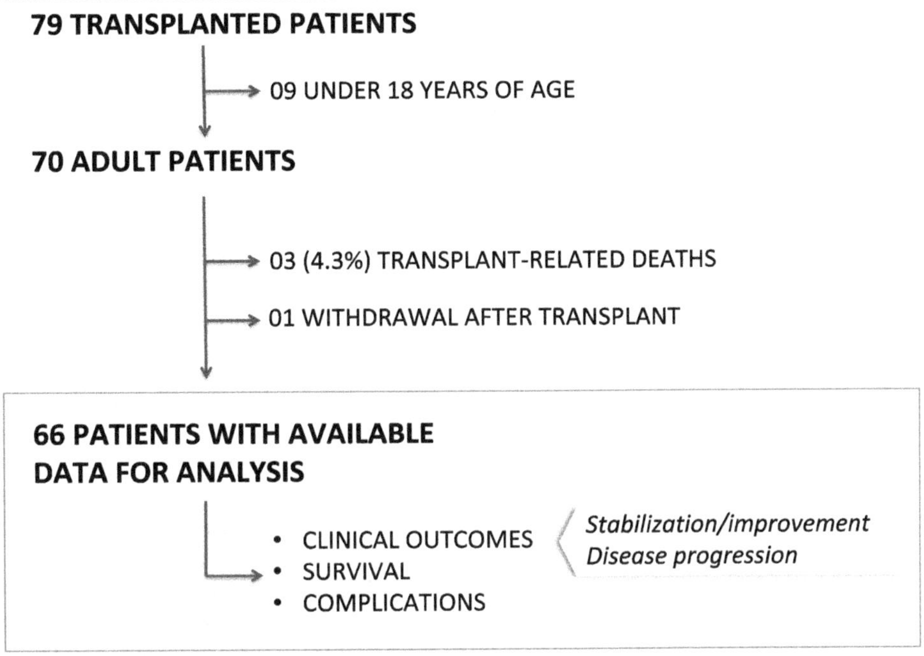

Fig. 2 Number of patients included in the retrospective study. From the initial 79 patients transplanted from 2009 to 2016, nine were under 18 years of age and were therefore excluded. Three patients died due to transplant-related complications (sepsis, complications of acute acalculous cholecystitis and acute cyclophosphamide-induced cardiotoxicity) and therefore did not have follow-up data. One patient voluntarily left the study after transplantation and was lost to follow-up (alive in December 2019, as confirmed by phone call)

in the neutropenic phase of HSCT, but infections were clinically identified in only 8 (11%) of the patients. After engraftment, cytomegalovirus (CMV) reactivations were detected by polymerase chain reaction in 10 (14%) of the patients in the immediate post-transplantation period (up to 60 days after HSCT), and were more frequent in patients treated with fludarabine and melphalan (4 out of 5 patients) than in the cyclophosphamide-treated patients (6 out of 62). None of the patients developed clinical manifestations of CMV disease. Two patients who had systemic lupus erythematosus (SLE) overlapping with the SSc presented improvement of both autoimmune diseases after HSCT, however some manifestations of SLE (hemolytic anemia and thrombocytopenia in one patient, and pericarditis in the other) reactivated approximately 24 months after transplant.

Survival

At 3, 5 and 8-year follow-up, the overall survival rates (95% confidence interval, CI) were 91.8% (81.2–97.1), 85.9% (73.8–93.4) and 81% (64.3–89.1) and the progression-free survival rates (CI) were 71.8%(61.1–83.4), 71.8% (60.1–82.9) and 70.5% (59.2–81.4), respectively (Fig. 3). There were three transplant-related deaths within 100 days after HSCT. One patient with extensive gastrointestinal involvement at baseline died 23 days after autologous HSCT due to sepsis by *Acinetobacter baumannii*. A second patient with advanced disease, but no evidence of cardiac involvement at enrolment died 60 days post-transplantation due to complications after an episode of acute cyclophosphamide-induced cardiac toxicity. A third patient presented an acute episode of acalculous cholecystitis and required emergency laparotomy during transplantation, while still in the neutropenic phase. In the post-operatory period, she presented a mixed septic and cardiogenic shock, which led to death 1 week after HSCT. Over long-term follow-up, nine additional patients died due to disease reactivation and organ failure, mostly cardiopulmonary, and one patient died due to central nervous system complications of thrombocytopenic thrombotic purpura (described in Table 2).

Disease outcomes

Before HSCT, median (range) mRSS was 24 (8–51), and significantly improved after the procedure, from 6 months until the 5-year follow-up time point (Fig. 4a). Forced vital capacity (Fig. 4b) and DLCO (Fig. 4c) percentages stabilized after HSCT in the 66 SSc patients that had follow-up data after HSCT. However, when separately analyzed, the subgroup of 51 patients with progressing interstitial lung disease (presenting more than 10% decline in FVC or DLCO in the 6 months preceding enrolment for HSCT) presented improvements in both FVC and DLCO predicted percentages after HSCT (Fig. 4d and e). In total, 17 patients had disease

Table 1 Patient baseline characteristics and transplant details

Total number of adult patients	70
Median (range) age (years)	35.9 (19–59)
Gender (%)	57 (81.4%) female
Disease subtype	67 (95.7%) diffuse
Median (range) disease duration (years)[a]	2 (1–7)
Organ involvement:	
Skin n (%)	70/70 (100%)
Interstitial lung disease, n (%)	59/70 (84.2%)
Pulmonary hypertension, n (%)	4/70 (5.7%) mild
Heart involvement, n (%)	32/70 (45.7%)[b]
Gastrointestinal, n (%)	57/62 (92%)
Kidney n	0
Positive anti-SCl70 antibodies, n (%)	43/64 (67.2%)
Previous immunosuppressive treatment:	
Methotrexate, n (%)	26/70 (37.1%)
Cyclophosphamide, n (%)	48/70 (68.6%)
Mycophenolate mofetil, n (%)	13/70 (18.6%)
Rituximab, n (%)	4/70 (5.7%)
Transplant regimen:	
Cyclophosphamide + ATG	65 (92.8%)
Fludarabine + Melphalan + ATG	5 (7.2%)

Baseline (pre-transplant) clinical characteristics of patients enrolled in the study
IV intravenous infusion, *ATG* anti-thymocyte globulin
[a]Disease duration from first non-Raynaud's phenomenon clinical manifestation until transplant
[b]Patients with severe heart involvement were excluded from transplant

reactivation after HSCT, 15 of which required further immunosuppressive treatment (Table 2). Worsening of the interstitial lung disease, verified by high-resolution computed tomography and decline in pulmonary function, was the most frequently detected reactivation, usually treated with rituximab and/or mycophenolate mofetil. Skin and myopathy reactivations were treated with methotrexate, and gastrointestinal worsening was treated with prokinetic agents and nutritional support. Two patients required jejunostomies for feeding.

Discussion

Hematopoietic stem cell transplantation for autoimmune diseases has been practiced for at least 20 years worldwide. To date, more than 2000 transplants have been reported by tenths of transplant centers [4]. At our center, the experience with HSCT has begun in 2001, with an initial focus on systemic lupus erythematosus and multiple sclerosis [30, 31]. Later, we started to consistently enroll patients with severe and progressive SSc. Here, we describe the clinical outcomes of 70 adult SSc patients treated at a single center, from 2009 and 2016, under similar transplant protocols.

Most patients in our study presented progressive interstitial lung involvement as indication for HSCT. When the whole cohort of patients was analyzed, we observed stabilization of pulmonary function, which agrees with most international studies [2, 5, 20–28]. However, when the subgroup of patients with progressive interstitial lung disease as indication for HSCT was analyzed separately, we were able to detect significant improvement of FVC and DLCO after HSCT. In accordance, a systematic review of the literature compiled data from the main clinical trials and found improvement in FVC at 1 and 2 years after HSCT [32].

Recently, we have reported quantitative computed tomography outcomes of our SSc patients, showing that in patients that improve lung function the volume of diseased lung parenchyma decreases after HSCT, when compared to pre-transplant measurements [33]. We believe that functional improvement reflects a control in the inflammatory component of interstitial lung disease, which is an early manifestation of diffuse SSc. Indeed, some authors suggest that patients should be transplanted early in disease course, aiming to achieve higher reversibility of organ involvement [21, 22]. In our study, the median disease duration of our patients, at enrolment, was 2 years, indicating that at least half were enrolled still at early stages of disease. On the other hand, we included patients up to 7 years of disease duration, but duration of disease did not strongly correlate with skin and lung function outcomes (data not shown), indicating that other factors, yet to be determined, might be participating.

The most clinically detectable outcome of HSCT is the improvement of skin thickness, assessed by mRSS. This is a consistent finding across studies on HSCT for SSc, as skin thickness decreases significantly, especially in the first 6 months after HSCT [1, 2, 5, 20, 24, 32]. Rodnan's score has good correlation with dermal thickness, evaluated both through skin biopsies and ultrasound [34, 35]. In fact, histopathological analyses show a decline in dermal thickness at 1 year post-transplantation, which is not different from that of healthy controls at 5 years after HSCT [5]. An interesting aspect is that most patients in our cohort had been previously treated with intravenous cyclophosphamide, and yet had a good response to HSCT using high-dose cyclophosphamide. We were not able to observe differences in outcomes according to previous therapy, and even if cyclophosphamide is not usually indicated for skin involvement, we did observe considerable improvement of mRSS after HSCT.

Skin involvement in SSc has a negative impact on survival and on quality of life [36]. A previous study from our group, which included a subset of patients also enrolled in this present study, has shown that autologous HSCT improves functional outcomes of SSc patients,

Table 2 Complications and disease-related events after transplantation

Transplant-related complications[a]	N (%)
Nausea/vomiting	70 (100%)
Alopecia	70 (100%)
Neutropenic fever	65 (93%)
Bacterial pneumonia	5 (7%)
Cyclophosphamide-induced cardiac dysfunction	4 (6%)
Sepsis	2 (3%)
Melphalan-induced mucositis	2 (3%)
Central catheter-related pneumothorax	1 (1%)
Acalculous cholecystitis	1 (1%)
Polyomavirus-induced hemorrhagic cystitis (mild)	1 (1%)
CMV reactivation (no CMV disease)	10 (14%)
Transplant-related deaths (total):	3 (4%)
Sepsis, *Acinetobacter baumannii*	
Complications of acalculous cholecystitis Acute myocardial toxicity	
Disease reactivations	
Skin worsening	3 (4%)
Pulmonary function worsening	6 (9%)
Inflammatory myopathy	2 (3%)
Gastrointestinal progression/gastroparesis	4 (6%)
Other (SLE reactivation, cytopenia) requiring immunosuppression	2 (3%)
Disease-associated deaths (total):	9 (13%)
Acute lung exacerbation (3 patients)	
Gastrointestinal progression (2 patients)	
Cardiac insufficiency (2 patients)	
Scleroderma renal crisis (1 patient)	
Pulmonary embolism (1 patient)	
Non-disease related events	
Thrombotic thrombocytopenic purpura (death)	1 (1%)
Pregnancies in female transplanted patients	3 (5.5%)

Number of complications associated or not associated with the transplant procedure, including disease reactivation and long-term survival outcomes
CMV cytomegalovirus, *SLE* systemic lupus erythematosus (disease overlap)
[a]Complications associated to the procedure within 60 days after HSCT

including functional capacity measured by the 6-min walking distance, inspiratory and expiratory lung pressures, joint range-of-motion, hand function and mouth opening, as well as physical and mental aspects of quality of life [37]. We consider important to evaluate such outcomes, as they reflect the positive impact of HSCT on the daily life of patients. Although most of these functional assessments are closely related with skin involvement, functional capacity did not strongly correlate with pulmonary, skin or musculoskeletal outcomes, suggesting that the improvement is a combination of multiple effects of HSCT.

Patient outcomes after HSCT for autoimmune diseases have considerably improved over the years. Nevertheless, a number of adverse events associated with the procedure still persist. Systemic sclerosis, among the autoimmune diseases, has the highest transplant-related morbidity and mortality rates [4, 38], mostly due to baseline organ involvement by the disease. Our study reports three transplant-related deaths. In at least two of these events, patients were very ill and severely affected by the disease. In our retrospective perspective, more stringent patient selection might have avoided the fatal outcomes. Systemic sclerosis has a very narrow window of opportunity for HSCT and patients at end-stage disease should not be enrolled. This is part of the "learning curve" that follows medical and scientific progress [4, 38]. Fortunately, advances in patient selection and

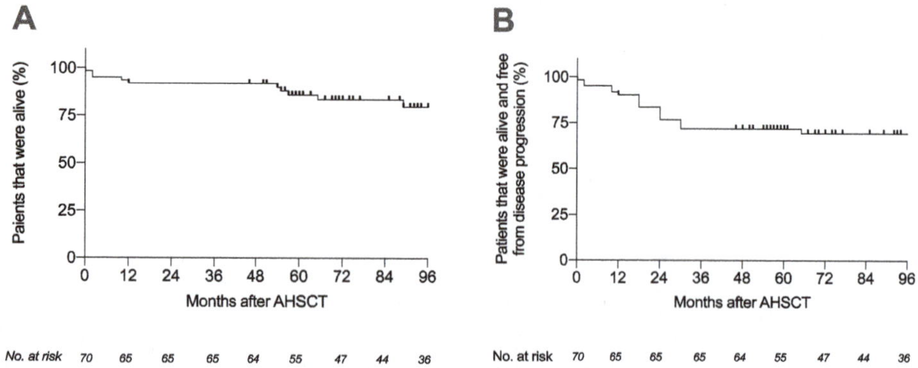

Fig. 3 Survival outcomes over 8-year follow-up after transplantation. **a** Overall survival; percentage of patients that were alive at each yearly follow-up time point. **b** Progression-free survival; percentage of patients that were alive and free from disease progression at each follow-up time point. Disease progression criteria are described in the Patients and Methods section. The numbers of patients at risk, at each time point, are described below each graph

management have enabled better survival rates and outcomes over the years [38].

Cardiac involvement plays a key role in patient safety, as SSc affects the heart in multiple and silent manners [20, 39]. Standard pre-transplantation evaluations with electro and echocardiography are not sufficiently accurate to identify SSc patients at risk during HSCT [20]. The combination of high dose cyclophosphamide, fluid overload and cytokine release inflicts excessive strain on the already dysfunctional cardiopulmonary system and may impose risks. Recently, the EBMT and partners have published recommendations for pre-transplantation evaluations of SSc patients [14]. In fact, at our center, cardiac failure events have declined, albeit not completely ceased, after we started to follow such guidelines, including cardiac MRI and right side catheterism with fluid overload in our pre-transplantation evaluation. In addition, in cases where the patient presented some

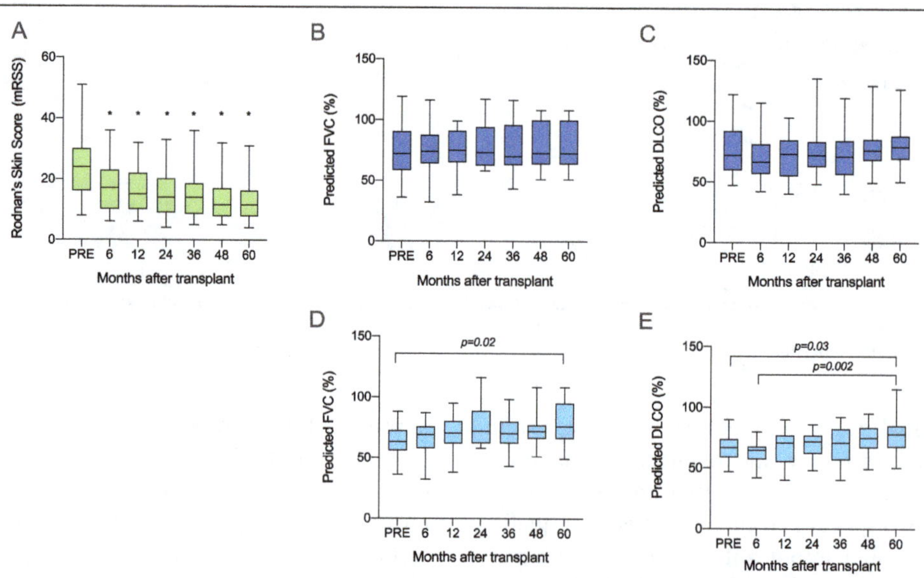

Fig. 4 Clinical Outcomes over 5-year follow-up after transplantation. **a** Modified Rodnan's Skin Score before and periodically after autologous hematopoietic stem cell transplantation (HSCT). * indicates significant diferences between baseline (PRE) and post-HSCT time points: PRE vs 6 months, $p = 0.007$; PRE vs 12 months, $p = 0.0006$; PRE vs 24, 36, 48 and 60 months, $p < 0.0001$. **b** Predicted forced vital capacity (FVC) percentages before and periodically after autologous HSCT in all patients included in the study. **c** Predicted percentages of diffusing capacity of lung carbon monoxide (DLCO) before and periodically after autologous HSCT in all patients included in the study. **d** Predicted FVC percentages before and periodically after autologous HSCT in the subset of patients with progressive interstitial lung disease at enrollment for transplantation. **e** Predicted percentages of diffusing capacity of lung carbon monoxide (DLCO) before and periodically after autologous HSCT in patients with progressive interstitial lung disease at enrollment for transplantation. Box plot limits indicate 25th to 75th percentiles; lines within boxes indicate the median and whiskers mark the 10th and the 90th percentiles

degree of cardiac damage, but not formally fulfilled the exclusion criteria, we chose an alternative transplant regimen, with fludarabine plus melphalan, instead of high dose cyclophosphamide. Although only a few patients have been included in this new regimen, we have observed a good profile of cardiac safety (data not shown), despite a possible increase in the incidence of mucositis and infectious events such as CMV reactivation. The number of patients transplanted with this alternative regimen is not large enough to enable comparisons regarding long-term efficacy in controlling disease progression. A similar strategy has been recently published, aiming to decrease the total dose of cyclophosphamide in patients with high SSc-associated cardiac risk [40].

The patients enrolled in our study have a severe disease profile, as most have diffuse skin involvement, positive anti-SCl 70 antibodies and progressive interstitial lung disease. We also included patients with overlapping SLE, and although SLE is also a primary indication for HSCT [4], it adds complexity and risk to the procedure. Patients with similar characteristics are also described by most trials on HSCT for SSc [1, 2, 20–23]. In face of the severity of the disease, these patients have benefited from HSCT, despite the toxicity of the procedure. On the other side, transplant-related mortality is closely related to the degree of organ involvement by the disease, especially cardiopulmonary and gastrointestinal [20, 38]. Therefore, adequate patient selection is key to ensure enrollment within the adequate window of opportunity. The main challenge is to identify patients with a disease severe enough to require HSCT, but still not too advanced in order to tolerate transplant-related toxicity. In this context, scientific dissemination and educational events are essential to increase rheumatologist awareness that HSCT may be an option for patients with the right profile of disease.

Conclusions

In this study, we show a Brazilian experience of HSCT as a therapeutic strategy for patients with SSc. The survival and disease outcomes here described are in accordance with those reported by other international transplant centers. Conventional treatment options for SSc have still limited efficacy in promoting disease control, and HSCT stands as an alternative for selected patients with severe and progressive disease.

Abbreviations

AST/ALT: Aspartate aminotransferase/alanine transaminase; ASTCT: American Society for Transplant and Cell Therapy; ATG: Anti-thymocyte globulin; CI: Confidence interval; CMV: Cytomegalovirus; DLCO: Diffusing capacity for carbon monoxide; EULAR: European League Against Rheumatism; FVC: Forced Vital Capacity; G-CSF: Granulocyte-colony stimulating factor; HIV: Human immunodeficiency virus; HSCT: Hematopoietic stem cell transplantation; HTLV: Human T-lymphotropic virus; mRSS: Modified Rodnan's Skin Score; SBTMO: Brazilian Society of Bone Marrow Transplantation; SD: Standard Deviation; SSc: Systemic sclerosis

Acknowledgements

The authors thank the multidisciplinary team of the Hospital das Clínicas da Faculdade de Medicina de Ribeirão Preto – Universidade de São Paulo for their work in patient care and also the Ribeirão Preto Regional Blood Center staff for processing and cryopreservation of the progenitor hematopoietic cells. Their contributions have made this manuscript possible.

Authors' contributions

AHN – made significant contributions to acquisition, interpretation and analysis of the data, and drafted the manuscript; MYKV, DAM, JBED, TGZ, MFCO and LFW contributed to data acquisition; MSG, DCZS, GMD and VCL contributed to the analysis and interpretation of the data; MCO designed the study, supervised data acquisition, interpretation and analysis and substantially revised the manuscript. All authors approve the submitted version of this manuscript. All authors agree both to be personally accountable for the author's own contributions and to ensure that questions related to the accuracy or integrity of any part of the work, even ones in which the author was not personally involved, are appropriately investigated, resolved, and the resolution documented in the literature.

Author details

[1]Graduate Program in Internal Medicine, Ribeirão Preto Medical School, University of São Paulo, Ribeirão Preto, Brazil. [2]Center for Cell-Based Therapy, Ribeirão Preto Medical School, University of São Paulo, Ribeirão Preto, Brazil. [3]Hospital das Clínicas da Faculdade de Medicina de Ribeirão Preto, Ribeirão Preto Medical School, University of São Paulo, Ribeirão Preto, Brazil. [4]Graduate Program in Oncology, Stem Cells and Cell Therapy, Ribeirão Preto Medical School, University of São Paulo, Ribeirão Preto, Brazil. [5]Graduate Program in Basic and Applied Immunology, Ribeirão Preto Medical School, University of São Paulo, Ribeirão Preto, Brazil. [6]Ribeirão Preto School of Nursing, University of São Paulo, Ribeirão Preto, Brazil. [7]Department of Internal Medicine, Ribeirão Preto Medical School, University of São Paulo, Avenida dos Bandeirantes 3900, Ribeirão Preto, SP 14048-900, Brazil.

References

1. Del Papa N, Pignataro F, Zaccara E, Maglione W, Minniti A. Autologous hematopoietic stem cell transplantation for treatment of systemic sclerosis. Front Immunol. 2018;9:2390.
2. Henes J, Oliveira MC, Labopin M, Badoglio M, Scherer HU, Del Papa N, et al. Autologous stem cell transplantation for progressive systemic sclerosis: a prospective non-interventional study from the European Society for Blood and Marrow Transplantation Autoimmune Disease Working Party. Haematologica. 2020. https://doi.org/10.3324/haematol.2019.230128.
3. Sullivan KM, Majhail NS, Bredeson C, Carpenter PA, Chatterjee S, Crofford LJ, et al. Systemic sclerosis as an indication for autologous hematopoietic cell transplantation: position statement from the American Society for Blood and Marrow Transplantation. Biol Blood Marrow Transplant. 2018;24:1961–4.
4. Snowden JA, Badoglio M, Labopin M, Giebel S, McGrath E, Marjanovic Z, et al. Evolution, trends, outcomes, and economics of hematopoietic stem cell transplantation in severe autoimmune diseases. Blood Adv. 2017;1:2742 55.
5. Nash RA, McSweeney PA, Crofford LJ, Abidi M, Chen C-S, Godwin JD, et al. High-dose immunosuppressive therapy and autologous hematopoietic cell transplantation for severe systemic sclerosis: long-term follow-up of the US multicenter pilot study. Blood. 2007;110:1388–96.
6. Binks M, Passweg JR, Furst D, McSweeney P, Sullivan K, Besenthal C, et al. Phase I/II trial of autologous stem cell transplantation in systemic sclerosis: procedure related mortality and impact on skin disease. Ann Rheum Dis. 2001;60:577–84.
7. Burt RK, Oyama Y, Traynor A, Quigley K, Brush M, Rodriguez J, et al. Hematopoietic stem cell transplantation for systemic sclerosis with rapid improvement in skin scores: is neoangiogenesis occurring? Bone Marrow Transplant. 2003;32(Suppl 1):S65–7.
8. Del Papa N, Onida F, Zaccara E, Saporiti G, Maglione W, Tagliaferri E, et al. Autologous hematopoietic stem cell transplantation has better outcomes than conventional therapies in patients with rapidly progressive systemic

sclerosis. Bone Marrow Transplant. 2017;52:53–8.
9. Farge D, Marolleau JP, Zohar S, Marjanovic Z, Cabane J, Mounier N, et al. Autologous bone marrow transplantation in the treatment of refractory systemic sclerosis: early results from a French multicentre phase I-II study. Br J Haematol. 2002;119:726–39.
10. Farge D, Passweg J, van Laar JM, Marjanovic Z, Besenthal C, Finke J, et al. Autologous stem cell transplantation in the treatment of systemic sclerosis: report from the EBMT/EULAR Registry. Ann Rheum Dis. 2004;63:974–81.
11. Henes JC, Schmalzing M, Vogel W, Riemekasten G, Fend F, Kanz L, et al. Optimization of autologous stem cell transplantation for systemic sclerosis -- a single-center longterm experience in 26 patients with severe organ manifestations. J Rheumatol. 2012;39:269–75.
12. Oyama Y, Barr WG, Statkute L, Corbridge T, Gonda EA, Jovanovic B, et al. Autologous non-myeloablative hematopoietic stem cell transplantation in patients with systemic sclerosis. Bone Marrow Transplant. 2007;40:549–55.
13. Burt RK, Oliveira MC, Shah SJ. Cardiac assessment before stem cell transplantation for systemic sclerosis. JAMA. 2014;312:1803.
14. Farge D, Burt RK, Oliveira MC, Mousseaux E, Rovira M, Marjanovic Z, et al. Cardiopulmonary assessment of patients with systemic sclerosis for hematopoietic stem cell transplantation: recommendations from the European Society for Blood and Marrow Transplantation Autoimmune Diseases Working Party and collaborating partners. Bone Marrow Transplant. 2017;52:1495–503.
15. Snowden JA, Sharrack B, Akil M, Kiely DG, Lobo A, Kazmi M, et al. Autologous haematopoietic stem cell transplantation (aHSCT) for severe resistant autoimmune and inflammatory diseases - a guide for the generalist. Clin Med. 2018;18:329–34.
16. Muraro PA, Douek DC, Packer A, Chung K, Guenaga FJ, Cassiani-Ingoni R, et al. Thymic output generates a new and diverse TCR repertoire after autologous stem cell transplantation in multiple sclerosis patients. J Exp Med. 2005;201:805–16.
17. Arruda LC, Clave E, Moins-Teisserenc H, Douay C, Farge D, Toubert A. Resetting the immune response after autologous hematopoietic stem cell transplantation for autoimmune diseases. Curr Res Transl Med. 2016;64:107–
18. Arruda LCM, Malmegrim KCR, Lima-Júnior JR, Clave E, Dias JBE, Moraes DA, et al. Immune rebound associates with a favorable clinical response to autologous HSCT in systemic sclerosis patients. Blood Adv. 2018;2:126–41.
19. Assassi S, Wang X, Chen G, Goldmuntz E, Keyes-Elstein L, Ying J, et al. Myeloablation followed by autologous stem cell transplantation normalises systemic sclerosis molecular signatures. Ann Rheum Dis. 2019;78:1371–8.
20. Burt RK, Oliveira MC, Shah SJ, Moraes DA, Simoes B, Gheorghiade M, et al. Cardiac involvement and treatment-related mortality after non-myeloablative haemopoietic stem-cell transplantation with unselected autologous peripheral blood for patients with systemic sclerosis: a retrospective analysis. Lancet. 2013;381:1116–24.
21. Burt RK, Shah SJ, Dill K, Grant T, Gheorghiade M, Schroeder J, et al. Autologous non-myeloablative haemopoietic stem-cell transplantation compared with pulse cyclophosphamide once per month for systemic sclerosis (ASSIST): an open-label, randomised phase 2 trial. Lancet. 2011;378:498–506.
22. van Laar JM, Farge D, Sont JK, Naraghi K, Marjanovic Z, Larghero J, et al. Autologous hematopoietic stem cell transplantation vs intravenous pulse cyclophosphamide in diffuse cutaneous systemic sclerosis: a randomized clinical trial. JAMA. 2014;311:2490–8.
23. Sullivan KM, Goldmuntz EA, Keyes-Elstein L, McSweeney PA, Pinckney A, Welch B, et al. Myeloablative autologous stem-cell transplantation for severe scleroderma. N Engl J Med. 2018;378:35–47.
24. Shouval R, Furie N, Raanani P, Nagler A, Gafter-Gvili A. Autologous hematopoietic stem cell transplantation for systemic sclerosis: a systematic review and meta-analysis. Biol Blood Marrow Transplant. 2018;24:937–44.
25. Kowal-Bielecka O, Fransen J, Avouac J, Becker M, Kulak A, Allanore Y, et al.13. Update of EULAR recommendations for the treatment of systemic sclerosis. Ann Rheum Dis. 2017;76:1327–39.
26. Oliveira MC, Elias JB, Moraes DA, Simões BP, Rodrigues M, Ribeiro AAF, et al. A review of hematopoietic stem cell transplantation for autoimmune diseases: multiple sclerosis, systemic sclerosis and Crohn's disease. Position paper of the Brazilian Society of Bone Marrow Transplantation. Hematol Transfus Cell Ther. 2020:S2531 1379(20)30032 8.
27. Subcommittee for Scleroderma Criteria of the American Rheumatism Association Diagnostic and Therapeutic Criteria Committee. Preliminary criteria for the classification of systemic sclerosis (scleroderma). Arthritis Rheum. 1980; 23:581–90.
28. van den Hoogen F, Khanna D, Fransen J, Johnson SR, Baron M, Tyndall A, et al. 2013 classification criteria for systemic sclerosis: an American college of rheumatology/European league against rheumatism collaborative initiative. Ann Rheum Dis. 2013;72:1747–55.
29. Clements PJ, Lachenbruch PA, Ng SC, Simmons M, Sterz M, Furst DE. Skin score. A semiquantitative measure of cutaneous involvement that improves prediction of prognosis in systemic sclerosis. Arthritis Rheum. 1990;33:1256–63.
30. Voltarelli JC, Stracieri ABPL, Oliveira MCB, Godoi DF, Moraes DA, Pieroni F, et al. Transplante de células-tronco hematopoéticas em doenças reumáticas. Parte 2: experiência brasileira e perspectivas futuras. Rev Bras Reumatol. 2005;45:301–12.
31. Voltarelli JC, Ouyang J. Hematopoietic stem cell transplantation for autoimmune diseases in developing countries: current status and future prospectives. Bone Marrow Transplant. 2003;32(Suppl 1):S69–71.
32. Eyraud A, Scouppe L, Barnetche T, Forcade E, Lazaro E, Duffau P, et al. Efficacy and safety of autologous haematopoietic stem cell transplantation in systemic sclerosis: a systematic review of the literature. Br J Dermatol. 2018;178:650–8.
33. Wada DT, de Almeida FA, de Moraes DA, Dias JBE, Baddini-Martinez J, Oliveira MC, et al. Automatic quantitative computed tomography evaluation of the lungs in patients with systemic sclerosis treated with autologous stem cell transplantation. J Clin Rheumatol. 2020;26(7S Suppl 2):S158–64.
34. Ruaro B, Sulli A, Pizzorni C, Paolino S, Smith V, Alessandri E, et al. Correlations between blood perfusion and dermal thickness in different skin areas of systemic sclerosis patients. Microvasc Res. 2018;115:28–33.
35. Chen C, Cheng Y, Zhu X, Cai Y, Xue Y, Kong N, et al. Ultrasound assessment of skin thickness and stiffness: the correlation with histology and clinical score in systemic sclerosis. Arthritis Res Ther. 2020;22:197.
36. Park EH, Strand V, Oh YJ, Song YW, Lee EB. Health-related quality of life in systemic sclerosis compared with other rheumatic diseases: a cross-sectional study. Arthritis Res Ther. 2019;21:61.
37. Costa-Pereira KR, Guimarães AL, Moraes DA, Dias JBE, Garcia JT, de Oliveira-Cardoso EA, et al. Hematopoietic stem cell transplantation improves functional outcomes of systemic sclerosis patients. J Clin Rheumatol. 2020;26(7S Suppl 2):S131–8.
38. Farge D, Labopin M, Tyndall A, Fassas A, Mancardi GL, Van Laar J, et al. Autologous hematopoietic stem cell transplantation for autoimmune diseases: an observational study on 12 years' experience from the European Group for Blood and Marrow Transplantation Working Party on Autoimmune Diseases. Haematologica. 2010;95:284–92.
39. Denton CP, Khanna D. Systemic sclerosis. Lancet. 2017;390:1685–99.
40. Burt RK, Han X, Quigley K, Arnautovic I, Shah SJ, Lee DC, et al. Cardiac safe hematopoietic stem cell transplantation for systemic sclerosis with poor cardiac function: a pilot safety study that decreases neutropenic interval to 5 days. Bone Marrow Transplant. 2021;56:50–9.

21

Surgical treatment for lumbar spinal stenosis: A single-blinded randomized controlled trial

Luiz Claudio Lacerda Rodrigues[1,2] and Jamil Natour[1*]

Abstract

Objective: To evaluate the effectiveness of surgery for the management of patients with symptomatic lumbar spinal stenosis.

Methods: Sixty-three patients with lumbar canal stenosis were randomized into two groups: the intervention group (IG) and control group (CG). IG patients underwent surgery and both groups participated in the same physical therapy program twice a week for a period of 12 weeks and were followed up at 1 year. The primary endpoint was visual analogue scale for pain, and the secondary endpoints were function (6-min walk test, Roland Morris and Oswestry questionnaires), quality of life (SF-36 questionnaire) and satisfaction with treatment (Likert scale).

Results: No significant difference between groups was observed for pain over time ($p = 0.145$). Significant differences between groups, in favor of the IG, were observed for the Oswestry score ($p = 0.006$) and vitality domain score of the SF-36 ($p = 0.047$). Function in the Roland Morris and 6-min walk test and the role of the physical domain of SF-36 also showed significant differences between the groups; however, these differences occurred due to a worsening of the IG in the short term, and the medium-term. The Likert scale demonstrated greater satisfaction with the IG treatment compared to control group.

Conclusions: Lumbar stenosis surgery did not improve pain in short and medium terms. Function and vitality were better in the group that underwent surgery in the medium term, and patients were more satisfied with the surgical treatment.

Trial registration: Clinicaltrials.gov (NCT02879461).

Keywords: Lumbar stenosis, Surgery, Back pain, Function, Spine, Quality of life

Introduction

Lumbar canal stenosis was first described by Antoine Portal in 1803. However, the first association of changes in the diameter of the spinal canal with clinical features and neurogenic claudication was performed by Verbiest [1, 2].

Neurogenic claudication, characterized by low back pain or weakness in the lower limbs, progressively worsening with an orthostatic position or walking, and improving after stopping, sitting or tilting the body forward, is the most common symptom of lumbar canal stenosis. The less common symptom is, unilateral radiculopathy [3].

Lumbar canal stenosis can be confused with many diseases, such as vascular claudication, tumors, peripheral neuropathy and knee or hip osteoarthritis [4]. The diagnosis is clinical, accompanied by findings in the imaging tests that confirm the narrowing of the spine canal [5].

Lumbar canal stenosis is among the most common causes of spinal surgery in individuals over 65 years. Functional disability and pain lead many patients to surgery after insufficient results are obtained with clinical

* Correspondence: jnatour@unifesp.br
[1]Rheumatology Division, Universidade Federal de São Paulo – Escola Paulista de Medicina (Unifesp-EPM), Sao Paulo, SP 04023900, Brazil

treatment. Even before adequate clinical treatment, many patients appeal to surgery, believing that it is a definitive a solution [6].

This is a large surgery, often involving laminectomy, arthrodesis and instrumentation, with a high cost to the health system.

The scientific literature, however, fails to demonstrate the advantages of surgical treatment. There are studies of poor methodological quality and those generally comparing different surgical techniques and not comparing surgical treatment with clinical treatment [7–11].

The aim of this study was to determine the effectiveness of surgery in the management of patients with symptomatic lumbar spinal stenosis.

Methods

A single-blind parallel randomized controlled trial was conducted with a 48-week follow-up period. Sixty-three patients of both genders, between 50 and 75 years old, were selected from the outpatient clinic and randomized into intervention group (IG) or control group (CG) using electronic randomization. Opaque envelopes were used to keep the secret of allocation. The study was approved by the institution's ethics committee and registered in clinicaltrials.gov (NCT02879461).

All the procedures were in accordance with the ethical standards of the responsible committee on human experimentation and with the Declaration of Helsinki and all patients agreed to participate and signed the informed consent form.

Only patients with up to three vertebral levels of lumbar canal stenosis were included in the study. The clinical diagnosis included the presence of claudication with less than 100 m of walking and at least two of the following complaints in the lower limbs: pain, weakness, numbness, and tingling that worsen with gait and improve with rest, whether they are associated with low back pain for at least 6 months [12].

The presence of lumbar canal stenosis was confirmed when the lumbar canal area was smaller than 100 mm^{2}, based on the Hamanishi criteria [13], measured on the lumbar spine MRI following L3 to S1, performed in a 1 Tesla device (Philips, Giroscan). The examination was performed with the patient in dorsal decubitus and with cushion on the knees to maintain flexion of the hip and knees. To avoid interference in the measurements of spinal canal due to angulation, all cuts were performed parallel to the discs, accepting an angulation difference of at most 5° [14].

The spinal canal diameter measurement was based on the laterolateral (a) and anteroposterior (b) diameter, always on the largest axis, with data provided by a computer program (OSIRIX® 2010) in the scanned image. These values were divided by two, individually, and multiplied by the value of π (PI) [3, 15]. The result obtained was multiplied by a constant that varied between 0.8 (when the spinal canal was circular), 0.7 (spinal canal elliptical), 0.6 in the presence of facet compression and 0.5 when compression was made by the disc and facets. Thus, (a / 2) X (b / 2) x π (constant) = area [13].

Patients were excluded if they showed the following: diabetes mellitus, hypertension or decompensated heart disease; systemic diseases affecting the lower limbs; neuromuscular diseases; patients with previous surgery on the spine; cognitive deficits that interfere with the ability to understand or interpret the questionnaires; spondylolisthesis, except degenerative; scoliosis with a Cobb angle greater than 10°; hip or knee disorders that could interfere with gait; total or partial arthroplasty in the hip or knee and lumbar canal stenosis in more than three levels.

The IG patients the underwent lumbar decompression surgery using the isolated posterior approach associated with arthrodesis, instrumented with the aid of radioscopy and always by the same senior surgeon. The arthrodesis was stimulated with the placement of a bone graft in the transverse processes and the use of pedicular screw implants without a cage. The surgery was done 1 week after the baseline evaluation. Patients in IG and CG were evaluated 4 weeks after baseline (T4 assessment) and both groups started physical therapy after this evaluation.

In the physical therapy program patients performed 5 exercises. All the exercises were performed in supine position with hips and knees flexed, feet resting on the bed and upper limbs resting along the body. Following the physical therapy program was detailed:

- Exercise 1: After deep inspiration, the patient contracts the muscles of the abdomen and buttocks, making a retroversion for 5 s, relax and restart. Strengthens abdominals and buttocks isometrically, 3 sets of 10 repetitions;
- Exercise 2: Performs gluteus contraction and hip lift (bridge). Strengthens buttocks and stabilizes the lumbar spine, 3 sets of 10 repetitions;
- Exercise 3: Pull one thigh interlacing the hands in the posterior region of the thigh, approaching the knee to the thorax, holding for 30 s and repeating with the other thigh, alternately performing the movement. Stretches lumbar paravertebral muscles, 10 repetitions on each side;
- Exercise 4: Pull both thighs at the same time, interlacing the hands in the posterior region of the thigh, approaching the knee to the thorax, and holding for 30 s. Stretches lumbar paravertebral muscles, 10 repetitions;
- Exercise 5: Using a stretching strap, hold the strap with both hands, place the strap on the arch of the

left foot and raise the left foot, straightening the left leg and keeping the right foot on the floor. Hold for 30 s. Stretches hamstring muscles, 10 repetitions on each side.

Patients in both groups took acetaminophen 750 mg up to three times daily for 90 days based on pain and patient's criteria.

Evaluations were performed by a blinded assessor at baseline (T0), after 4 (T4), 12 (T12 - end of physiotherapy), 24 (T24) and 48 (T48) weeks.

Patients were clinically evaluated at each time point to detect possible clinical or surgical complications, such as disabling pain, respiratory and surgical site infection, deep venous thrombosis and vascular complications.

The primary outcome was pain in the last week. This was measured using a visual analogue scale (VAS) ranging from 0 cm (no pain) to 10 cm (unbearable pain) [16];

Secondary outcomes were:

- Function - measured using the Roland-Morris questionnaire [17], with scores ranging from 0 to 24 points (lower scores denote better function); the Oswestry questionnaire [18], with scores ranging from 0 to 5 points (lower scores denote better function) and the 6-min walk test (6MWT) following the American Thoracic Society guidelines [19].
- General health. - assessed using the short form 36 (SF-36) questionnaire, with overall scores ranging from 0 to 100, and higher scores denote better general health [20].
- Patient satisfaction with treatment - measured with a Likert scale. The following question was asked: "How do you feel about your treatment?". The patient could select one of the five answer options: 5: much better; 4: a little better; 3: unchanged; 2: a little worse or 1: much worse.

Statistical analysis

Sample size was calculated for the repeated-measure analysis of variance (ANOVA) with two repetitions per situation, using the VAS for pain as the main parameter, with a standard deviation (SD) of 2 cm. For the determination of a minimal effect of 2 cm, a 5% α error, 20% β error and SD (σ) of 2 cm were established. The calculation determined a sample of 26 patients per group. Considering a possible loss of 20%, 63 patients were selected.

The following tests were used in data analysis:

✓ $\chi 2$, Student's t test and Mann–Whitney were used to determine the homogeneity of the sample at the initial evaluation.

✓ Repeated-measures ANOVA with Bonferroni adjustments were used to determine differences in the outcomes between groups over time.

✓ Pearson correlation were used to determine a correlation between pain and other baseline parameters like age, BMI and canal diameter.

Using intention-to-treat analysis, data from all patients initially enrolled were analyzed. For cases in which there was an interruption of treatment, the patients were first asked to come in and perform only the evaluations. For patients who refused to return for the evaluations, the last data collected were repeated in the subsequent evaluations.

Results

Sixty-three patients were randomized, 31 patients in the IG and 32 in the CG. The flowchart of the study is presented in Fig. 1.

The mean age of the IG patients was 60.7 years and the CG was 60.2 years. The IG had 8 men and 23 women, the CG had 8 men and 24 women ($p = 0.941$). The demographic data of the sample at the initial evaluation were shown in Table 1. The diameter of the vertebral canal was evaluated at the time of inclusion (Table 1).

During surgery, arthrodeses of different segments were performed. In three patients, one level was set, in eight patients, two levels were set, and in 20 patients, there were three levels.

No significant difference, using repeated measures ANOVA, were found between the groups for pain using the VAS (Table 2, Fig. 2), and in the following domains of SF-36: physical functioning; bodily pain; general health; social functioning; and role emotional and mental health (Table 2).

For function and quality of life, significant difference between groups were found for the following parameters:

- Oswestry ($p = 0.006$) - IG presented worsening in T4 and improvement from T12 to T48 remaining better than CG at the end the study. Significant differences between groups were found at T24 ($p = 0.011$) and T48 ($p = 0.009$), Table 2 and Fig. 2;
- Roland Morris ($p = 0.005$) - IG presented worsening in T4 and improvement after T12 reaching scores similar to CG in T48. Significant differences between groups were found at T4 ($p = 0.001$) and T12 ($p = 0.001$), Table 2 and Fig. 2;
- 6-min walk test ($p < 0.001$) - IG presented worsening in T4 and improvement after T12 reaching scores similar to CG in T48. Significant differences between the groups were found at T4 ($p = 0.001$) and T12 ($p = 0.024$), Table 2 and Fig. 2;

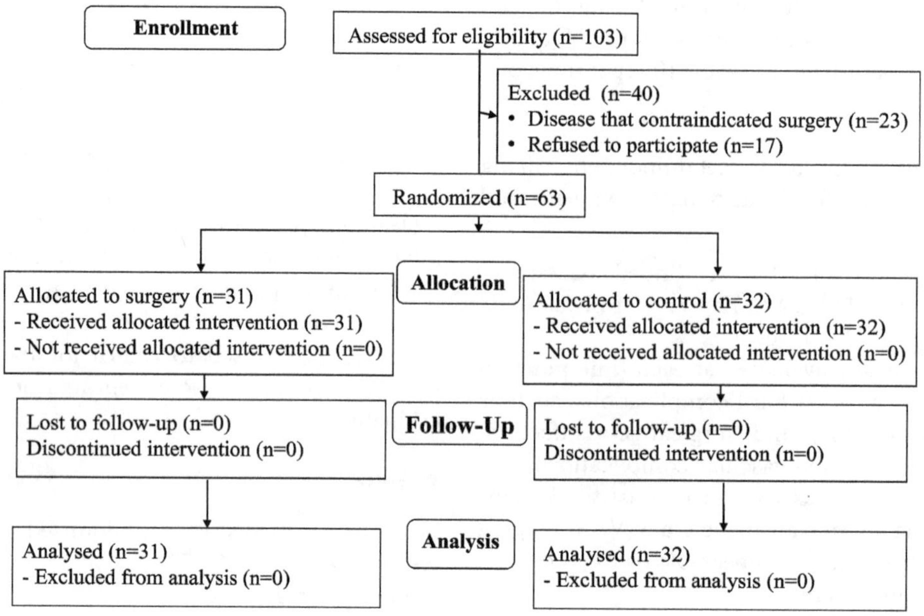

Fig. 1 Study flowchart

- Role physical domain of SF-36 ($p = 0.023$) - IG presented worsening in T4 and improvement after T12 reaching scores similar to CG in T48. Significant differences between groups were found at T4 ($p = 0.003$) and T24 ($p = 0.007$), Table 2 and Fig. 2;
- Vitality domain of SF-36 ($p = 0.047$) - IG presented improvement compared to CG. Significant differences between the groups were found at T4 ($p = 0.023$), T24 ($p = 0.014$) and T48 ($p = 0.25$), Table 2 and Fig. 2.

For treatment satisfaction, a significant difference between the groups was found based on the Likert scale ($p = 0.024$). Analyzing data from the groups separately, we find that at all evaluated times, more patients from the IG choose the "slightly better" alternative: in T4, 80.6% of the IG versus 21.9% of the CG chose this option; in T12 83.9% versus 34.4; in T24 71% versus 18.8 and in T48 58.1% versus 31.3 (Table 3).

Paracetamol use was similar between groups over time with a mean of 163 ± 49.88 tablets for the CG and 174 ± 50.84 for the IG ($p = 0.371$).

Table 1 Demographic data of sample cohorts at baseline

	Intervention group ($n = 31$)	Control group ($n = 32$)	*P* intergroup
Gender – n (%)			0.714
Female	23 (74.2)	25 (78.1)	
Male	8 (25.8)	7 (21.9)	
Age – mean (SD)	60.71 (7.41)	60.22 (7.27)	0.423
Height – mean (DP)	161.87 (10.06)	163.63 (11.45)	0.521
Weight – mean (SD)	76.74 (13.34)	71.03 (11.79)	0.077
Systemic hypertension – n (%)	21 (67.7)	16 (50)	0.151
Diabetes – n (%)	6 (19.3)	9 (28.1)	0.413
Canal diameter in mm^2 – mean (SD)			
L3/L4	94.26 (15.31)	100.34 (14.19)	0.206
L4/L5	81.87 (10.64)	81.44 (12.63)	0.725
L5/S1	84.13 (9.29)	86.25 (11.28)	0.191

Data present as number (percentage) or mean (standard deviation)

Table 2 Pain, function and quality of life data over time

	T0			T4		T12		T24		T48		
	IG	CG	P intergroup	IG	CG	IG	CG	IG	CG	IG	CG	*P* interaction
VAS	4.35 (3.21)	4.47 (2.91)	0.890	*5.10 (2.52)*	*5.28 (2.93)*	*3.81 (1.74)*	*4.41 (2.95)*	*3.61 (2.85)*	*6.00 (5.91)*	*3.32 (2.77)*	*4.59 (3.10)*	0.145
ODI	47.81 (19.36)	47.50 (18.68)	0.468	*50.19 (22.18)*	*46.25 (21.60)*	*42.45 (20.58)*	*46.06 (20.36)*	*34.90 (22.23)*	*45.84 (22.51)*	*35.74 (20.03)*	*47.81 (16.69)*	**0.006** *
RM	14.42 (6.88)	14.72 (6.75)	0.274	*18.71 (5.31)*	*14.59 (6.61)*	*16.42 (5.01)*	*13.47 (7.09)*	*13.00 (6.50)*	*14.22 (7.11)*	*12.71 (6.53)*	*13.63 (7.07)*	**0.005** *
6MWT	287.16 (91.56)	293.56 (85.29)	0.766	*209.03 (83.04)*	*295.03 (86.32)*	*242.68 (93.35)*	*291.31 (86.28)*	*279.00 (66.77)*	*282.25 (110.18)*	*283.52 (62,34)*	*284.13 (77.79)*	**< 0.001** *
SF-36												
PF	30.16 (26.25)	32.50 (25.65)	0.722	*14.35 (14.36)*	*34.22 (28.17)*	*22.39 (26.77)*	*37.97 (25.74)*	*23.87 (25.78)*	*33.91 (31.00)*	*25.65 (25.58)*	*39.84 (27.95)*	0.123
RP	17.74 (31.09)	16.41 (30.85)	0.877	*1.61 (6.24)*	*27.34 (43.24)*	*11.58 (23.27)*	*17.97 (36.61)*	*9.68 (26.36)*	*33.00 (46.40)*	*19.35 (37.48)*	*22.66 (41.81)*	**0.023** *
BP	38.61 (21.74)	36.88 (21.64)	0.856	*33.35 (24.74)*	*37.00 (23.55)*	*41.52 (25.27)*	*40.53 (23.12)*	*45.81 (26.26)*	*36.53 (21.40)*	*46.10 (25.74)*	*39.59 (20.75)*	0.210
GH	56.03 (24.70)	53.13 (27.15)	0.647	*64.58 (25.53)*	*57.19 (24.95)*	*66.97 (23.96)*	*54.97 (23.67)*	*69.35 (25.55)*	*55.38 (23.44)*	*62.29 (28.20)*	*55.75 (24.38)*	0.285
Vit	48.23 (25.51)	49.22 (27.18)	0.891	*50.16 (32.31)*	*46.56 (32.21)*	*63.23 (26.32)*	*48.44 (29.69)*	*63.87 (24.35)*	*45.94 (32.54)*	*61.45 (27.09)*	*47.97 (29.21)*	**0.047** *
SF	57.66 (34.26)	57.41 (32.66)	0.158	*60.08 (29.65)*	*60.94 (33.26)*	*68.15 (30.25)*	*65.63 (30.78)*	*73.39 (27.53)*	*58.98 (36.09)*	*69.35 (28.66)*	*66.41 (30.85)*	0.249
RE	40.86 (48.87)	42.71 (48.81)	0.876	*45.16 (50.59)*	*76.04 (42.53)*	*54.84 (50.59)*	*76.04 (42.53)*	*55.91 (49.73)*	*74.67 (42.44)*	*49.46 (50.09)*	*76.00 (42.58)*	0.145
MH	61.55 (30.65)	60.75 (27.33)	0.890	*62.42 (30.29)*	*61.25 (29.47)*	*60.77 (30.05)*	*62.88 (27.66)*	*64.77 (26.28)*	*59.63 (32.47)*	*63.74 (29.28)*	*65.00 (27.26)*	0.771

Data presented as the mean (SD)
IG intervention group, *CG* control group, *VAS* visual analogue scale, *ODI* Oswestry, *RM* Roland Morris, *6MWT* six minute walk test, *PF* Physical functioning, *RP* Role physical, *BP* Bodily pain, *GH* General health, *Vit* Vitality, *SF* Social functioning, *RE* Role emotional, *MH* Mental health
* *p* value statistically significant

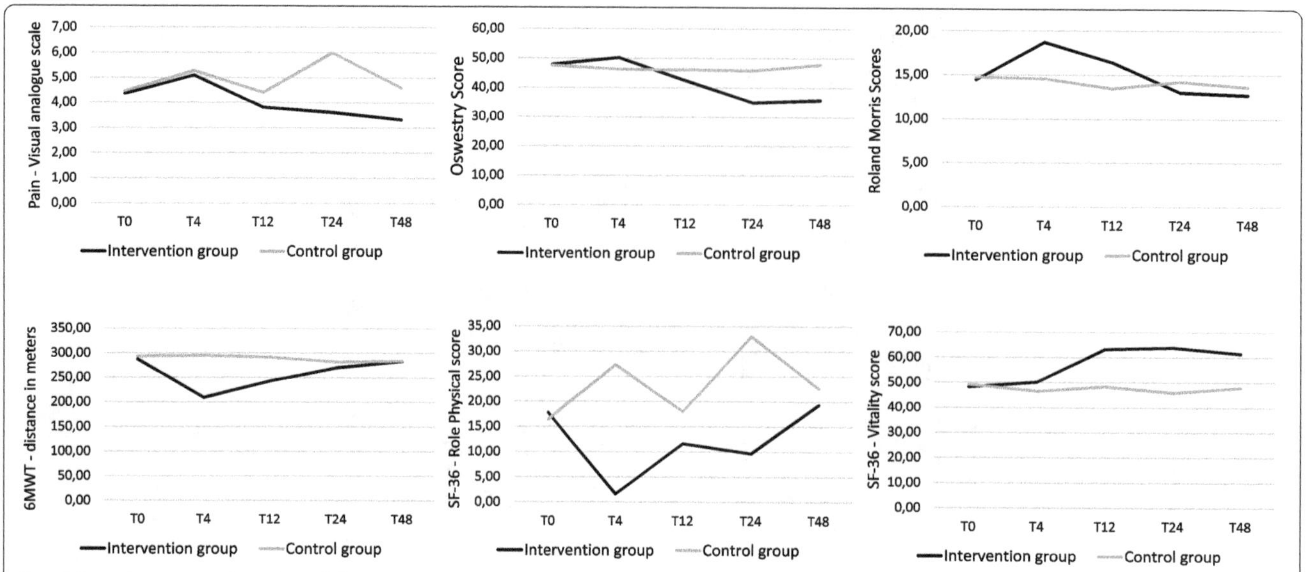

Fig. 2 Pain, function and quality of life scores over time

Regarding correlation, using the Pearson test we found low correlation with no statistical evidence between pain and: age ($r = 0{,}066$, $p = 0{,}605$), IMC ($r = 0{,}007$, $p = 0{,}953$), canal diameter L3/L4 ($r = 0{,}085$, $p = 0{,}507$), canal diameter L4/L5 ($r = 0{,}119$, $p = 0{,}350$) and canal diameter L5/S1 ($r = 0{,}235$, $p = 0{,}604$).

Discussion

The findings of our study show that canal stenosis surgery associated with physical therapy does not improve pain in the short and medium terms, but there is an improvement in function and vitality in the medium term, and patients report satisfaction with the treatment.

In the literature, the vast majority of studies are open and show follow-up data for patients after surgery, with varied surgical techniques used, evaluating whether to perform surgery, the placement of spacers or different laminectomy techniques [7–10]. However, we did not find studies comparing the association of surgical treatment with physiotherapy with physical therapy alone, as in our study.

All of our patients underwent a physiotherapy program created by our team to strengthen the abdominal muscles and stretch the posterior trunk and lower limb muscles because similar exercise programs are performed in daily practice and are indicated for the management of these patients by many authors.

Many outcomes reported in the literature for the evaluation of patients with lumbar spinal stenosis have positive and negative attributes, so a combination of questionnaires or tests may be necessary to properly capture the impact of lumbar stenosis on a patient's pain, disability, and quality of life. As pain is usually the main complaint of lumbar spinal stenosis, we chose this parameter as the main one on this study, and the other questionnaires as Roland Morris, Oswestry, SF-36 and 6 minute walk test were used as secondary outcomes.

It is important to note that in our study, pain worsened in the two groups between the baseline and first reevaluation, and this can be explained by surgery in the IG; however we find it difficult to explain the

Table 3 Patient satisfaction with treatment over time

	T4		T12		T24		T48		
	IG	CG	IG	CG	IG	CG	IG	CG	**P interaction 0.024**
Much better	0	1 (3.1)	2 (6.5)	4 (12.5)	3 (9.7)	2 (6.3)	7 (22.6)	6 (18.8)	
Slightly better	25 (80.6)	7 (21.9)	26 (83.9)	11 (34.4)	22 (71)	6 (18.8)	18 (58.1)	10 (31.3)	
Unchanged	6 (19.4)	12 (37.5)	2 (6.5)	8 (25)	3 (9.7)	13 (40.6)	5 (16.1)	7 (21.9)	
Slightly worse	0	11 (34.4)	1 (3.2)	9 (28.1)	2 (6.3)	10 (31.1)	1 (3.2)	9 (28.1)	
Much worse	0	1 (3.1)	0	0	1 (3.2)	1 (3.1)	0	0	

Data presented as n (%); *IG* intervention group, *CG* control group; data presented as n (%)

same behavior in the CG because the patients had not yet begun physical therapy.

During the physiotherapy period, both groups improved in pain, and after the end of the physiotherapy, the patients of the IG continued to improve, with an improvement of approximately 1 cm in VAS for pain. By contrast, the CG presented a worsening in the 3 months after the end of the physiotherapy, followed by an improvement until the end of the study. Despite these small differences between groups, we found no statistically or clinically significant difference between the groups over time for the pain parameter.

Other studies showed mixed results regarding pain measured by the VAS. Ulrich et al., described improvement at 6 months, maintained for 12 months, and showing a more stable evolution, but his work was in older patients and without a control group [21]. Skolasky et al., showed that after 6 months, surgical patients had an improvement of pain with a 2 cm drop in VAS. This drop remained during the follow-up of 12 months, with 63% of his patients improving more than 2 cm. After 1 year, patients were better than baseline in both groups [22]. Ahmad et al. compared two surgical techniques, and also showed an improvement of 2 cm in VAS [23]. In assessing clinically treated patients, Schneider et al. showed that the VAS of the patients did not change, similar to our study [24].

For function, we found significant differences in the three instruments used to measure it. Oswestry showed a statistically and clinically significant improvement in favor of IG. In T24, the improvement was 12.9 points and in T48 it was 12.07 points. Some authors consider 12.8 points as a clinically important difference for the patient with low back pain [25, 26].

In other studies, superior improvements were observed. Ahmad et al. found an improvement of 23 points in the Oswestry in the operated patients, despite their study cohort [23]. Hemansen et al. compared three different decompression techniques, finding an improvement of approximately 20 points in Oswestry, regardless of the technique used [27]. Skolasky et al. did a prospective, but not controlled, analysis for a period of 12 months and observed improvement in the Oswestry at 3 months postoperative, maintaining the values at 6 months and with an improvement of 20 points in the final evaluation [22].

For function with both the Roland Morris questionnaire and the 6MWT questionnaire, we found a difference between the groups over time, but this was due to a worsening of the GI in T4, shortly after surgery and before starting physical therapy, and then both parameters were improved. At the end of the study, there were no differences between both groups. Again, worsening in the IG can be explained by the surgical intervention, which did not occur in the CG.

Compared with other studies, Ulricha et al., in a prospective multicenter cohort study, evaluated Roland Morris in patients undergoing surgery with a 1 year follow-up. In this period, he observed that there was a drop of 7 points in the questionnaire, with one difference being the average age at work of 82 years [21].

Regarding 6MWT, Försth et al., in an randomized controlled trial (RCT), obtained divergent results after fusion surgery because their patients showed an improvement of more than 100 m after 12 months of surgery [28]. Yamashita et al., in 2003, followed patients after laminectomy surgery in an open-label study and demonstrated that operated patients had no improvement in the ability to ambulate after surgery [29]. Slätis et al. showed in an RCT that the ambulatory or control patients' ambulatory ability did not change after 1 year of surgery, consistent with the results of this research [30]. Malmivaara et al., in an RCT comparing surgical and non-surgical treatment, showed that after 2 years of follow-up, their patients who underwent surgical treatment were better at pain and limitations, but their ability to walk remained unchanged [31]. Rodrigues et al., in an RCT comparing the use of oral corticosteroids with placebo in patients with canal stenosis, also showed that after 6 months of evolution, no improvement was observed in both groups and that the placebo group had, on average, an increase of only 10 m in relation to the initial evaluation [32].

In the quality of life questionnaire, the differences found in role physical fluctuated, with improvement and worsening of both groups over time, but with no difference between them at the end of the study. By contrast, vitality showed an improvement of approximately 15% in the GI in T12, T24 and T48 ($p = 0.023$, $p = 0.014$ and $p = 0.25$, respectively) comped with the control group, which may also have influenced the improvement of function and satisfaction with treatment.

Westein et al. performed an RCT comparing surgical and non-surgical treatment in patients with canal stenosis and did not detect improvement in the SF-36 questionnaire, as well as in the other evaluation instruments used [33]. In another RCT comparing surgical and non-surgical treatment in patients with degenerative spondylolisthesis, Westein et al. described positive results with surgery in the pain and physical function domains in the SF-36, different from that observed in our study [34].

The transient worsening of the operated group in some variables could be explained by the expected limitations and pain in the postoperative period, without, however, being perpetuated. These, as well as other results, demonstrate the safety of the surgery because the patients were not worse than before and there were no clinical complications resulting from the surgery.

Patient satisfaction, measured with the Likert scale, showed an advantage for those operated on. The functional improvement experienced by these patients may have generated the perception of more satisfaction with the treatment, despite not having less pain. It is impossible to blind patients, which may also explain this difference because operated patients would tend to value a major medical intervention with all of the additional care that they naturally received in relation to the CG.

El-Abed et al. showed in their case-control study that patients who underwent surgery significantly improved their evaluation [35]. Many studies using the Likert-type scale as an evaluation tool were not identified. In summary, the operated patients were more satisfied with the treatment than the control group.

The surgery performed in all patients of this study is a lumbar decompression using a posterior approach associated with arthrodesis. As our patients were relatively young, if we performed only decompression surgery without arthrodesis, we would probably have many patients with instability. Thus, we chose to perform arthrodesis after decompression to unify the procedure to all patients, once only older patients with a lot of arthrosis in the spine would not be left with an unstable spine without instrumented arthrodesis. So, it is important to say that our results do not be generalized to patients undergoing decompression surgery without arthrodesis.

The selection of patients may influence the results; however, we selected patients who are usually submitted for this type of surgery based on internationally accepted inclusion criteria. Other population, with different diseases duration, degree of disability, impairment of canal stenosis, or another age group, deserve further studies. Another limitation of our study is related to the disease duration, patients were included if have chronic pain (more than 6 months), but we do not ask about disease duration in the baseline. A longer duration of the disease usually leads to more disabilities and is an important parameter that may have influenced the results of this study.

Conclusion

In conclusion, lumbar stenosis surgery had no effect on pain improvement in the short and medium terms. Function and vitality were better in the group that underwent surgery in the medium term, and patients were more satisfied with the surgical treatment. Further studies should be performed, and surgery should be indicated with caution in patients like ours.

Clinical messages

- Patients who underwent surgery for lumbar canal stenosis associated with physical therapy for 12 weeks and followed by 1 year showed no improvement in pain when compared to the control group who did only physical therapy;
- The function, vitality and satisfaction with the treatment were better in patients undergoing surgery in the medium term.
- Lumbar stenosis surgery had no effect on pain in short and medium term.

Abbreviations

IG: Intervention group; CG: Control group; VAS: Visual analogue scale; 6MWT: 6-min walk test; SF-36: Short form 36; ANOVA: Analysis of variance; SD: Standard deviation; RCT: Randomized controlled trial

Acknowledgements

Not applicable.

Authors' contributions

Rodrigues LCL – Conceptualization, Methodology, Data collection, Writing-Original draft preparation and Editing; Jamil Natour – Conceptualization, Methodology, writing-reviewing and editing. The author(s) read and approved the final manuscript.

Author details

Rheumatology Division, Universidade Federal de São Paulo – Escola Paulista de Medicina (Unifesp-EPM), Sao Paulo, SP 04023900, Brazil. [2]Faculdade de Medicina Santa Marcelina, Sao Paulo, Brazil.

References

1. Verbiest H. A radicular syndrome from developmental narrowing of the lumbar vertebral canal. J Bone Joint Surg (Br). 1954;36:230–7.
2. Verbiest H. The significance and principles of computerized axial tomography in idiopathic developmental stenosis of the bony lumbar vertebral canal. Spine. 1979;4(4):369–78. https://doi.org/10.1097/00007632-197907000-00005.
3. Naylor A. Factors in the development of the spinal stenosis syndrome. J Bone Joint Surg (Br). 1978;61:319–28.
4. Thomas SA. Spinal stenosis: history and physical examination. Phys Med Rehabil Clin N Am. 2003;14(1):29–9. https://doi.org/10.1016/S1047-9651(02)00049-9.
5. Blau JN, Lond MB. Intermittent claudication of the cauda equina. Lancet. 1961;277(7186):1081–6. https://doi.org/10.1016/S0140-6736(61)92310-8.
6. Deyo RA, Gray DT, Kreuter W, Mirza S, Martin B. United States trends in lumbar fusion surgery for degenerative conditions. Spine. 2005;30(12):1441–5. https://doi.org/10.1097/01.brs.0000166503.37969.8a.
7. Shabat S, Arizon Z, Folman Y, Leitner J, David R, Pevzner E, et al. Long-term outcomes of decompressive surgery for lumbar spinal stenosis in octogenarians. Eur Spine J. 2008;17(2):193–8. https://doi.org/10.1007/s00586-007-0514-8.
8. Airaksinen O, Hermo A, Saari T. Surgical treatment of lumbar spinal stenosis: patients' postoperative disability and working capacity. Eur Spine J. 1994; 3(5):261–4. https://doi.org/10.1007/BF02226576.
9. Hurri H, Slätis P, Soini J, Tallroth K, Alaranta H, Laine T, et al. Lumbar spinal stenosis: assessment of long-term outcome 12 years after operative and conservative treatment. J Spinal Disord. 1998;11(2):110–5.
10. Atlas S, Keller RB, Robson D, Deyo RA, Singer DE. Surgical and nonsurgical management of lumbar spinal stenosis: four-years outcomes from the Maine lumbar spine study. Spine. 2000;25(5):556–62. https://doi.org/10.1097/00007632-200003010-00005.
11. Atlas SJ, Keller RB, Wu YA, Deyo RA, Singer DE. Long-term outcomes of surgical and nonsurgical management of lumbar spine study. Spine. 2005; 30(8):936–43. https://doi.org/10.1097/01.brs.0000158953.57966.c0.
12. Arbit E, Pannullo S. Lumbar stenosis: a clinical review. Clin Orthop Relat Res. 2001;384:137–43. https://doi.org/10.1097/00003086-200103000-00016
13. Hamanishi C, Matukura N, Fujita M, Tomihara M, Tanaka S. Cross-sectional area of the stenotic lumbar dural tube measured from the transverse views of magnetic resonance imaging. J Spinal Disord. 1994;7(5):388–93.

14. Madsen R, Jensen TS, Pope M, Sørensen JS, Bendix T. The effect of body position and axial load on spinal canal morphology: an MRI study of central spinal stenosis. Spine. 2008;33:61–7.
15. Lee CK, Rauschning W, Glenn W. Lateral lumbar spinal canal stenosis: classification, pathologic anatomy and surgical decompression. Spine. 1988; 13:313–20.
16. Zanoli G. Outcome assessment in lumbar spine surgery. Acta Orthop Suppl. 2005;76(318):5–47.
17. Nusbaum L, Natour J, Ferraz MB, Goldenberg J. Translation, adaptation and validation of the Roland-Morris questionnaire-Brazil Roland-Morris. Braz J Med Biol Res. 2001;34(2):203–10. https://doi.org/10.1590/S0100-879X2001 000200007.
18. Vigatto R, Alexandre NM, Correa Filho HR. Development of a Brazilian Portuguese version of the Oswestry Disability Index: cross-cultural adaptation, reliability, and validity. Spine. 2007;32:481–6.
19. ATS Committee on Proficiency Standards for Clinical Pulmonary Function Laboratories. ATS statement: guidelines for the six-minute walk test. Am J Respir Crit Care Med. 2002;166:111–7.
20. Ciconelli RM, Ferraz MB, Santos W, Meinão I, Quaresma MR. Tradução Para Língua Portuguesa E Tradução Do Questionário Genérico De Avaliação De Qualidade De Vida SF-36 (Brasil SF-36). Rev Bras Reumatol. 1999;39:143–50.
21. Ulrich NH, Kleinstück F, Woernle CM, Antoniadis A, Winklofer S, Burgstaller JM, et al. Clinical outcome in lumbar decompression surgery for spinal canal stenosis in the aged population: a prospective Swiss multicenter cohort study. Spine. 2015;40:415–22.
22. Skolasky RL, Wegener ST, Maggard AM, Riley LH 3rd. The impact of reduction of pain after lumbar spine surgery: the relationship between changes in pain and physical function and disability. Spine. 2014;39:1426–32.
23. Ahmad S, Hamad A, Bhalla A, Turner S, Balain B, Jaffray D. The outcome of decompression alone for lumbar spinal stenosis with degenerative spondylolisthesis. Eur Spine J. 2017;26(2):414–9. https://doi.org/10.1007/s00586-016-4637-7.
24. Schneider MJ, Terhorst L, Murphy D, Stevans JM, Hoffman R, Cambron JS. Exploratory analysis of clinical predictors of outcomes of nonsurgical treatment in patients with lumbar spinal stenosis. J Manip Physiol Ther. 2016;39(2):88–94. https://doi.org/10.1016/j.jmpt.2016.01.001.
25. Johnsen LG, Hellum C, Nygaard OP, Storheim K, Brox JI, Rossvoll I, et al. Comparison of the SF6D, the EQ 5D, and the Oswestry disability index in patients with chronic low back pain and degenerative disc disease. BMC Musculoskelet Disord. 2013;14(1):148. https://doi.org/10.1186/1471-24 74-14-148.
26. Copay AG, Glassman SD, Subach BR, Berven S, Schuler TC, Carreon LY. Minimum clinically important difference in lumbar spine surgery patients: a choice of methods using the Oswestry disability index, medical outcomes study questionnaire short form 36, and pain scales. Spine J. 2008;8(6):968–74. https://doi.org/10.1016/j.spinee.2007.11.006.
27. Hermansen E, Romild UK, Austevoll IM, Solberg T, Storheim K, Brox JI, et al. Does surgical technique influence clinical outcome after lumbar spinal stenosis decompression? A comparative effectiveness study from the Norwegian registry for spine surgery. Eur Spine J. 2017;26(2):420–7. https://doi.org/10.1007/s00586-016-4643-9.
28. Försth P, Ólafsson G, Carlsson T. A randomized, controlled trial of fusion surgery for lumbar spinal stenosis. N Engl J Med. 2016;374(15):1413–23. https://doi.org/10.1056/NEJMoa1513721.
29. Yamashita K, Hayashi J, Ohzono K, Hiroshima K. Correlation of patient satisfaction with symptom severity and walking ability after surgical treatment for degenerative lumbar spinal stenosis. Spine. 2003;28:2477–81.
30. Slätis P, Malmivaara A, Heliövaara M, Sainio P, Herno A, Kankare J, et al. Long-term results of surgery for lumbar spinal stenosis: a randomised controlled trial. Eur Spine J. 2011;20(7):1174–81. https://doi.org/10.1007/s00586-010-1652-y.
31. Malmivaara A, Slätis P, Heliövaara M, Sainio P, Kinnunen H, Kankare J, et al. Surgical or nonoperative treatment for lumbar spinal stenosis? A randomized controlled trial. Spine. 2007;32:1–8.
32. Rodrigues LC, Natour J. A double-blind, randomized controlled, prospective trial assessing the effectiveness of oral corticoids in the treatment of symptomatic lumbar canal stenosis. J Negat Results Bioemed. 2014;13(1):13. https://doi.org/10.1186/1477-5751-13-13.
33. Weinstein JN, Tosteson TD, Lurie JD, Tosteson ANA, Blood E, Hanscom B, et al. Surgical versus nonsurgical therapy for lumbar spinal stenosis. N Engl J Med. 2008;358(8):794 10. https://doi.org/10.1056/NEJMoa0707136
34. Weinstein JN, Lurie JD, Tosteson TD, Hanscom B, Tosteson ANA, Blood EA, et al. Surgical versus nonsurgical treatment for lumbar degenerative spondylolisthesis. N Engl J Med. 2007;356(22):2257–70. https://doi.org/10.1 056/NEJMoa070302.
35. El-Abed K, Barakat M, Ainscow D. Multilevel lumbar spinal stenosis decompression: midterm outcome using a modified hinge osteotomy technique. J Spinal Disord Tech. 2011;24(6):376–80. https://doi.org/10.1097/BSD.0b013e3182014aa1.

22

The effects of COVID-19 fear and anxiety on symptom severity, sleep quality, and mood in patients with fibromyalgia

Damla Cankurtaran[*], Nihal Tezel, Buse Ercan, Sadik Yigit Yildiz and Ece Unlu Akyuz

Abstract

Background: During the COVID-19 pandemic, individuals faced psychological stress caused by fear and anxiety due to the high transmission and mortality rate of the disease, the social isolation, economic problems, and difficulties in reaching health services. Fibromyalgia (FM) is a chronic centralized pain sensitivity disorder. Psychological, physical and/or autoimmune stressors were found to increase FM symptoms. This pilot study aimed to evaluate the COVID-19 fear and anxiety level, and to examine their effect on disease severity, sleep quality, and mood in FM patients compared to control group.

Methods: This pilot study conducted as a cross-sectional study, and included 62 participants. Participants were divided into two groups: FM patient group ($n = 31$) and control group ($n = 31$). Symptom severity, sleep quality, and mood were determined using the Revised Fibromyalgia Impact Questionnaire (FIQR), Pitsburg Sleep Quality Index (PSQI), and Hospital Anxiety Depression Scale (HADS), respectively. In order to evaluate the level of COVID-19 fear and anxiety, the Fear of COVID-19 Scale (FCV-19S) and Coronavirus Anxiety Scale (CAS) were used compared to control group.

Results: FIQR, PSQI, HAD-A, HAD-D, FCV-19S and CAS scores were significantly higher in the FM group ($p = 0.01$). A positive significant correlation was found between FCV-19S and CAS results and FIQR, PSQI, and HAD-anx results in FM patients ($p < 0.05$).

Conclusion: This pilot study showed that, the individuals with FM can be more affected by psychological stress, and this situation negatively affects the symptom severity, sleep quality, and mood in FM patients, so these patients should be closely monitored in terms of psychological stressors and their effects during pandemics. More studies with more participants are necessary to describe the challenges lived by fibromyalgia population.

Keywords: Fibromyalgia, COVID-19, Fear of COVID-19 scale, Coronavirus anxiety scale, Symptom severity

Introduction

The World Health Organization (WHO) announced the start of an epidemic related to the novel coronavirus disease (COVID-19) that caused viral pneumonia in Wuhan, China, in December 2019. Since then, COVID-19 has spread all over the world and WHO declared it to be a pandemic in March 2020 [1]. Previous studies have shown that individuals' well-being was adversely affected by prior pandemic periods [2–4]. During the COVID-19 pandemic, individuals faced psychological stress caused by fear and anxiety due to the high transmission and mortality rate of the disease, the social isolation which resulted from quarantine to prevent rapid transmission, economic problems, and difficulties in reaching health

* Correspondence: damlacengizftr@gmail.com
Department of Physical Medicine and Rehabilitation, University of Health Sciences Diskapi Yildirim Beyazit Training and Research Hospital, Altındag, 06080 Ankara, Turkey

services [5, 6]. Previous studies have found an increase in mental disorders such as anxiety, depression, and post-traumatic stress disorder during the COVID-19 pandemic [5–7].

Fibromyalgia (FM) is a chronic centralized pain sensitivity disorder with widespread, wandering, increasing-decreasing pain attacks accompanied by fatigue, sleep disturbance, mood disorders, and somatic symptoms [8]. In controlled studies in the literature, psychological, physical and/or autoimmune stressors were found to increase FM symptoms [9]. Anxiety and psychological stress cause an increase in symptom severity in FM patients and adversely affect their quality of life [10, 11].

There are studies in the literature examining the effect of the lockdown period on FM symptoms but there is no study examining the effect of COVID-19 fear and anxiety in FM patients (disease severity, sleep quality, and mood) [9, 12]. Therefore, our study aimed to evaluate the COVİD-19 fear and anxiety level, and to examine their effect on disease severity, sleep quality, and mood in FM patients.

Materials-method

Ethical statement

This study was approved by the local institutional ethics committee of our hospital (Approval number: 102/17) and was conducted in accordance with the Declaration of Helsinki guidelines. Signed informed consent was obtained from each participant prior to data collection.

Study design and participants

This pilot study conducted as a cross-sectional study, and included 62 participants. Participants were divided into two groups as the FM patient group ($n = 31$) and control group ($n = 31$). The FM group included patients between the ages of 18–65, who applied to the physical medicine and rehabilitation outpatient clinic between December 15, 2020, and February 1, 2021, who had been diagnosed with primary FM for more than 1 year according to the 2016 American College of Rheumatology criteria, and who had not been changed drug or dose for 3 months, and who had been clinically stable for at least 3 months. Patients with secondary FM or was changed drug or dose within 3 months, mood disorders, history of medication with any antidepressant or anxiolytic drugs, advanced musculoskeletal problems, additional rheumatologic diseases, COVİD-19 infection history, severe metabolic, endocrine, cardiovascular, pulmonary, genitourinary, gastrointestinal, progressive or non-progressive central or peripheral neurological diseases; and patients who underwent some type of therapy like yoga, meditation or other alternative therapies were not included in the study. The control group was selected from healthy volunteers (relatives or clinic staff) with no manifestation of disease and ages between the ages of 18–65.

Data collection

Data related to demographic characteristics such as age, gender, height, weight, body mass index, professions, educational status, and marital status were obtained from the participants. In addition, symptom severity, sleep quality, and mood were determined using the Revised Fibromyalgia Impact Questionnaire (FIQR), Pitsburg Sleep Quality Index (PSQI), and Hospital Anxiety Depression Scale (HADS), respectively. In order to evaluate the level of COVID-19 fear and anxiety, the Fear of COVID-19 Scale (FCV-19S) and Coronavirus Anxiety Scale (CAS) were used.

Revised fibromyalgia impact questionnaire (FIQR)

FIQR was used to evaluate FM physical functionality and the severity of its symptoms. The questionnaire focuses on three areas including function, overall impact, and symptoms. The total score ranges from 0 to 100, and higher scores indicate worse functionality and increased symptom severity [13].

Hospital anxiety depression scale (HADS)

HADS is a scale developed specifically to evaluate mood disorders such as anxiety and depression. The scale includes a total of 14 questions, 7 of which belong to the anxiety subscale, and the remaining 7 questions belong to the depression subscale. Each question is scored between 0 and 3, and both the depression and anxiety subscale scores range from 0 to 21. Higher scores indicate more severe anxiety and depression [14].

Pitsburg sleep quality index (PSQI)

The PSQI is a scale consisting of 19 self-reported questions and 7 items that evaluate sleep quality. The total score of the survey is obtained from the sum of the 7-item scores. The scores range from 0 to 21, and lower scores indicate better sleep quality [15].

Fear of COVID-19 scale (FCV-19S)

FCV-19S is a short, 7-question questionnaire developed to evaluate the level of fear and anxiety related to COVID-19 virus. Each question is evaluated with a five-point Likert type scale (1 = strongly disagree to 5 = strongly agree) [16]. The Turkish adaptation of the questionnaire was made by Satıcı et al. [17]. The cut-off value in FCV-19S is determined as 16.5, and scores higher than this value have a significant predictive power on anxiety, health-related anxiety, and post-traumatic stress disorder [18].

Coronavirus anxiety scale (CAS)

CAS is another 5-question questionnaire developed by Lee et al. to evaluate the psychological effects of the pandemic period. Validity and reliability checks of the

Turkish adaptation of the scale have been conducted Each question is scored using a 5-point time anchored scale (0 ¼ not at all to 4 ¼ nearly every day over the last 2 weeks) [19, 20].

Comparisons

COVID-19 fear and anxiety were compared between the FM and control groups, and the relationship between the level of COVID-19 fear and anxiety and FM symptom severity, sleep quality, and mood was investigated in the FM group.

Statstical analyses

`Data analyses were conducted using Statistical Package for the Social Sciences (SPSS 22.0 for Windows) software. The variables were investigated using visuals (histograms and probability plots) and Shapiro-Wilks test to determine whether they are normally distributed. In reporting descriptive statistics, data were expressed as mean ± standard deviation (SD) and median (minimum-maximum) for continuous variables, and as frequencies and percentages (%) for nominal and categorical variables. The χ^2 tests, Fisher's exact or Likelihood ratio tests were used to compare nominal variables and categorical variables between the groups. In addition, the independent samples T tests and Mann-Whitney U tests were used to compare the continuous values between the groups. The relationship between FCV-19S, CAS and FIQR, PSQI, and HADS in the FM group were examined by Spearman correlation analysis. A p-value less than 0.05 ($p < 0.05$) was accepted as statistically significant.

Results

No significant differences were found between the two groups in terms of age, gender, BMI, marital status, education level, occupation, and comorbidities ($p > 0.05$). Table 1 shows comparison of general characteristics of the participants of the two groups.

FIQR, PSQI, HADS-A, HADS-D, FCV-19S and CAS scores were significantly higher in the FM group compared to the control group ($p = 0.01$) (Table 2).

A positive significant correlation was found between FCV-19S and CAS results and FIQR, PSQI, and HAD-anx results in FM patients ($p < 0.05$) (Table 3). No significant correlation was found between the HAD-dep and FCV-19S and CAS results ($r = 0.316$, $p = 0.084$; $r = 0.339$, $p = 0.062$, respectively).

A high level of positive significant correlation was found between FCV-19S and CAS results for all patients ($r = 0.778$, $p < 0.001$).

Table 1 Comprasion of general characterristics of participants between two groups

	FM group $n = 31$	Control Group $n = 31$	P
Age (years)			
Median ± SD	45.9 ± *9.33*	41.91 ± *9.17*	0.06[a]
Gender *n(%)*			
Female/male	28 (90.3)/3 (9.7)	26 (83.9)/5 (16.1)	0.71[b]
BMI (kg/cm^2)			
Median ± SD	28.59 ± *5.22*	26.49 ± *3.55*	0.18[a]
Education Status *n(%)*			
Illiterate	2 (6.5)	0	
Primary school	12 (38.7)	15 (48.4)	0.13[c]
Middle school	7 (22.6)	2 (6.5)	
High school	5 (16.1)	5 (16.1)	
Univesity	5 (16.1)	9 (29.0)	
Mariatal status *n(%)*			
Marrage	22 (71.0)	20 (64.5)	
Single	7 (22.6)	9 (29.0)	0.85[c]
Divorcee	2 (6.5)	2 (6.5)	
Professions *n(%)*			
Unemployed /housewife	20 (64.5)	18 (58.07)	
Worker	7 (22.6)	5 (16.1)	0.28[c]
Student	1 (3.2)	0	
Officier	2 (6.5)	8 (25.8)	
Other	1 (3.2)	0	
Comorbidities *n(%)*			
No	20 (64.5)	25 (80.6)	
HT	2 (6.5)	3 (9.7)	
DM	2 (6.5)	2 (6.5)	0.20[c]
HT + DM	2 (6.5)	0	
Hipothyroidism	2 (6.5)	0	
Other	3 (9.7)	1	

FM fibromiyalgia, *SD* standard deviation, *BMI* body mass index, *HT* hypertension, *DM* Diabetes mellitus, [a] independent sample t test, [b] Fisher exact test, [c] Likelihood ratio test, bold values show $p < 0.05$

Discussion

It was not find similar study the relates the effect of COVID-19 anxiety and fear on symptom severity, sleep quality, and mood in FM patients. The results of ongoing research revealed that the COVID-19 fear and anxiety levels in FM patients were higher than healthy patients. In FM patients, COVID-19 fear and anxiety were found to be associated with symptom severity, sleep quality, and anxiety level.

Although the cause of FM is still not fully understood, central sensitization in the central nervous system, which is associated with the development of increased sensitivity to pain signals, is the most accepted mechanism [21]. Although the main symptom of FM is pain, it is a heterogeneous picture that seriously disrupts the quality of life, including physical and mental fatigue, impaired sleep quality, headache, irritable bowel syndrome,

Table 2 Comprassion of results of Fibromiyalgia Impact Questionnare, Pitsburg Sleep Quality Index, Hospital Anxiety and Depression Scale, Fear of COVİD-19 Scale, and Coronavirus Anxiety Scele between two groups

	FM group $n = 31$	Control Group $n = 31$	p
FIQR			
median (min-max)	69.13 (25.22–94.22)	18.33 (10.95–73.98)	**0.01**[a]
PSQI			
median (min-max)	10 (5–15)	4 (1–14)	**0.01**[a]
HADS-A			
median (min-max)	9 (4–20)	6 (1–17)	**0.01**[a]
HADS-D			
median (min-max)	10 (1–17)	5 (1–18)	**0.01**[a]
FCV-19S			
median ± SD	20.96 ± *8.86*	14.67 ± *7.13*	**0.01**[b]
CAS			
median (min-max)	5 (0–18)	0 (0–18)	**0.01**[a]

FIQR Fibromiyalgia impact questionnare-revised, *PSQI* Pitsburg sleep quality index, *HADS-A* Hospital anxiety and depression scale-anxiety subscale, *HADS-D* Hospital anxiety and depression scale-depression subscale, *FCV-19S* Fear of coronavirus-19 scale, *CAS* Coronavirus anxiety scale, [a] Mann-Withney U test, [b] independent sample t test, bold values show $p < 0.05$

cognitive disorders, and psychological problems [10]. The most common psychological problems in FM patients are anxiety and depression. Anxiety disorders are found in between 13 and 64% and depression in between 20 and 80% of FM patients [10]. In one study, 80% of FM patients reported poor sleep quality [22].

The whole world faced an unexpected pandemic in 2020, leading to negative psychological effects in the general population such as depression, stress, sleep disturbance, anger, and anxiety about one's own health and the health of their relatives, phobias, and avoidance behavior [7]. Specifically, infected people, individuals with a high risk of infection (including the elderly, people with compromised immune function, and those living or cared for in public places), individuals with pre-existing medical or psychiatric illnesses, and those who had substance use problems were found to have an increased risk for adverse psychosocial outcomes [23].

Table 3 Realiation between Fibromiyalgia Impact Questionnare, Pitsburg Sleep Quality Index, Hospital Anxiety and Depression Scale, and Fear of COVİD-19 Scale, Coronavirus Anxiety Scele in Fibromiyalgia Group

$n = 31$	FCV-19S		CAS	
	r	P	r	p
FIQR	0.724	**< 0.01**	0.558	**0.001**
PSQI	0.416	**0.020**	0.439	**0.014**
HADS-anx	0.712	**0.001**	0.423	**0.018**
HADS-dep	0.316	0.084	0.339	0.062

FIQR Fibromiyalgia impact questionnare-revised, *PSQI* Pitsburg sleep quality index, *HADS* Hospital anxiety and depression scale, *FCV-19S* Fear of coronavirus-19 scale, *CAS* Coronavirus anxiety scale, *r* correlation cofficients, *p* values show statistical significance, bold values show $p < 0.05$, *p* values calculated with Spearman correlation test

During the pandemic period, new scales have been developed to evaluate the fear and anxiety associated with COVID-19 infection, which has a high transmission and mortality rate [16, 24, 25]. Among those scales, FCV-19S and CAS were used in our study. This study aimed to evaluate the level of fear and anxiety more accurately by using two separate scales and a significant correlation was found between the two scales.

Although the pandemic period has caused fear and anxiety in all individuals, previous studies have shown that those with pre-existing mood disorders were affected more by the negative psychological factors caused by the epidemic [26]. In our study, COVID-19-related fear and anxiety levels were found to be significantly higher in FM patients than the control group.

This study examined the effect of COVID-19 fear and anxiety on FM symptoms, sleep quality, and anxiety-depression levels. The results showed that COVID-19 fear and anxiety negatively affected FM symptom severity, sleep quality, and anxiety levels in FM patients.

In a study conducted by Hruschak et al., in which 150 patients with FM, chronic spine, and post-surgical chronic pain were included, patients' self-reported pain severity was found to be higher after 4–8 weeks of social isolation compared to the pre-pandemic period. Furthermore, psychological factors such as anxiety, depression, sleep disorders, and stress were found to be associated with worse pain. In addition, the presence of FM was found to be an independent risk factor for greater pain during social isolation [27].

In a study comparing the symptom severity of FM patients in the pre-pandemic period with the lockdown period due to the COVID-19 pandemic, a significant difference was found in the total FIQR scores and pain, depression, and anxiety subdomains during the lockdown period compared to the pre-pandemic period. Additionally, a significant increase was found in the Generalized Anxiety Disorder-7 score during the lockdown period [9]. In a letter to editor, 67% of 32 FM patients reported that their general health status (well-being) worsened during the pandemic period [12].

Anxiety and depression are two closely related conditions [28]. However, our study found no relationship between depression levels and anxiety due to COVID-19. COVID-19 causes acute stress in the daily life of individuals. The severity of depression has been shown to be related to the duration of exposure to the stressor [29]. Given that our study is a cross-sectional study, more studies with longer follow-ups are needed to evaluate this relationship.

This pilot study is limited due to its small sample size and cross-sectional design.

Conclusion

Particular attention should be paid to patients with previous psychological disorders such as FM patients during pandemic periods. Because these individuals are more affected by psychological stress than other individuals, and this situation negatively affects the symptom severity, sleep quality, and mood in FM patients. The patients should be closely monitored in terms of psychological stressors and their effects especially using telemedicine applications, and necessary precautions should be taken immediately. We still continue to see the effects of the COVID-19 pandemic. Therefore, more studies with more participants are necessary to describe the challenges lived by fibromyalgia population.

Acknowledgments

We are grateful to all our participants.

Authors' contributions

Each named author has substantially contributed to the research and/or drafting of the manuscript. The author(s) read and approved the final manuscript.

References

1. World Health Organization website. https://www.who.int/ (accessed 15th January 2021).
2. Sim K, Chua HC. The psychological impact of SARS: a matter of heart and mind. CMAJ. 2004;170(5):811–2. https://doi.org/10.1503/cmaj.1032003.
3. Wu P, Fang Y, Guan Z, Fan B, Kong J, Yao Z, et al. The psychological impact of the SARS epidemic on hospital employees in China: exposure, risk perception, and altruistic acceptance of risk. Can J Psychiatr. 2009;54(5):302 11. https://doi.org/10.1177/070674370905400504.
4. Kim CW, Song HR. Structural relationships among public's risk characteristics, trust, risk perception and preventive behavioral intention: the case of MERS in Korea. Crisisnomy. 2017;13:85–95.
5. Dubey S, Biswas P, Ghosh R, Chatterjee S, Dubey MJ, Chatterjee S, et al. Psychosocial impact of COVID-19. Diabetes Metab Syndr. 2020;14(5):779–88. https://doi.org/10.1016/j.dsx.2020.05.035.
6. Xiong J, Lipsitz O, Nasri F, Lui LMW, Gill H, Phan L, et al. Impact of COVID-19 pandemic on mental health in the general population: a systematic review. J Affect Disord. 2020;277:55–64. https://doi.org/10.1016/j.jad.2020.08.001.
7. Talevi D, Socci V, Carai M, Carnaghi G, Faleri S, Trebbi E, et al. Mental health outcomes of the CoViD-19 pandemic. Riv Psichiatr. 2020;55(3):137–44. https://doi.org/10.1708/3382.33569.
8. Mohabbat AB, Mohabbat NML, Wight EC. Fibromyalgia and chronic fatigue syndrome in the age of COVID-19. Mayo Clin Proc Innov Qual Outcomes. 2020;4(6):764–6. https://doi.org/10.1016/j.mayocpiqo.2020.08.002.
9. Batres-Marroquín AB, Medina-García AC, Vargas Guerrero A, Barrera-Villalpando MI, Martínez-Lavín M, Martínez-Martínez LA. Effect of COVID-19 pandemic lockdown on fibromyalgia symptoms. J Clin Rheumatol. 2020; Publish Ahead of Print. https://doi.org/10.1097/RHU.0000000000001685.
10. Di Tella M, Ghiggia A, Tesio V, Romeo A, Colonna F, Fusaro E, et al. Pain experience in fibromyalgia syndrome: the role of alexithymia and psychological distress. J Affect Disord. 2017;208:87–93. https://doi.org/10.1016/j.jad.2016.08.080
11. Galvez-Sánchez CM, Montoro CI, Duschek S, Del Paso GAR. Pain catastrophizing mediates the negative influence of pain and trait-anxiety on health-related quality of life in fibromyalgia. Qual Life Res. 2020;29(7):1871–81. https://doi.org/10.1007/s11136-020-02457-x.
12. Cavalli G, Cariddi A, Ferrari J, Suzzi B, Tomelleri A, Campochiaro C, et al. Living with fibromyalgia during the COVID-19 pandemic: mixed effects of prolonged lockdown on the well-being of patients. Rheumatology (Oxford). 2021;60(1):465–7. https://doi.org/10.1093/rheumatology/keaa738.
13. Bennett RM, Friend R, Jones KD, Ward R, Han BK, Ross RL. The revised fibromyalgia impact questionnaire (FIQR): validation and psychometric properties. Arthritis Res Ther. 2009;11(4):R120. https://doi.org/10.1186/ar2783.
14. Zigmond AS, Snaith RP. The hospital anxiety and depression scale. Acta Psychiatr Scand. 1983;67(6):361–70. https://doi.org/10.1111/j.1600-0447.1983.tb09716.x.
15. Climent-Sanz C, Marco-Mitjavila A, Pastells-Peiró R, Valenzuela-Pascual F, Blanco-Blanco J, Gea-Sánchez M. Patient reported outcome measures of sleep quality in fibromyalgia: a COSMIN systematic review. Int J Environ Res Public Health. 2020;17(9):2992. https://doi.org/10.3390/ijerph17092992.
16. Ahorsu DK, Lin CY, Imani V, Saffari M, Griffiths MD, Pakpour AH. The fear of COVID-19 scale: development and initial validation. Int J Ment Heal Addict. 2020:1–9. https://doi.org/10.1007/s11469-020-00270-8.
17. Satici B, Gocet-Tekin E, Deniz ME, Satici SA. Adaptation of the fear of COVID-19 scale: its association with psychological distress and life satisfaction in Turkey. Int J Ment Heal Addict. 2020:1–9. https://doi.org/10.1007/s11469-020-00294-0.
18. Nikopoulou VA, Holeva V, Parlapani E, Karamouzi P, Voitsidis P, Porfyri GN, et al. Mental health screening for COVID-19: a proposed cutoff score for the Greek version of the fear of COVID-19 scale (FCV-19S). Int J Ment Heal Addict. 2020:1–14. https://doi.org/10.1007/s11469-020-00414-w.
19. Evren C, Evren B, Dalbudak E, Topcu M, Kutlu N. Measuring anxiety related to COVID-19: a Turkish validation study of the coronavirus anxiety scale. Death Stud. 2020;3:1–7. https://doi.org/10.1080/07481187.2020.1774969.
20. Lee SA. Coronavirus anxiety scale: a brief mental health screener for COVID-19 related anxiety. Death Stud. 2020;44(7):393–401. https://doi.org/10.1080/07481187.2020.1748481.
21. Cagnie B, Coppieters I, Denecker S, Six J, Danneels L, Meeus M. Central sensitization in fibromyalgia? A systematic review on structural and functional brain MRI. Semin Arthritis Rheum. 2014;44(1):68–75. https://doi.org/10.1016/j.semarthrit.2014.01.001.
22. Wu YL, Chang LY, Lee HC, Fang SC, Tsai PS. Sleep disturbances in fibromyalgia: a meta-analysis of case-control studies. J Psychosom Res. 2017; 96:89–97. https://doi.org/10.1016/j.jpsychores.2017.03.011.
23. Pfefferbaum B, North CS. Mental health and the Covid-19 pandemic. N Engl J Med. 2020;383(6):510–2. https://doi.org/10.1056/NEJMp2008017.
24. Lee SA, Mathis AA, Jobe MC, Pappalardo EA. Clinically significant fear and anxiety of COVID-19: a psychometric examination of the coronavirus anxiety scale. Psychiatry Res. 2020;290:113112. https://doi.org/10.1016/j.psychres.2020.113112.
25. Arpaci I, Karataş K, Baloğlu M. The development and initial tests for the psychometric properties of the COVID-19 phobia scale (C19P-S). Personal Individ Differ. 2020;164:110108. https://doi.org/10.1016/j.paid.2020.110108.
26. Yao H, Chen JH, Xu YF. Patients with mental health disorders in the COVID-19 epidemic. Lancet Psychiatry. 2020;7(4):e21. https://doi.org/10.1016/S2215-0366(20)30090-0.
27. Hruschak V, Flowers KM, Azizoddin DR, Jamison RN, Edwards RR, Schreiber KL. Cross-sectional study of psychosocial and pain-related variables among patients with chronic pain during a time of social distancing imposed by the coronavirus disease 2019 pandemic. Pain. 2021;162(2):619–29. https://doi.org/10.1097/j.pain.0000000000002128.
28. Beard C, Millner AJ, Forgeard MJ, Fried EI, Hsu KJ, Treadway MT, et al. Network analysis of depression and anxiety symptom relationships in a psychiatric sample. Psychol Med. 2016;46(16):3359–69. https://doi.org/10.1017/S0033291716002300.
29. Ramezanzadeh F, Aghssa MM, Abedinia N, Zayeri F, Khanafshar N, Shariat M, et al. A survey of relationship between anxiety, depression and duration of infertility. BMC Womens Health. 2004;4(1):9. https://doi.org/10.1186/1472-6874-4-9.

23

Intestinal microbiota and active systemic lupus erythematosus

Juliana Rosa Pires Vieira[1], Andréa Toledo de Oliveira Rezende[1*], Marcos Rassi Fernandes[1,2] and Nilzio Antonio da Silva[1,3]

Abstract

Background: Systemic Lupus Erythematosus (SLE) is an autoimmune disease, characterized by being multi-systemic and, therefore, reaching various organs and affecting mainly young women. Its pathogenesis comprehends many factors, including the interaction between microbiota and immune system. This systematic review assessed the relationship between intestinal microbiota and SLE in activity, highlighting microbiota representative patterns regarding quantity and diversity.

Methods: This study considered researches carried out in patients with SLE, with no restriction of age or gender, which fulfilled the classification criteria of either Systemic Lupus International Collaborating Clinic (SLICC), American College of Rheumatology (ACR) or European League Against Rheumatism (EULAR) and used the Systemic Lupus Erythematosus Disease Activity Index (SLEDAI) to classify disease in activity or remission were included. The search was carried out from October, 2020 to January, 2021 using the following databases: Medline via Pubmed, Scopus, and Embase. Five papers were included with a total of 288 participants with SLE.

Results: Regarding microbiota in patients with SLE in activity, there was significant increase in the following genera: *Lactobacillus, Streptococcus, Megasphaera, Fusobacterium, Veillonella, Oribacterium, Odoribacter, Blautia*, and *Campylobacter.* On the other hand, decrease in *Faecalibacterium* and *Roseburia genera* as well as *Ruminococcus gnavus* species was observed in remission cases, showing differences between the microbiota profile in SLE in activity and in remission.

Conclusions: Results suggest that dysbiosis may be involved in the disease activity process.

Trial registration: CRD42021229322.

Keywords: Microbiota, Systemic lupus erythematosus, Inflammation, Dysbiosis, SLE

Introduction

Systemic Lupus Erythematosus (SLE) is an autoimmune, chronic, and multi-systemic disease that affects mainly young women [1]. This condition has as main feature intolerance to autoantigens [2] resulting in numerous antibodies and inflammatory recruitment of T cells, producing pro-inflammatory cytokines [3].

The cause of SLE is unknown, however its predisposing factors are: (a) genetic, e.g. CSK and IRF7 genes; (b) immune, comprehending the production of B cells that produce antibodies and T cells; and (c) hormonal, related to estrogen increase. Additionally, environmental and/or psychological factors are also triggers, such as sunlight exposure, drugs, intestinal microbiota, Epstein-Barr virus, cytomegalovirus, smoking, sedentary lifestyle, and stress [4–8].

Among the abovementioned factors, intestinal microbiota plays a fundamental role in metabolic function, epithelium barrier maintenance, immune system

* Correspondence: rezende.andrea@hotmail.com
[1]Postgraduate Program in Health Sciences, School of Medicine of the Universidade Federal de Goiás (UFG), Goiânia, Brazil

modulation and homeostasis, as well as protection against infection by pathogenic agents. On the other hand, intestinal balance is preserved by a complex cellular network that acts on the development of innate and adaptive immune response [9].

Therefore, intestinal microbiota may be important on the development and maintenance of SLE symptoms [6]. Immune responses against intestinal microorganisms could exacerbate preexistent inflammation and imbalance of intestinal regulating T cells (Treg/Th17), which could attack intestinal microbiota and amplify dysbiosis. This process leads to a vicious cycle in which the disease states continues [9].

In view of that, it is necessary an in-depth study for better understanding the role of intestinal microbiota in SLE etiopathogenesis and activity, focusing on the following questions: (a) does intestinal microbiota present distinctive characteristics, assessed by quantity and diversity, in patients with SLE in activity?; (b) is there dysbiosis in the microbiota of SLE in activity?; (c) is the pattern of intestinal bacteria different in SLE in activity and SLE in remission?

It is important to highlight that this is the first systematic review addressing the relationship between microbiota and active SLE. In this context, this paper aimed to verify whether there is a relationship between intestinal microbiota composition and SLE activity. The hypothesis is that there are representative patterns and dysbiosis in the microbiota composition of patients with SLE in activity, distinct of those from SLE patients in remission.

Methods

This study was conducted and reported in line with the *Preferred Reporting Items for Systematic Reviews and Meta-Analyses* (PRISMA) [10]. The review adopted the PECO structure (Population, Exposure, Comparator, and Outcome) recommended for systematic reviews [11]. The PECO structure was defined as 'P' (patients with SLE), 'E' (intestinal microbiota composition), 'C' (SLE in remission and healthy control group), and 'O' (SLE in activity). This systematic review was registered with the *International Prospective Register of Systematic Reviews* (PROSPERO) [12] under number CRD42021229322.

Eligibility criteria

This review included observational studies (cross-sectional, cohort, and case-control) which analyzed the intestinal microbiota composition in patients with SLE. Publications concerning cases with SLE, with no restriction of age or gender, which fulfilled the classification criteria of either Systemic Lupus International Collaborating Clinic (SLICC) [13], European League Against Rheumatism (EULAR) or American College of Rheumatology (ACR) [14] and considered the Systemic Lupus Erythematosus Disease Activity Index (SLEDAI) [15] to classify disease in activity or in remission were included. Researches that used only animals were excluded, however studies which included both animals and SLE patients were considered, and it is important to highlight that this review described only data from humans. Studies that assessed composition of microbiota based on stool sample using culture-dependent methods either real-time polymerase chain reaction (PCR), fluorescence in situ hybridization (FISH) or pyrosequencing for bacterial 16S ribosomal ribonucleic acid (rRNA) genes were considered. There was no restriction on language and publication year.

Ecological studies, case reports or case series, literature reviews, randomized clinical trials, dissertation, thesis and conference summaries, as well as duplicate articles and unavailable data even after contacting the authors were excluded. Researches in patients with intestinal and metabolic diseases that somehow affect intestinal microbiota, in addition to articles that did not provide measures for microbiota composition were also be excluded.

Databases

Searches were carried out from October, 2020 to January, 2021 using the following databases: Medline via Pubmed, Scopus, and Embase. The search strategy applied MeSH terms in PubMed, Emtree terms in Embase, and both terms in Scopus. Relevant keywords about SLE and microbiota were also used, aiming to encompass all articles on this issue.

The search was adapted for each database, and the following strategy was used in Pubmed:

1. = "lupus erythematosus, systemic" [MeSH] OR "systemic lupus erythematosus" OR "lupus erythematosus disseminates"
2. = microbiota [MeSH] OR microbiotas OR "microbial community" OR "community, microbial" OR "microbial communities" OR "microbial community composition" OR "community composition, microbial" OR "composition, microbial community" OR "microbial community compositions" OR "microbial community structure" OR "community structure, microbial" OR "microbial community structures" OR microbiome OR microbiomes OR "human microbiome" OR "human microbiomes" OR "microbiome, human
3. = dysbiosis [MeSH] OR recurrence [MeSH] OR "severity of Illness Index"[MeSH] OR relapse OR "disease severity"
4. = 1 AND 2 AND 3

Review process

The search was performed by two independent researchers (JRPV and ATOR), who grouped the articles and deleted the duplicated ones using Mendeley software. Then, these researchers individually selected the articles using Rayyan software, afterwards read the titles, the abstracts and, finally, the entire article, according to the eligibility criteria, and so articles were included. Disagreements about inclusion were discussed and resolved by a third senior reviewer (MRF).

Data extraction

In order to assess the risk of bias, Downs & Black Scale [16] was used, it consists of an instrument with 27 items, however only 16 items are applicable to observational studies (questions 1–3, 5–7, 9–12, 17, 18, 20, 21, 25, 26). This systematic review was based on the following aspects: a) objective clearly stated; b) main outcomes clearly described; c) sample characteristics clearly defined; d) distribution of principal confounders clearly described; e) main findings clearly defined; f) random variability in estimates provided; g) losses to follow-up described; h) probability values reported; i) sample target representative of population; j) sample recruitment representative of population; k) analyses adjusted for different follow-up duration; l) statistical tests appropriately used; m) accurate primary outcomes; n) patient sample recruited from the same population; o) adequate adjustment for confounders; and p) losses of sample to follow-up considered. The punctuation was applied for each manuscript according to the number of items considering the total percentage (0 to 17 points[1]). Low bias risk was defined as total score > 70%.

The Grading of Recommendations, Assessment, Development, and Evaluation (GRADE) [17] was applied to assess the quality of the evidence of the selected studies. For each study, the quality was ultimately assigned one of the following four grades: high quality (four filled circles), moderate quality (three filled circles), low quality (two filled circles), or very low quality (one filled circle). Following this approach, observational studies were lower (beginning with two circles), some items may compromise the quality of evidence, such as: risk of bias, imprecision, inconsistency, indirectness, and publication bias. Conversely, the quality of evidence may increase (additional filled circles) when the effects are sufficiently relevant, when all plausible biases would underestimate the effect, or when a dose-response gradient is present [18].

Data were extracted from articles that presented information related to intestinal microbiota and SLE in activity or remission and, then, they were inserted in a standardized form prepared by the authors. The following aspects were considered: author, year/country where the study was carried out, type of study, participants, microbiota analysis method, SLEDAI cut-off score ≥ 8 was used to define active SLE, and outcomes.

[1]Item number 5 can present two scores.

Results

The search resulted in 500 papers, out of which 327 were duplicates, 146 titles did not include the terms 'microbiota' and 'SLE', and 12 abstracts were not related to the subject. Subsequently, ten papers were eliminated after being read entirely as they did not meet the eligibility criteria. Therefore, five papers were selected for the systematic review (Fig. 1).

These papers were considered as low bias risk, three of them scored 80% at Downs & Black Scale while the remaining two papers received a score of 76%. In relation to GRADE, two papers obtained moderate quality and the other three, low quality. The individual results of the studies can be found in (Table 1).

The total number of participants considering the five studies was 530, out of which 195 had SLE in activity, 93 SLE in remission, and 222 healthy controls. Concerning participants' gender, two studies considered both genders and three studies prioritized female. Regarding the country where they were carried out, three are from China [19–21], one from the United States [7], and one from Spain [3]. All of them used DNA extraction in stool samples through RNAr 16S sequencing as analysis method of fecal microbiota (Table 2).

Either SLICC, EULAR or ACR classification criteria were applied in all of the researches as well as SLEDAI, which was applied to assess the disease activity index. Concerning the type of study, two of them was cross-sectional and three was cohort.

Three of the studies were focused on the relationship between microbiota and SLE in activity, one focused on microbiota of SLE in remission, and one focused on both.

With respect to intestinal microbiota composition and its main characteristics in patients with SLE in activity, studies highlighted greater amount of bacteria from the following genera: *Lactobacillus* (*Lactobacillus mucosae* species) [7, 21], *Streptococcus* (*Streptococcus anginosus* species), *Megasphaera*, *Fusobacterium*, *Veillonella* (*Veillonella díspar* species), *Oribacterium* [21], *Odoribacter* [7], and *Blautia* (*Lachnospiraceae* family) [7, 19]. Besides, *Streptococcus* and *Campylobacter* genera standed out as positively correlated with SLEDAI [7, 21].

Regarding phyla, high level of *Proteobacterias* (*Epsilonproteobacteria* class, *Campylobacterales* order and *Campylobacter* genus) [20, 7], *Bacteroidetes* (*Prevotella* genus), and *Actinobacteria* (*Rhodococcus* and *Eggerthella*

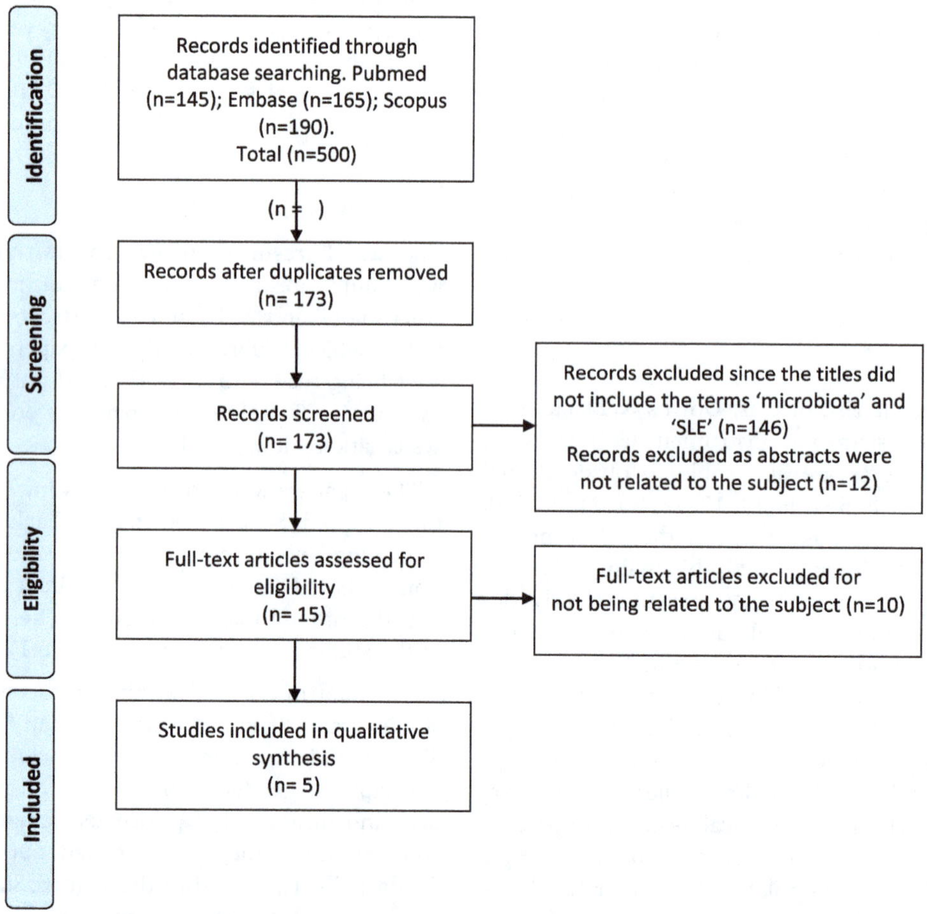

Fig. 1 PRISMA Flow Diagram of search and study selection

Table 1 Methodological quality assessment and strength of evidence

Study (year)	Conflict of Interests	Ethical Approval	Downs and Black checklist																		GRADE
			A	B	C	D	E	F	G	H	I	J	K	L	M	N	O	P	Total	Score#	
Chen at al. 2020	No	Yes	1	1	1	0	1	1	1	1	1	1	1	1	1	1	0	1	14	80%	●●●○
He at al. 2016	No	Yes	1	1	1	0	1	1	–	1	1	1	1	1	1	1	0	–	12	80%	●●○○
Li at al. 2019	No	Yes	1	1	1	0	1	1	1	1	1	1	1	1	1	1	0	1	14	80%	●●●○
Luo at al. 2018	No	*	1	1	1	0	1	1	1	1	1	1	1	1	1	0	0	1	13	76%	●●○○
Hevia at al. 2014	*	Yes	1	1	1	0	1	1	–	1	1	1	–	1	1	–	0	–	10	76%	●●○○

Downs and Black checklist: A) objective clearly stated; B) main outcomes clearly described; C) sample characteristics clearly defined; D) distribution of principal confounders clearly described; E) main findings clearly defined; F) random variability in estimates provided; G) lost to follow-up described; H) probability values reported; I) sample target representative of population; J) sample recruitment representative of population; K) analyses adjusted for different follow-up duration; L) statistical tests appropriately used; M) primary outcomes valid/reliable; N) sample recruited from the same population; O) adequate adjustment for confounding; and P) losses of sample to follow-up taken into account (corresponding to questions 1–3, 5–7, 9–12, 17,18, 20, 21, 25,26). Questions G and P were applied only for longitudinal studies. Questions K and N were applied only for case-control and longitudinal studies

Score reaches 100% with 13, 15, and 17 points for cross-sectional, case-control, and longitudinal studies, respectively

*, not reported, –, not applied

GRADE, Grading of Recommendations, Assessment, Development and Evaluations; one filled circle, very low quality; two filled circles, low quality; three filled circles, moderate quality; four filled circles, high quality

Table 2 Characteristics of the studies included in the systematic review

Author/ year Location	Type of Study	Participants	Gender	Method of Microbial Analysis	SLEDAI cut-off score used to define active SLE	Results
Chen et al. 2020 China	prospective cohort	117 patients with untreated SLE, 52 patients with SLE post-treatment; 115 healthy controls.	Female and Male	DNA of stool samples using RNAr 16S sequencing	Not informed	• Disease activity and microbial diversity decreased significantly after treatment. • ↓ microbial richness and uniformity in untreated SLE compared with control group. • Seven species[1] of markers enriched in patients with untreated SLE and reduced after treatment. • Post-treatment microbial composition is more similar to that in control group.
He et al. 2016 China	cross-sectional	45 patients untreated SLE and 48 healthy controls	Female	DNA of stool sample using RNAr 16S sequencing	Not informed	• ↑ phyla: *Bacteroidetes, Actinobacteria* and *Proteobacteria*. • ↓ phyla: *Firmicutes* in individuals with untreated SLE.
Li et al. 2019 China	prospective cohort	19 patients with SLE in activity, 21 in remission, and 22 healthy controls.	Female	DNA of stool sample using RNAr 16S sequencing	Active SLE patients: SLEDAI ≥8	• Dysbiosis and constitution of microbial community was different in SLE in activity and SLE in remission, however, microbial diversity is the same. • ↓ *Bifidobacterium* genus and *Ruminococcus.gnavus* species in active SLE when compared with SLE in remission. • ↑ six genera[2] as well as *Proteobacteria* phylum in SLE in activity compared to healthy controls. • *Lactobacillus* genus associated with more serious diseases.
Luo et al. 2018 USA	prospective cohort	14 patients with SLE in activity and 17 healthy controls	Female and Male	DNA of stool sample using RNAr 16S sequencing	Active SLE patients: SLEDAI ≥8	• ↓ microbial diversity in SLE in activity. • ↑ *Proteobacteria* phylum, ↑ *Odoribacter* and *Blautia* genera and an unnamed genus (*Rikenellaceae* family) in SLE in activity. • *Firmicutes* and *Bacteroidetes* ratios did not differ in microbiota between SLE and non-SLE.
Hevia et al. 2014 Spain	cross-sectional	20 patients with SLE in remission and 20 healthy controls	Female	DNA of stool sample using RNAr 16S sequencing	Active SLE patients: SLEDAI ≥8	• Dysbiosis in SLE in activity compared to SLE in remission • ↑ three genera[3] and *Bacteroidetes* phylum, ↓*Firmicutes* ratio in patients with SLE in remission. • ↑ *Lachnospiraceae* and *Ruminococcaceae* in healthy controls

↑ greater quantity or enrichment
↓lower quantity or depleted
Notes: [1]*Clostridium sp. ATCC BAA-442, Atopobium rimae, Shuttleworthia satelles, Actinomyces massiliensis, Bacteroides fragilis, Clostridium leptum,* and one non-classified *Escherichia.*
[2] *Lactobacillus, Streptococcus, Megasphaera, Fusobacterium, Veillonella* and *Oribacterium.*
[3]*Dialister, Pseudobutyrivibrio,* and *Bifidobacterium.*

genera) was observed in patients with SLE who were not treated [19].

Seven markers species enhanced in patients with untreated SLE and which were reduced after treatment were found: *Clostridium sp. ATCC BAA-442, Atopobium rimae, Shuttleworthia satelles, Actinomyces massiliensis, Bacteroides fragilis, Clostridium leptum,* and non-classified *Escherichia* [19]. Furthermore, some species are positively correlated with SLEDAI, such as: *Ruminococcus torques, Lactobacillus salivarius* [19], *Lactobacillales* [21], and *Clostridium sp. ATCC BAA-442* [19]. However, healthy controls presented greater quantity of *Lachnospiraceae* and *Ruminococcaceae* families [3].

Considering bacteria found in reduced amount in SLE in activity, those belonging to *Tenericutes* and *Mollicutes* phyla, *Faecalibacterium* (*prausnitzii*), *Roseburia, Bifidobacterium* genera, and *Ruminococcus gnavus* species [21] are mentioned. Decrease in *Firmicutes* phylum as well as *Pseudobutyrivibrio* and *Dialister* genera [20] was observed in patients with untreated SLE.

Focusing on the dysbiosis issue, researches highlighted that microbial richness and uniformity was reduced in SLE in activity, although the number of species was maintained [19]. Besides, there was decrease in diversity after treatment and SLEDAI reduction [19]. However, it was observed that diversity and species metrics were significantly higher in healthy controls than in patients with SLE in activity [21].

Concerning the microbiota of patients with SLE in remission, attenuation in ratio *Firmicutes/Bacteroidetes* was inferred, with decrease of *Firmicutes* and increase of *Bacteroidetes* considering the overall bacterial level [3]. Exacerbated amount of *Dialister, Pseudobutyrivibrio,* and *Bifidobacterium* genera was also verified [3]. Differences in the microbial community constitution were observed between SLE in activity and in remission, such as *Bifidobacterium* genus increased in stool samples from patients with SLE in remission compared with those in activity [21]. Besides, *Ruminococcus gnavus* species was reduced, while *Streptococcus, Lactobacillales de Bacillie,* and *Streptococcus anginosus* species were enriched in patients with SLE in activity when compared with the group in remission. However, both groups were similar regarding diversity [21].

Discussion

This is the first systematic review that verified whether there is a relationship between intestinal microbiota composition and SLE in activity considering representative patterns, dysbiosis, and heterogeneity in active and in remission clinical conditions. This study evidenced particular characteristics in microbial profile in patients with SLE in activity, presenting different aspects when compared with those in remission. It was also noticed that there is intestinal dysbiosis, especially in SLE in activity.

Considering bacterial genera that were positively correlated with SLE in activity, pro-inflammatory bacteria were highlighted, such as *Streptococcus, Megasphaera* [21] as well as heterogeneity of intestinal microbiota. It was observed that bacterial diversity was reduced [21] in relation to microbial richness and uniformity, but not in relation to the number of species [19] . This supports studies that reported pro-inflammatory bacteria as responsible for releasing substances which aggravates the level of systemic inflammation [22] related to the intestinal disorder of autoimmune diseases [23–25].

Most of human infections are caused by opportunist pathogens that typically compose patient's normal microbiota, when there is significant amount of these pathogenic bacteria a disorder in the natural microbiota can be induced, thus circumventing the defense mechanisms and generating clinical symptoms [26]. The mucous immunological system is responsible for eliminating pathogens, therefore an inadequate immune response imbalances intestinal homeostasis, triggers dysbiosis and contributes to local and systemic inflammation as well as metabolic dysfunction [27].

Patients with SLE in activity present specific dysbiosis in microbiota and its related metabolic pathways [21] as a consequence of altered immunological function [3]. Therefore, changes in balanced microbiota composition, i.e. dysbiosis, may play an important role in promoting chronic inflammation in autoimmune diseases [24, 25] resulting in exacerbation, rapid progression, and disease worsening [28].

In relation to anti-inflammatory bacteria found in this review, it was observed decrease mainly in the phylum *Tenericutes* and *Mollicutes,* responsible for the modulation of the immune system. These types of bacteria can induce regulatory T cells, allowing the host to tolerate the amount of antigens in the intestine, thus preventing inflammation [29]. In addition, anti-inflammatory bacteria ferment carbohydrate, releasing butyrate, a fatty acid able to inhibit the production of pro-inflammatory cytokines, such as IL-12 and TNF-α [30].

When the interaction between anti and pro-inflammatory bacteria is altered, resulting in disruption of homeostasis, there is a dysbiosis [29]. This may result in local infection, inflammation and invasiveness [31] as well as complications that may lead SLE to the active condition. This is in line with researches that support that many autoimmune diseases, including SLE, were associated with intestinal microbiota dysbiosis, intestinal barrier dysfunction, and microbial translocation [32].

Concerning the pattern of intestinal bacteria in SLE in remission this review corroborates other studies related to imbalance in the ratio between *Bacteroidetes* and *Firmicutes* [31]. Approximately 90% of bacterial microbiota is composed of these two genera, which act in host metabolism and immunity [22], and their disproportion is correlated with clinical conditions [33]. *Firmicutes* are essential in the absorption of fatty acids and energy from carbohydrates while *Bacteroidetes* play a role in the absorption of polysaccharides [28].

Therefore, although another research indicates that microbiota composition in SLE post-treatment is similar to healthy control groups [19], SLE patients present *Firmicutes/Bacteroidetes* ratio next to 2.5 times lower [28]. This shows changes in intestinal microbiota may be pointed out even in SLE in remission [31], demonstrating association between dysbiosis and lupus [28].

Regarding differences in intestinal bacteria patterns, it was observed reduction in anti-inflammatory bacteria and enrichment of the pro-inflammatory ones in patients with SLE in activity when compared with those in remission [21]. This emphasizes that although they present similar diversity [21], the microbiota profile is different between both groups.

The relationship between microbiota and autoimmune diseases is relatively recent, so few studies (just five) were eligible to this systematic review, identifying investigation gaps. It is necessary in-depth studies to provide better understanding of aspects related not only to etiopathogenesis but also to the inflammatory process during SLE progression.

However, the main characteristic of this study was to raise an issue that has been insufficiently studied in literature. The results presented herein may be a source of encouragement for future studies focused on microbiota as a biomarker of activity in SLE, supporting medical community to elaborate investigation sequences and disease treatment.

The limitations of this review include the low number of SLE patients (288) and methodological diversity related to gender, some considered male and female patients while others prioritized female.

Conclusion

This systematic review evidenced representative microbiota patterns in SLE in activity, with greater amount of pathogenic bacteria and reduction of commensal bacteria, therefore indicating that there may be a relation between intestinal microbiota dysbiosis and disease activity. Besides, differences concerning intestinal microbiota pattern between SLE in activity and in remission were presented.

Abbreviations

ACR: American College of Rheumatology; **EULAR**: European League Against Rheumatism; **GRADE**: Grading of Recommendations, Assessment, Development and Evaluations; **MeSH**: Medical Subject Headings; **PECO**: Population, Exposure, Comparator and Outcome; **PRISMA**: Preferred Reporting Items for Systematic Reviews and Meta-Analyses; **PROSPERO**: International prospective register of systematic reviews; **SLE**: Systemic Lupus Erythematosus; **SLEDAI**: Systemic Lupus Erythematosus Disease Activity; **SLICC**: Systemic Lupus International Collaborating Clinic

Acknowledgements

We thank Capes for the doctorate degree scholarship of A.T.O. Rezende.

Authors' contributions

ATOR and JRP: outline development, paper writing, contribution to the methodologic aspect, database searches, and data analysis. MRF and NAS: manuscript preparation guidance, concept creation, and article design (objectives, theme and title). ATOR, JRP, MRF and NAS: reading and approval of the final manuscript.

Author details

[1]Postgraduate Program in Health Sciences, School of Medicine of the Universidade Federal de Goiás (UFG), Goiânia, Brazil. [2]Department of Orthopedics/Traumatology, School of Medicine of the Universidade Federal de Goiás (UFG), Goiânia, Brazil. [3]Rheumatology Service of Hospital das Clínicas, School of Medicine of the Universidade Federal de Goiás (UFG), Goiânia, Brazil.

References

1. Esmaeili S-A, Mahmoudi M, Momtazi AA, Sahebkar A, Doulabi H, Rastin M. Tolerogenic probiotics: potential immunoregulators in systemic lupus erythematosus. J Cell Physiol. 2017;232(8):1994–2007. https://doi.org/10.1002/jcp.25748.
2. Zhang H, Liao X, Sparks JB, Luo XM. Dinâmica da microbiota intestinal em auto-imune lúpus. Appl Environ Microbiol. 2014;80(24):7551–60. https://doi.org/10.1128/AEM.02676-14.
3. Hevia A, Milani C, López P, Cuervo A, Arboleya S, Duranti S, et al. Intestinal dysbiosis associated with systemic lupus erythematosus. MBio. 2014;5(5).
4. López P, Sánchez B, Margolles A, Suárez A. Intestinal dysbiosis in systemic lupus erythematosus: cause or consequence? Curr Opin Rheumatol. 2016; 28(5):515–22. https://doi.org/10.1097/BOR.0000000000000309.
5. González S, Gutiérrez-Díaz I, López P, Suárez A, Fernández-Navarro T, Sánchez BMA. Microbiota and oxidant-antioxidant balance in systemic lupus erythematosus. Nutr Hosp. 2017;34(4):934–41. https://doi.org/10.20960/nh.546.
6. Neuman H, Koren O. The gut microbiota: a possible factor influencing systemic lupus erythematosus. Curr Opin Rheumatol. 2017;29(4):374–7. https://doi.org/10.1097/BOR.0000000000000395.
7. Luo XM, Edwards MR, Mu Q, Yu Y, Vieson MD, Reilly CM, et al. Gut microbiota in human systemic lupus erythematosus and a mouse model of lupus. Appl Environ Microbiol. 2018;84(4):1–10.
8. Mu Q, Zhang H, Luo XMXM. SLE: Another Autoimmune Disorder Influenced by Microbes and Diet? Front Immunol. 2015;6(NOV):608.
9. López P, De Paz B, Rodríguez-Carrio J, Hevia A, Sánchez B, Margolles A, et al. Th17 responses and natural IgM antibodies are related to gut microbiota composition in systemic lupus erythematosus patients. Sci Rep. 2016;6:1–12.
10. Moher D, Shamseer L, Clarke M, Ghersi D, Liberatî A, Petticrew M, et al. Preferred reporting items for systematic review and meta-analysis protocols (PRISMA-P) 2015 statement. 2015.
11. Morgan RL, Whaley P, Thayer KASH. Identifying the PECO: a framework for formulating good questions to explore the association of environmental and other exposures with health outcomes. Environ Int. 2018;121(Pt 1): 1027–31. https://doi.org/10.1016/j.envint.2018.07.015.
12. Booth A, Clarke M, Dooley G, Ghersi D, Moher D, Petticrew M, et al. The nuts and bolts of PROSPERO: an international prospective register of systematic reviews. Syst Rev. 2012;1(1):2. https://doi.org/10.1186/2046-4053-1-2.
13. Petri M, Orbai AM, Alarcõn GS, Gordon C, Merrill JT, Fortin PR, et al. Derivation and validation of the systemic lupus international collaborating clinics classification criteria for systemic lupus erythematosus. Arthritis Rheum. 2012;64(8):2677–86. https://doi.org/10.1002/art.34473.
14. Aringer M, Costenbader K, Daikh D, Brinks R, Mosca M, Ramsey-Goldman R, et al. 2019 European league against rheumatism/American College of Rheumatology Classification Criteria for systemic lupus erythematosus. Arthritis Rheum. 2019;71(9):1400–12. https://doi.org/10.1002/art.40930.
15. Parker B, Bruce IN. Clinical markers, metrics, indices, and clinical trials. Ninth Edit. Vol. 4, Dubois' Lupus Erythematosus and Related Syndromes. Elsevier Inc.; 2018. 614–630 p.
16. Downs SH, Black N. The feasibility of creating a checklist for the assessment of the methodological quality both of randomised and non-randomised studies of health care interventions. J Epidemiol Community Health. 1998; 52(6):377–84. https://doi.org/10.1136/jech.52.6.377.
17. Guyatt G, Oxman AD, Akl EA, Kunz R, Vist G, Brozek J, et al. GRADE guidelines. J Clin Epidemiol. 2011;64(4):383–94. https://doi.org/10.1016/j.jclinepi.2010.04.026.
18. Balshem H, Helfand M, Schünemann HJ, Oxman AD, Kunz R, Brozek J, et al. GRADE guidelines: 3. Rating the quality of evidence. J Clin Epidemiol. 2011; 64(4):401–6. https://doi.org/10.1016/j.jclinepi.2010.07.015.
19. Chen B, Jia X, Xu J, Zhao L, Ji J, Wu B, et al. The gut microbiota of non-treated patients with SLE defines an autoimmunogenic and proinflammatory profile. Arthritis Rheum. 2020:2.
20. He Z, Shao T, Li H, Xie Z, Wen C. Alterations of the gut microbiome in Chinese patients with systemic lupus erythematosus. Gut Pathog. 2016;8(1): 1–7.
21. Li Y, Wang H-F, Li X, Li H-X, Zhang Q, Zhou H-W, et al. Disordered intestinal microbes are associated with the activity of systemic lupus erythematosus. Clin Sci. 2019;133(7):821–38. https://doi.org/10.1042/CS20180841.
22. Tremaroli V, Bäckhed F. Functional interactions between the gut microbiota and host metabolism. Nature. 2012;489(7415):242–9. https://doi.org/10.1038/nature11552.
23. van der Meulen TA, Harmsen HJM, Bootsma H, Spijkervet FKL, Kroese FGM, Vissink A. The microbiome–systemic diseases connection. Oral Dis. 2016; 22(8):719–34. https://doi.org/10.1111/odi.12472
24. Lynch SV, Pedersen O. The human intestinal microbiome in health and disease. N Engl J Med. 2016;375(24):2369–79. https://doi.org/10.1056/NEJMra1600266

25. Proal AD, Albert PJ, Marshall TG. The human microbiome and autoimmunity. Curr Opin Rheumatol. 2013;25(2):234–40. https://doi.org/10.1097/BOR.0b013e32835cedbf.
26. Ara L, Castro S. Colonization of the intestinal microbiota and its influence on health host. Univ Ciências da Saúde, Brasília [Internet]. 2016;14(1):85–96. Available from: https://www.publicacoesacademicas.uniceub.br/cienciasaude/article/view/3629
27. Shin N, Whon TW, Bae J. Proteobacteria: microbial signature of dysbiosis in gut microbiota. Trends Biotechnol [Internet]. 2015;1–8. Available from: https://www.sciencedirect.com/science/article/pii/S0167779915001390 (27).
28. Yacoub R, Jacob A, Wlaschin J, Mcgregor M, Richard J, Alexander JJ. Lupus: The microbiome angle. Immunobiology [Internet]. 2017; Available from: https://www.sciencedirect.com/science/article/pii/S0171298517302115
29. Macdonald TT, Monteleone G. Regulation of homeostasis and inflammation in the intestine. YGAST [Internet]. 2011;140(6):1768–75 Available from: https://doi.org/10.1053/j.gastro.2011.02.047.
30. Magalhaes JG, Tattoli I, Girardin SE. The intestinal epithelial barrier : How to distinguish between the microbial flora and pathogens 2007;19:106–15. Available from: https://www.sciencedirect.com/science/article/pii/S1044532307000024
31. De Luca F, Shoenfeld Y. The microbiome in autoimmune diseases. Clin Exp Immunol. 2019;195(1):74–85. https://doi.org/10.1111/cei.13158.
32. Mu Q, Kirby J, Reilly CM, Luo XM. Leaky gut as a danger signal for autoimmune diseases. Front Immunol. 2017;8(MAY):598.
33. Maranduba CMDC, De Castro SBR, De Souza GT, Rossato C, Da Guia FC, Valente MAS, et al. Intestinal microbiota as modulators of the immune system and neuroimmune system: Impact on the host health and homeostasis. J Immunol Res. 2015;2015.

24

Quality of referrals to a rheumatology service before and after implementation of a triage system with telemedicine support

Deise Marcela Piovesan[1*], Vanessa Barrili Busato[1], Romulo Gomes da Silveira[1], Aline Defaveri do Prado[1], Cynthia Goulart Molina-Bastos[2,3], Sheila Hickmann[1], Guilherme Kopik Bongiorno[1], Camila de David Cruz[1], Sheron Zamboni[1], Julio César Simon[1], Marcelo Rodrigues Gonçalves[2,3] and Markus Bredemeier[1]

Abstract

Purpose: To evaluate the quality of referrals for a first Rheumatology consultation at a tertiary care center in a southern Brazilian capital (Porto Alegre, RS), having as background findings from a similar survey performed in 2007/2008. Since then, our state has implemented referral protocols and a triage system with teleconsulting support exclusively for referrals from locations outside the capital, permitting a comparison between patients screened and not screened by the new system.

Methods: Physicians of the Rheumatology Service at Hospital Nossa Senhora da Conceição prospectively collected information regarding first visits over a 6-month period (Oct 2017 to March 2018). We recorded demographic characteristics, diagnostic hypotheses, date of referral, and the municipality of origin (within the state of Rio Grande do Sul). We considered adequate referrals from primary health care when a systemic autoimmune inflammatory disease (SIRD) was suspected at first evaluation by the attending rheumatologist.

Results: Three hundred fifty-seven patients/appointments were eligible for analysis (193 from the capital and 164 from small and medium towns). In 2007/2008, suspected SIRD occurred in 76/260 (29.2%) and 73/222 (32.9%) among patients from the capital and outside counties, respectively ($P = 0.387$). In 2017/2018, suspected SIRD occurred in 75/193 (38.9%) and 111/164 (67.7%) in patients from the capital and outside counties, respectively (difference: 28.8, 95% CI: 19.0 to 38.9, $P < 0.001$), indicating a marked improvement in referrals submitted to the new triage system.

Conclusion: The quality of Rheumatology referrals in our state improved over the 10-year interval under study, particularly among patients from locations submitted to referral protocols and teleconsulting support.

Keywords: Telemedicine, Referral, Waiting time, Access to care, Telerheumatology

* Correspondence: deise.piovesan@hotmail.com
[1]Rheumatology Service at Hospital Nossa Senhora da Conceição (HNSC), Grupo Hospitalar Nossa Senhora da Conceição (GHC), Avenida Francisco Trein, 596, 3 Andar, Porto Alegre, Rio Grande do Sul, Brazil

Introduction

The long waiting time for consultations with specialists is one of the most significant limitations of the Brazilian public health system (*Sistema Único de Saúde*, SUS). The difference between supply and demand in Rheumatology consultations is leading to a long list of patients waiting for an appointment [1].

In rheumatic inflammatory diseases, the time from first symptoms to the initiation of treatment is one of the main factors related to prognosis [2]. Besides the personal impact caused by the delay in treatment, there is an economic burden associated with the morbidity of rheumatic diseases that the early initiation of the treatment could minimize [3]. In Brazil, rheumatic diseases are an important cause of public healthcare expenditures. The indirect cost for patients with rheumatoid arthritis was estimated at US$ 2423.51 per patient per year [4]. Early access to care for patients with a systemic inflammatory rheumatic disease (SIRD) is a current challenge in Brazil as well as in developed countries [5].

Rheumatology tertiary care centers should prioritize care for patients with systemic inflammatory rheumatic diseases (SIRDs) instead of diseases manageable at the primary care level [6]. In a previous study, performed at our Rheumatology Clinic at Hospital Nossa Senhora da Conceição/Grupo Hospitalar Conceição (HNSC/GHC) in 2007–2008, we evaluated 487 referrals from the capital and outside counties of our state (Rio Grande do Sul) [1]. We observed that only approximately 30% of the patients referred to Rheumatology (from both origins) had SIRDs, and there was no adequate prioritization of severe or urgent cases. In 2016, a project of the Federal University of Rio Grande do Sul [UFRGS] introduced a telemedicine system (TelessaúdeRS/UFRGS) for referrals to Rheumatology in the State of Rio Grande do Sul, in partnership with the Brazilian Ministry of Health and the State Health Department [7]. However, this system was initially introduced only for referrals from outside counties, excluding those from the capital. This created the opportunity to observe the effect of telemedicine in the quality of referrals independently from other changes that could have influenced public healthcare over time, given that the only significant difference in the referral processes was the introduction of this telemedicine system. So, our aim in the present study is to evaluate the impact of telemedicine in the quality of referrals to Rheumatology tertiary care, comparing the cases from outsides counties (screened by the telemedicine system) and cases from the capital (unscreened cases), having as background the data collected in 2007/2008 [1], when there was no regulation of referrals at all.

Material and methods

We performed a cross-sectional study at the Rheumatology Service of (HNSC/GHC). The study was approved by the Ethics Committee of the HNSC and registered under the number 04529218.0.0000.5530 of the CAAE (Certificate of Presentation for Ethical Appreciation).

The TelessaúdeRS/UFRGS™ project identified the most common rheumatic diseases referred for specialized medical consultations. Family physicians and rheumatologists created referral protocols for each of these conditions. The protocols, available for the primary care physicians, defined the minimal required information that must be provided in the referral document and the clinical criteria to ask for a specialized care appointment [7, 8]. All requests for specialized care appointments are analyzed by the medical regulatory team, reviewing the adequacy of the request according to requirements of the protocol. After that, the medical regulatory team decides to authorize the referral or request additional information from the primary care provider. Whenever the team agrees with the necessity of referral to the Rheumatology specialist, they classify it according to the priority degree, also based on the protocol. When the request does not fulfill the criteria for referral, a telephone consultation (provided by TelessaúdeRS™ via a free telephone hotline) was indicated. Teleconsulting was given by a trained primary health care physician or the rheumatologist itself (both members of the TelessaúdeRS™ staff). Anyhow, the rheumatologist was always available for consultation if necessary [7–9]. Once the use of the protocol was approved by the State Health Secretariat of Rio Grande do Sul, the regulatory process was applied to every new referral from outside counties. Besides that, the team also retrospectively revised the waiting list of patients from outside counties and applied the new system to these referrals [9]. This system was not applied to patients referred from the state capital during the period covered by this report.

For the present study, we collected data from patients scheduled for first Rheumatology consultations from October 01, 2017, to March 31, 2018. All patients attending first appointments and referred from primary health care (PHC) were considered eligible. Using a standard research protocol, we gathered the following data from the referral document elaborated at the PHC unit: the place of origin, date of referral from the PHC unit, and diagnostic hypotheses elaborated by the PHC physician. Further data collected during the consultation were attendance or not (in case of absenteeism), age, gender, diagnostic hypothesis formulated during the consultation by the rheumatologist (up to 3 could be recorded), urgency or not (we defined urgency if there was a risk of damage to a vital organ, rheumatoid arthritis with factors for worse prognosis or pregnancy), and the date of the consultation. If the date of referral was not reported on the PHC document, we asked the patient to choose a date according to his recall of the moment of referral. In rare cases, it was necessary to contact patients afterward by telephone or review medical records to clarify uncertain information. For analytical purposes, when the rheumatologist suspected any systemic inflammatory rheumatic disease (SIRD) during the first visit, the referral was considered adequate. The diseases classified as SIRD were rheumatoid arthritis, systemic lupus erythematosus, Sjögren's syndrome, systemic sclerosis, inflammatory myopathies, undifferentiated or overlapping autoimmune connective tissue diseases, spondyloarthritis (including ankylosing spondylitis, psoriatic arthritis, arthritis associated with inflammatory bowel disease, reactive arthritis, and undifferentiated spondyloarthritis), polymyalgia rheumatica, antiphospholipid syndrome, systemic vasculitis, and other less common autoimmune disorders (e.g., sarcoidosis, remitting seronegative symmetrical synovitis with pitting edema, and relapsing polychondritis). The research protocol and all study procedures were almost identical to those employed in our 2007/2008 study [1], making the results easily comparable.

Statistical analysis

Statistical analyses were performed using SPSS for Windows, version 20.0 (IBM Corporation, Armonk, NY, USA). Quantitative variables were graphically and statistically tested (with the Kolmogorov-Smirnov goodness-of-fit test) for normality of distribution. We describe categorical variables as numbers and percentages and tested associations using Pearson's chi-square test. Homogeneity of 2 × 2 tables across strata was evaluated with Woolf's test. We presented variables with a normal distribution as mean ± standard deviation (SD). We presented non-normal quantitative or ordinal variables as median and the 25th and 75th percentiles and performed between-group comparisons using the Mann-Whitney test. Two-tailed P values less than or equal to 0.05 were considered statistically significant.

Results

There were 500 Rheumatology first consultations schedules during the study period. Of these, 71 were already being treated in the Rheumatology unit; therefore, they were not considered first-time Rheumatology visits (these consultations were scheduled as first visits only for bureaucratic reasons). Of the remaining appointments, 72 did not attend, and 357 patients remained available for analysis; the characteristics of these patients are described in Table 1. Suspected SIRD by the rheumatologist occurred in approximately half of the cases. The date of referral was not reported in the official referral document of only 23 patients (6.4%). The mean ± SD waiting time was 10.5 ± 7.8 months.

Table 2 shows diagnostic hypotheses formulated by the PHC doctors. The most frequent hypothesis was rheumatoid arthritis (RA, 27.5%), followed by systemic lupus erythematosus (SLE, 15.4%). Referrals for suspected osteoarthritis and fibromyalgia, which generally do not require secondary or tertiary care, occurred in 5.0 and 4.5% of cases, respectively. Table 3 shows the most frequent diagnosis ascertained or suspected in the first consultations by the rheumatologist. RA was the main hypothesis in 20.4% of cases, followed by osteoarthritis (17.4%) and fibromyalgia (16.8%). SLE was suspected in 11.5% of the cases.

Table 4 describes the waiting time for rheumatologic consultation in the 2017/2018 and the 2007/2008 surveys. Comparing both surveys, there is a significant increase in the waiting time for rheumatologic consultation over the 10 years period under study.

Table 5 compares prevalence of suspected SIRD and urgent cases obtained in 2007/2008 with those observed in the present study (2017/2018). In general, the prevalence of suspected SIRD raised from approximately 30% in 2007/2008 to more than 50% in 2017/2018. In 2007/

Table 1 Demographic characteristics of eligible patients (total of 357 patients)

Female – n (%)	305 (85.4)
Age (years) – mean ± SD, range of values	53.0 ± 14.9, 13 to 85
Origin:	
Porto Alegre (capital) – n (%)	193 (54.1%)
Outside counties within the same state – n (%)	164 (45.9%)
Waiting time (months) - median (P25 - P75), range of values	12.1 (4.4–14.1), 0.23 to 63.8
Urgent need for an appointment (according to rheumatologist) – n (%)	78 (21.8)
Suspected SIRD according to the general practitioner– n (%)	220 (61.6)
Suspected SIRD according to the rheumatologist – n (%)	186 (52.1)
Referral date (obtained from the referencing document) – n (%)	334 (93.6)

SD standard deviation; *P25* 25th percentile; *P75* 75th percentile; *SIRD* systemic inflammatory rheumatic disease

Table 2 Frequency of diagnoses formulated by the general practitioner to justify referral ($n = 357$)

Diagnosis	n (%)
Rheumatoid arthritis	98 (27.5%)
Systemic lupus erythematosus	55 (15.4%)
Undifferentiated arthralgia	41 (11.5%)
Unspecified inflammatory disease	23 (6.4%)
Osteoarthritis	18 (5.0%)
Fibromyalgia	16 (4.5%)
Psoriatic arthritis	15 (4.2%)
Ankylosing spondylitis	15 (4.2%)
Sjögren's syndrome	9 (2.5%)
Non-specific rheumatism	9 (2.5%)
Gout	6 (1.7%)
Systemic sclerosis	5 (1.4%)
Laboratory abnormalities	4 (1.1%)
Other diseases	43 (12.0%)

2008, the proportion of patients with a SIRD was similar in outside counties (32.9%) and in the capital (29.2%), as well as the frequency of urgent cases (44.7 and 42.3%, respectively). In 2017/2018, however, the prevalence of SIRDs was significantly higher in patients from interior towns (67.7%) comparing to those from the capital (38.9%) (difference in prevalence, 28.8, 95% CI, 18.1 to 38.9%, $P < 0.001$), suggesting a positive impact of the triage system in the quality of referrals. In the same direction, in 2017/2018, urgent cases represented 29.9% of cases from outside counties versus 15.0% of cases from the capital (difference in prevalence, 14.9, 95% CI, 5.7 to 23.3%, $P = 0.001$).

Table 3 Diagnostic hypotheses formulated by the rheumatologist at first consultations ($n = 357$)

Diagnosis	n (%)
Rheumatoid arthritis	73 (20.4%)
Osteoarthritis	62 (17.4%)
Fibromyalgia	60 (16.8%)
Systemic lupus erythematosus	41 (11.5%)
Spondyloarthritis	18 (5.0%)
Psoriatic arthritis	15 (4.2%)
Periarthritis	14 (3.9%)
Sjögren's Syndrome	10 (2.8%)
Gout	9 (2.5%)
Systemic sclerosis	5 (1.4%)
Systemic vasculitis	5 (1.4%)
Osteoporosis	5 (1.4%)
Juvenile idiopathic arthritis	4 (1.1%)
Uveitis	4 (1.1%)
Low back pain	3 (0.8%)
Behçet's disease	2 (0.6%)
Anti-phospholipid syndrome	2 (0.6%)
Sarcoidosis	2 (0.6%)
Dermato- or polymyositis	2 (0.6%)
Eosinophilic fasciitis	1 (0.3%)
Other diseases	20 (5.6%)

Discussion

In this cross-sectional study, we observed a significant improvement in the quality of referrals to Rheumatology consultations in the state of Rio Grande do Sul over 10 years. Comparing the results of the 2007/2008 survey with those observed in the present study (2017/2018), we noticed more cases suspected of SIRDs in the latter (52.1%, versus 30.9% in the former). However, we found that the increase in the proportion of SIRDs was more marked in outside counties' referrals (from 33 to 68%) compared to referrals from the capital (from 29 to 39%) over these 10 years. This change may be explained partly by a general improvement in knowledge of the rheumatic diseases among PHC physicians. However, the more marked increase in the proportion of adequate referrals from outside counties suggest that much of this improvement is related to the application of the triage program and teleconsulting support system [7–9].

Previous studies had already demonstrated the benefits of referral screening processes for referrals to specialized care [5, 10]. In a Canadian study similar to ours, the implantation of triage for referrals promoted a reduction in waiting time for patients with suspected inflammatory arthritis (IA) and connective tissue diseases (CTD). In contrast, the waiting time for those with suspected non-IA and non-CTD increased [11]. Teleconsulting support seems to work as a continued medical education process, leading to reduced referrals to specialties and improving the quality of referrals [12]. In our country, Meyama et al. evaluated the impact of teleconsulting in referrals in Santa Catarina (another Southern Brazilian state). They found a decrease of more than 50 % in new solicitations of Rheumatology referrals after starting a mandatory teleconsulting program [12].

Interestingly, we observed a reduction in cases classified as urgent in 2017/2018 compared to the 2007/2008 survey. A difference in the classification methodology can probably explain this finding. In 2007/2008, cases were classified as urgent based on subjective rheumatologist's evaluation without following clear pre-specified criteria. However, in the present survey, we used stricter criteria (pregnancy, risk of vital organ damage, and RA with poor prognosis) to define an urgent case.

We noticed that the waiting time for consultation increased considerably during the time frame encompassed by this study. A possible explanation for this

Table 4 Comparison of waiting time (months) of patients referred for first Rheumatology consultations in 2007/2008 (482 patients) and 2017/2018 (357 patients)

	Mean ± SD	Median (P25-P75), range of values	*P* Value*
2007/2008	7.8 ± 11.1	3.8 (1.5–10.0), 0.1 to 96.0	< 0.001
2017/2018	10.5 ± 7.8	12.1 (4.4–14.1), 0.2 to 63.8	

* Mann-Whitney test. *SD* standard deviation; *P25* 25th percentile; *P75* 75th percentile

observation is that we collected the data from October 01, 2017, to March 31, 2018, just a year and a half after the changes in the referral system. Given that data from TelessaúdeRS/UFRGS™ shows a decrease in about 30% of referrals after the triage system with protocols was implemented [9], it is likely that the waiting time of our 2017/2018 sample reflects patients already waiting for a long time for a rheumatology consultation before the implementation of the system. To illustrate that, when Telessaúde started the process, there were more than 7000 cases on the waiting list for Rheumatology appointments (unpublished data). Advances in the treatment of rheumatic diseases and the knowledge of the importance of early treatment to obtain better outcomes may also have stimulated a larger number of referrals, increasing the waiting list, and consequently, the waiting time.

There was a significant disparity in the suspicion of fibromyalgia and osteoarthritis among primary care physicians and rheumatologists in the present study. Of the 357 patients referred, only 9.5% (34 patients) had one of these diseases as an initial suspicion by the primary care physician (the screening system accepted these cases, according to the protocol, because they were considered refractory to management in primary care or the diagnosis was doubtful). On the other hand, one of these two diseases was the first hypothesis in 122 patients (34.2%) at the first rheumatology visit. Cases of fibromyalgia and osteoarthritis can usually be managed at the primary care level [6]. The low prevalence of SIRDs and the high frequency of musculoskeletal symptoms in the general population represent a challenge to the general practitioner to identify such patients timely. Equipping him with the necessary knowledge to recognize these patients more safely is crucial for improving the referral process [13]. Measures such as lectures, discussion with the rheumatologist, and educational material are strategies that have already demonstrated benefits on the quality and quantity of referrals [5].

The present study has several strengths. There are no similar studies evaluating referral from primary care to Rheumatology and the impact of applying referral protocols with telemedicine support in our environment. The high number of first consultation visits (the largest in the state of Rio Grande do Sul at that time, compared to other tertiary care centers) in our service allowed us to obtain a significant and representative number of individuals from different origins for the analysis.

Our study also has limitations. The observational design of our research has well-known limitations in comparison to experimental studies. So,we cannot absolutely affirm that the improvement in referral quality is explained only by changes in the referral process. Another limitation is that we did not assess the effects of the different components of the referral process (triage with protocol and teleconsulting) independently. For analytical purposes, we considered as appropriate only referrals suspected of SIRDs. We know that some patients with other diseases (such as gout, osteoarthritis, and

Table 5 Comparison of features of patients referred to first Rheumatology consultations in 2007/2008 (482 patients) and 2017/2018 (357 patients)

	Porto Alegre (Capital)	Outside Counties	*P* Value*	*P* value of homogeneity test**
Hometown				–
2007/2008 – n (%)	260 (53.9)	222 (46.1)	–	
2017/2018 – n (%)	193 (54.1)	164 (45.9)	–	
Urgent cases				0.016
2007/2008 – n (%)	110/260 (42.3)	98/219 (44.7)†	0.591	
2017/2018 – n (%)	29/193 (15.0)	49/164 (29.9)	0.001	
Systemic inflammatory rheumatic diseases				< 0.001
2007/2008 – n (%)	76/260 (29.2)	73/222 (32.9)	0.387	
2017/2018 – n (%)	75/193 (38.9)	111/164 (67.7)	< 0.001	

*Pearson qui-square test comparing capital and outside counties. **Woolf's test for homogeneity of 2 × 2 tables across strata; a statistically significant difference indicates heterogeneity. †For 3 cases, information on urgency was missing

fibromyalgia) may sometimes require specialized diagnostic evaluation and treatment, particularly in refractory cases. Even so, the increased proportion of SIRDs among referred patients represents greater adequacy in the referral process, as these patients could hardly be adequately treated at the primary level of care. In such cases, intravenous infusions, immunosuppressants, and specialized tests available only in more advanced levels of care are often required. We based the diagnosis of a SIRD on the first clinical evaluation by the rheumatologist and previous medical exams brought by the patients. Therefore, some initial diagnoses may have changed during medical follow-up. Another potential limitation is that we analyzed only patients referred to the HNSC/ GHC Rheumatology Service, not including patients referred to other services. However, considering that the schedule of appointments for different Rheumatology services occurs in a centralized and non-regionalized manner and the large number of patients received by our service, our sample can be considered representative of referrals to Rheumatology in our state.

Conclusions

Considering the present results, we conclude that the quality of referrals to specialist consultation in Rheumatology improved in our state over 10 years. Most of this progress can probably be attributed to applying the triage system with protocols and telemedicine support. However, further changes are still necessary to reduce the waiting time for consultations and attain higher referral quality. Continuous and coordinated efforts among rheumatologists, general practitioners, and health managers are needed to optimize access to rheumatologic assistance.

Acknowledgments

We thank Elise Botteselle Oliveira (Teleconsulting Team Coordinator) and Rudi Roman (Referral Program Team Coordinator) from TelessaudeRS for their invaluable assistance.

Authors' contributions

DMP worked on the conception, analysis, and interpretation of data, drafting the article and approval of the version to be published. VBB worked on the conception, data collecting, analysis, and approval of the version to be published. RGS worked on the conception, data collecting, analysis, and approval of the version to be published. ADP worked on the conception, drafting the article, and approval the version to be published. CGMB worked on interpreting data, drafting the article, and approval the version to be published. SH worked conception, data collecting, and approval of the version to be published. GKB worked on the conception, data collecting, and approval of the version to be published. CDC worked on the conception, data collecting, and approval of the version to be published. SZ worked on the conception, data collecting, and approval of the version to be published. JCS worked on conception, data collecting, and approval of the version to be published. MR worked on the interpretation of data, drafting the article, and approval of the version to be published. MB worked on the conception, analysis, and interpretation of data, preparing the article and approval of the version to be published.

Author details

[1]Rheumatology Service at Hospital Nossa Senhora da Conceição (HNSC), Grupo Hospitalar Nossa Senhora da Conceição (GHC), Avenida Francisco Trein, 596, 3 Andar, Porto Alegre, Rio Grande do Sul, Brazil. [2]Federal University of Rio Grande do Sul (UFRGS), Porto Alegre, Rio Grande do Sul, Brazil. [3]TelessaúdeRS, Federal University of Rio Grande do Sul (UFRGS), Porto Alegre, Rio Grande do Sul, Brazil.

References

1. Simon JS, Maltichk M, da Silva EE, Lima VRB, Bredemeier M. Evaluation of the waiting time for rheumatology consultations at a tertiary care center of Porto Alegre – RS. Rev AMRIGS. 2008;52(4):303–8.
2. Hyrich KL. Patients with suspected rheumatoid arthritis should be referred early to rheumatology. BMJ. 2008;336(7637):215–6. https://doi.org/10.1136/bmj.39381.597454.AE.
3. Cross M, Smith E, Hoy D, Carmona L, Wolfe F, Vos T, et al. The global burden of rheumatoid arthritis: estimates from the global burden of disease 2010 study. Ann Rheum Dis. 2014;73(7):1316–22. https://doi.org/10.1136/annrheumdis-2013-204627.
4. de Azevedo ABC, Ferraz MB, Ciconelli RM. Indirect costs of rheumatoid arthritis in Brazil. Value Health J Int Soc Pharmacoeconomics Outcomes Res. 2008;11(5):869–77. https://doi.org/10.1111/j.1524-4733.2008.00332.x.
5. Villeneuve E, Nam JL, Bell MJ, Deighton CM, Felson DT, Hazes JM, et al. A systematic literature review of strategies promoting early referral and reducing delays in the diagnosis and management of inflammatory arthritis. Ann Rheum Dis. 2013;72(1):13–22. https://doi.org/10.1136/annrheumdis-2011-201063.
6. Hosie GAC. Series on education: teaching rheumatology in primary care. Ann Rheum Dis. 2000;59(7):500–3. https://doi.org/10.1136/ard.59.7.500.
7. Gonçalves MR, Umpierre RN, D'Avila OP, et al. Expanding primary care access: a telehealth success story. Ann Fam Med. 2017;15(4):383. https://doi.org/10.1370/afm.2086.
8. Deise Marcela Piovesan, Dimitris RucksVarvakiRados, Elise Botteselle de Oliveira, et al. Reference protocols for adult rheumatology. Published online 2017. https://www.ufrgs.br/telessauders/documentos/protocolos_resumos/protocolo_ses_reumatologia_20170911_v015_cvc.pdf.
9. Katz N, Roman R, Rados DV, Oliveira EB, Schmitz CAA, Gonçalves MR, et al. Access and regulation of specialized care in Rio Grande do Sul: the RegulaSUS strategy of TelessaúdeRS-UFRGS. CiencSaude Coletiva. 2020;25(4):1389–400. https://doi.org/10.1590/1413-81232020254.28942019.
10. Bignell K, Bender C, Lichtenstein A, et al. Improving access in rheumatology: evaluating the validity of a paper triage process involving an advanced practice physiotherapist through a retrospective chart review. Physiother Theory Pract. 2020;36(1):203–10. https://doi.org/10.1080/09593985.2018.1482978.
11. Farrer C, Abraham L, Jerome D, Hochman J, Gakhal N. Triage of rheumatology referrals facilitates wait time benchmarks. J Rheumatol. 2016;43(11):2064–7. https://doi.org/10.3899/jrheum.151235.
12. Maeyama MA, Calvo MCM. Integration of telehealth in regulation centers: teleconsulting as a mediator between primary care and specialized care. Rev Bras Educ Médica. 2018;42(2):63–72. https://doi.org/10.1590/1981-52712015v42n2rb20170125.
13. Mallen CD, Helliwell T, Scott IC. How can primary care physicians enhance the early diagnosis of rheumatic diseases? Expert Rev Clin Immunol. 2018;14(3):171–3. https://doi.org/10.1080/1744666X.2018.1429919.

25

Risk factors for the flare of systemic lupus erythematosus and its influence on prognosis

Xiaohong Zeng*, Ling Zheng, Hongbing Rui, Rihui Kang, Junmin Chen, Huaning Chen and Jizan Liu

Abstract

Objectives: To explore the risk factors for systemic lupus erythematosus (SLE) flare and their impact on prognosis.

Methods: The clinical characteristics, laboratory results, and treatment plans of 121 patients with SLE flare were retrospectively analyzed. Ninety-eight SLE outpatients with sustained remission during the same period were selected as controls. Logistic multivariate regression analysis was employed to screen for risk factors for SLE flare.

Results: Infection, thrombocytopenia, arthritis, anti-nucleosome antibodies positive, anti-β2-glycoprotein I (IgG) antibodies positive, and patient's self-discontinuation of medicine maintenance therapy might be risk factors for SLE flare. Patients who discontinued medicine maintenance therapy by themselves had a significantly higher rate of severe SLE flare than patients with regular medicine maintenance therapy ($P = 0.033$). The incidence of anemia associated with SLE ($P = 0.001$), serositis ($P = 0.005$), and pulmonary hypertension ($P = 0.003$) in patients who discontinued medicine maintenance therapy were significantly higher than patients with regular medicine maintenance therapy. SLE patients with regular medicine maintenance therapy for less than 3 years had a higher risk of pulmonary hypertension than those with regular medicine maintenance therapy longer than 3 years ($P = 0.034$).

Conclusions: The accompanying thrombocytopenia, arthritis, anti-nucleosome antibodies positive and anti-β2-glycoprotein I (IgG) antibodies positive at the onset of SLE may affect the prognosis of SLE. Patient's self-discontinuation of medicine maintenance therapy is the main cause of SLE flare, which may induce severe flare in SLE patients and lead to a significantly higher incidence of pulmonary hypertension.

Keywords: Systemic lupus erythematosus, Flare, Infection, Therapy, Pulmonary hypertension

Background

Systemic lupus erythematosus (SLE) is a serious chronic autoimmune disease, which can involve multiple organs and cause systemic damage. Although the treatment of SLE has been improving, most patients still go through alternating courses of flare and remission. Flare is an important factor for organ damage and poor prognosis of SLE [1], as the same time, it also brings heavy psychological burden to patients [2]. Therefore, remission achievement and its maintenance have become central in the management of SLE patients. At present, the cause of SLE flare is still unclear, but infection is considered to be a possible reason [3, 4], because it could lead to more frequent hospitalization and higher mortality [4]. In China, the main cause of death in SLE patients has changed from renal and central nervous system complications in 1980's to infections since 1996 to date [5, 6], which may be associated with the longer course of glucocorticoids and immunosuppressive treatments in SLE patients [6]. In recent years, several studies [7, 8]

* Correspondence: xiaohongzeng86@hotmail.com
Department of Rheumatology, the First Affiliated Hospital of Fujian Medical University, 20 Chazhong Road, Fuzhou 350005, Fujian, China

showed that patients could benefit from reducing or discontinuing the maintenance therapy with glucocorticoids, when SLE patients reached complete remission. Moreover, the recommendations for the management of SLE underline the importance of glucocorticoids progressive tapering until withdrawal [8]. However, only a few SLE patients without both glucocorticoids and immunosuppressants maintenance therapy could still stay at persistent remission [9–11]. A china cohort also showed that only 14.7% of patients successfully stopped both glucocorticoids and immunosuppressants during follow-up [9]. These suggest that the medicine maintenance therapy, especially the maintenance therapy of immunosuppressants in remission [11], is also related to SLE flare. So far, there is no relevant research on the correlation between medicine maintenance therapy and SLE flare, and it is unknown how long the medicine maintenance therapy needs to last. However, it is important to identify which patients are likely to have SLE flare, and what is the heterogeneity of the clinical manifestations or serum indicators in these patients, which is of great significance for the management of SLE patients in remission period. Therefore, this study retrospectively analyzed the clinical characteristics and treatments of patients with SLE flare in our center, to screen for risk factors for SLE flare and explore the impact for discontinuation of medicine maintenance therapy on the prognosis of SLE.

Study subjects

The clinical data of patients with SLE treated in the First Affiliated Hospital of Fujian Medical University from January 2013 to December 2018 were retrospectively analyzed. They met the SLE American College of Rheumatology (ACR) classification criteria [12]. Patients who met the following criteria were included in the SLE flare group: (1) patients aged 18 years or older, (2) patients were initially diagnosed with SLE in our hospital, (3) patients who achieved complete or clinical remission after initial treatment of SLE, (4) patients should be followed up at least three times a year, and (5) patients with SLE flare for the first time after complete or clinical remission and re-hospitalized for treatment. SLE patients who were followed up in outpatient clinic during the same period, met criteria 1 to 4 and were still in complete or clinical remission at the last follow-up were selected as the comparison group. Patients with pregnancy and other autoimmune diseases were excluded.

Methods

Definition of disease activity, remission and flare

SLE disease activity was measured based on the systemic lupus erythematosus disease activity index 2000 (SLEDAI-2 K) developed by the International Clinical Collaboration Group for SLE [13]. SLE organ damage was evaluated with the SLE damage index (SDI) developed by the Systemic Lupus Erythematosus International Collaborating Clinics (SLICC)/ACR [14].

Complete remission of SLE [15] was defined as SLEDAI-2 K of 0 in corticosteroid-free and immunosuppressant-free patients (antimalarials allowed), clinical remission as serological active clinical quiescent disease (SACQD) according to SLEDAI-2 K $\leq$ 4 in corticosteroid-free patients or patients on prednisone 1–5 mg/day, (stable immunosuppressants and antimalarials allowed) [15].

The definition of SLE flare, including the definitions of mild to moderate flare and severe flare, referred to the SELENA-SLEDAI flare index [16]. SLE flare was defined as one or more of the following: 1) the SLEDAI-2 K instrument score increase, 2) new or worse activity, medication changes, and new or worsening symptoms and organ damage attributable to lupus. Mild to moderate flares were defined as one or more of the following: a) greater than 3-point increment in SLEDAI-2 K instrument score, with total score less than 12; b) new or worsening discoid, photosensitive, or other rash attributable to lupus (including lupus profundus, cutaneous vasculitis, or bullous lupus), nasopharyngeal ulcers, pleuritis, pericarditis, arthritis, or fever not attributable to infection; c) increase in prednisone dosage but not greater than 0.5 mg/kg of body weight per day; and d) initiation of therapy with either hydroxychloroquine or nonsteroidal anti-inflammatory drugs, without an increase in prednisone dosage. Severe flares were defined as one or more of the following: a) SLEDAI-2 K instrument score greater than 12; b) new or worsening central nervous system involvement, vasculitis, glomerulonephritis, myositis, thrombocytopenia (platelet count $< 60 \times 10^9$cells/L), or hemolytic anemia (hemoglobin level < 70 g/L or decrease in hemoglobin level > 30 g/L over a 2-week period), each requiring doubling of corticosteroid dosage to a final dosage greater than 0.5 mg/kg per day or acute hospitalization; c) any manifestation requiring an increase in dosage of prednisone or equivalent drug to greater than 0.5 mg/kg per day, or initiation of therapy with cyclophosphamide, azathioprine, mycophenolate mofetil, or methotrexate; and d) hospitalization for lupus activity.

Patients with Pulmonary hypertension were diagnosed based on right heart catheterization or echocardiography (peak tricuspid regurgitation velocity > 3.4 m/s) [17], and those with left heart disease and pulmonary thrombosis were excluded.

Data collection

The following clinical data were collected: sex, age, disease duration, clinical symptoms, treatment plans, treatment duration and laboratory indicators, including complete blood count, urinalysis, liver and kidney function, antinuclear antibodies (ANA), anti-double-stranded

DNA antibodies (ds-DNA), anti-ribonucleoprotein (anti-RNP) antibodies, anti-Smith (anti-SM) antibodies, anti-Sjogren's syndrome A antibodies (anti-SSA), anti-Sjogren's syndrome B antibodies (anti-SSB), anti-nucleosome antibodies (AnuA), anti-ribosomal RNP antibody, anti-cardiolipin antibodies (aCL), anti-β2-glycoprotein I (anti-β2GPI) antibodies and lupus anticoagulants (LAs). ANA was measured by a standardized ELISA, the results were in the format of the absorbance value of sample / the cut off value (s/co). ANA in serum present in titer > 1.0 s/co defined as positive. While ds-DNA in serum present in titer > 100 IU/ml defined as positive, measured by a standardized ELISA. The SLEDAI-2 K score and SDI of all the patients at each hospitalization and outpatient follow-up were recorded, and the SDI increment (SDI_2-SDI_1), which was the difference between the SDI at the rehospitalization of a patient with flared SLE and the SDI at the last time of achieving complete or clinical remission of SLE, was calculated.

Statistical analysis

SPSS 20.0 was used for statistical processing. Quantitative data that conformed to the normal distribution were analyzed using Student's t-test. The Mann–Whitney U-test was used for data that were not normally distributed. Qualitative data were analyzed using the χ^2 test or Fisher's exact probability test. $P < 0.05$ represented statistical significance. Factors with $P < 0.1$ in univariate analysis were input into the multivariate model to screen for possible risk factors using the logistic multivariate regression analysis, in which test the significance was set to 5%. The Kaplan-Meier test was used to estimate the survival of all patients.

Results

Clinical manifestations, laboratory examinations, and treatments of the flared group and the comparison group

From January 2013 to December 2018, 121 patients were included in the SLE flare group, including 113 females and 8 males with an age of 39.9 ± 13.1 (mean ± SD) years and a disease duration of 93.2 ± 80.1 (mean ± SD) months. Ninety-eight patients were included in the comparison group, including 84 females and 14 males with an age of 42.7 ± 13.8 (mean ± SD) years and a disease duration of 78.6 ± 44.9 (mean ± SD) months. The SLE flare group had a significantly longer disease course than the comparison group ($P < 0.001$). At the initial onset of SLE, the SLEDAI-2 K score of the SLE flare group and the comparison group were 11.6 ± 4.1 (mean ± SD) and 10.4 ± 4.2 (mean ± SD) points, respectively, with no significant difference ($P > 0.05$). The incidence of infection in the SLE flare group was significantly higher than that in the comparison group (54/121 vs 2/98, $P < 0.001$) (Table 1). There was no significant difference ($P > 0.05$) in the incidence of clinical symptoms at the initial onset of SLE between the two groups of patients, which included fever, rash, arthritis, oral ulcer, hair loss, serositis, leukopenia, thrombocytopenia, lupus nephritis, Neuropsychiatric lupus, lupus pneumonia, cardiac damage, and lupus-related gastrointestinal damage. In the flared group, there were 6 patients with secondary antiphospholipid syndrome (APS), while none of the comparison group had APS ($P < 0.05$) (Table 1).

The autoantibody profile at the onset of SLE is laid out in Table 1. In the SLE flare group, the positive rates of anti-SM antibodies (28.9%), AnuA (38%), immunoglobulin G (IgG)-anticardiolipin (aCL) antibodies (5.0%), IgG-anti-β2-GPI antibodies (16.5%), and LA (10.7%) were higher than in the comparison group (all $P < 0.05$). (Table 1).

All patients received glucocorticoids (orally or intravenously) at the time of initial treatment. The starting dose of glucocorticoids in the flared group was 0.9 ± 0.9 mg/kg/d (mean ± SD), 23 of them had an initial starting dose of glucocorticoids exceeding 0.8 mg/kg/d, 98 patients used hydroxychloroquine for initial treatment, and 49 patients received combined immunosuppressants treatment, include cyclophosphamide (CTX), mycophenolate mofetil (MMF), azathioprine (AZA), methotrexate (MTX), cyclosporine A (CsA) and tacrolimus (FK-506) (Table 1). The starting dose of glucocorticoids in the comparison group was 0.9 ± 0.4 mg/kg/d (mean ± SD), and 21 patients had an initial starting dose of glucocorticoids exceeding 0.8 mg/kg/d, 91 patients used hydroxychloroquine for initial treatment, and 70 patients received combined immunosuppressants treatment. In the SLE flare group, only 5 patients achieved complete remission, while 7 patients achieved complete remission in the comparison group. There was no significant difference in the median time of achieving the clinical remission and glucocorticoid accumulation between the two groups. The application rate of immunosuppressants ($P < 0.001$) and hydroxychloroquine ($P = 0.017$) in the SLE flare group was lower than that in the comparison group (Table 1). During the follow-up period, the proportion of patients' self-discontinuation of medicine maintenance therapy in the SLE flare group was significantly higher than that in the comparison group (P < 0.001) (Table 1).

Logistic multivariate regression analysis of risk factors for SLE flare

A model for logistic multivariate regression analysis was established using SLE flare as the dependent variable and using factors with $P < 0.1$ in univariate analysis as independent variables, which included sex, disease duration, infection, arthritis, thrombocytopenia, antiphospholipid

Table 1 Clinical characteristics and treatment in patients with SLE flare or sustained remission of SLE

	SLE flare group ($n = 121$ Case)	comparison group ($n = 98$ Case)	*P*-value
Age (Year), mean (SD)	39.9(13.1)	42.7(13.8)	0.431
Gender (female/male)	113/8	84/14	0.072
Disease duration (Month), mean (SD)	*93.2(80.1)*	*78.6(44.9)*	*< 0.001**
Infection	*54(44.6)*	*2(2.4)*	*< 0.001**
Flare degree			
Mild and moderate SLE flare, n (%)	28 (23.1)		
Severe SLE flare, n (%)	93 (76.9)		
Initial symptom, n (%)			
Fever	36(29.8)	32(32.7)	0.662
Rash	68(56.2)	63(64.3)	0.268
Arthritis	67(55.4)	42(42.9)	0.078
oral ulcer	26(21.5)	21(21.4)	1.000
Hair loss	23(19.0)	14(14.3)	0.372
Serositis	24(19.8)	21(21.4)	0.867
Leucopenia [a]	18(14.9)	14(14.3)	1.000
Thrombocytopenia [b]	19(15.7)	7(7.1)	0.060
Lupus nephritis	31(25.6)	28(28.6)	0.648
Neuropsychiatric lupus	8(6.6)	7(7.1)	1.000
Lupus pneumonia	3(2.5)	0	0.255
Lupus related cardiac damage	0	1(1.0)	0.447
Lupus related gastrointestinal damage	3(2.5)	0	0.255
Antiphospholipid syndrome	*6(5.0)*	*0*	*0.034**
SLEDAI-2 k (score), mean (SD)	11.6(4.1)	10.4(4.2)	0.800
Initial serological indicators			
ANA (s/co), mean (SD)	4.6(2.7)	4.7(3.1)	0.336
ds-DNA (IU/ml), mean (SD)	490.8(260.1)	545.4(244.0)	0.919
Anti-RNP, n (%)	55(45.4)	42(42.9)	0.785
Anti-SM, n (%)	*35(28.9)*	*14(14.3)*	*0.014**
Anti-SSA, n (%)	82(67.8)	56(57.1)	0.122
Anti-SSB, n (%)	27(22.3)	21(21.4)	1.000
Anti-nu, n (%)	*46(38.0)*	*14(14.3)*	*< 0.001**
Anti-rRNP, n (%)	38(29.0)	21(21.4)	0.125
aCL-IgM, n (%)	4(3.3)	7(7.1)	0.226
aCL-IgG, n (%)	*6(5.0)*	*0*	*0.034**
Anti-β2GPI-IgG, n (%)	*20(16.5)*	*7(7.1)*	*0.040**
LA (n, %)	*13(10.7)*	*0*	*< 0.001**
Initial treatment			
The median time of achieving the clinical remission (Month), mean (SD)	3.17 ± 0.70	3.05 ± 0.65	0.661
SLE patients with Complete remission, n (%)	5(4.1)	7(7.1)	0.380
Glucocorticoid amount (mg/kg/d), mean (SD)	0.9(0.9)	0.9(0.4)	0.323
initial glucocorticoid amount > 0.8 mg/kg/d, n (%)	23(19.0)	21(21.4)	0.735
Glucocorticoid cumulative at the time of achieving clinical remission (mg), mean (SD)	1780.8 ± 1016.1	1808.0 ± 1049.3	0.416
Hydroxychloroquine, n (%)	*98(81.0)*	*91(92.9)*	*0.017**

Table 1 Clinical characteristics and treatment in patients with SLE flare or sustained remission of SLE *(Continued)*

	SLE flare group (n = 121 Case)	comparison group (n = 98 Case)	P-value
Immunosuppressive agent treatment, n (%)	*49(40.5)*	*70(57.9)*	*< 0.001**
CTX	13 (10.7)	21(21.4)	0.837
MMF	9 (7.4)	7(7.1)	0.275
AZA	10 (8.3)	17(17.3)	0.663
MTX	11 (9.1)	13(13.3)	0.647
FK-506	2 (1.7)	8(8.2)	0.194
CsA	4 (3.3)	4(4.1)	0.716
Treatment during follow-up			
patient's self-discontinuation of medicine maintenance therapy, n (%)	*65(53.7)*	*7(7.1)*	*< 0.001**
Regular maintenance therapy before SLE flare	*56(46.3)*	*91(93.8)*	*< 0.001**
Prednisone(≤5 mg/d)	8(6.6)	24(24.5)	/
Prednisone(≤5 mg/d) + HCQ	20(16.5)	32(32.7)	/
Prednisone(≤5 mg/d) + HCQ + MMF	6(5.0)	7(7.1)	/
Prednisone(≤5 mg/d) + HCQ + AZA	9(7.4)	11(11.2)	/
Prednisone(≤5 mg/d) + HCQ + MTX	10(8.3)	11(11.2)	/
Prednisone(≤5 mg/d) + HCQ + CsA	2(1.7)	3(3.0)	/
Prednisone(≤5 mg/d)HCQ + FK-506	1(0.8)	3(3.0)	/

N: Number of cases; *: P value < 0.05; a: white blood count < 4.0×10^9/L; b: platelet count < 100×10^9/L; *SLEDAI-2 K* Systemic lupus erythematosus disease activity index-2000; *ANA* antinuclear antibodies; ds-DNA: Anti double-stranded DNA antibody; *Anti-RNP* anti-ribonucleoprotein antibody; *Anti-SM* anti-Smith antibody; *Anti-SSA* anti-Sjogren's syndrome antigen A antibody; *Anti-SSB* anti-Sjogren's syndrome antigen B antibody; *Anti-nu* anti-nucleosome antibody; *Anti-rRNP* anti-ribosomal RNP antibody; *anti-β2GPI* anti-β2-glycoprotein I antibody; *aCL* anti-cardiolipin antibody; *IgG* immunoglobulin G; *IgM* immunoglobulin M; *LA* Lupus anticoagulant; *HCQ* Hydroxychloroquine; *CTX* Cyclophosphamide; *MMF* Mycophenolate mofetil; *AZA* Azathioprine; *MTX* Methotrexate; *CsA* Cyclosporine A; *FK-506* Tacrolimus

syndrome, anti-SM antibodies, AnuA, aCL (IgG), anti-β2-GPI (IgG), LA, use hydroxychloroquine for initial treatment, administration of immunosuppressants in initial treatment, patients' self-discontinuation of medicine maintenance therapy. The results showed that infection, arthritis, thrombocytopenia, AnuA and anti-β2-GPI (IgG) were risk factors for SLE flare, patient's self-discontinuation of medicine maintenance therapy after clinical remission of SLE would increase the risk of SLE flare, and the use of immunosuppressants and hydroxychloroquine in the initial treatment reduced SLE flare. (Table 2).

A subgroup analysis of patients with initial thrombocytopenia, which were divided into the Flare group and the Stable remission group (Table 3). There were no statistical differences in clinical symptoms and organ damages between the two groups. Glucocorticoid cumulative at the time of achieving clinical remission in the Flare group were less than that in the Stable remission group (1653.7 ± 942.4 mg vs 2384.7 ± 1390.0 mg, $P < 0.001$), and the proportion of using immunosuppressants in the Flare group were lower than that in the Stable remission group (9 cases, 47.4% vs 7 cases, 100%, $P = 0.023$). Among them, the use of cyclophosphamide

Table 2 Multiple logistic regression analysis of risk factors for SLE flare

Variable	OR	95%CI	P-value
Infection	**31.383**	**(6.494,151.695)**	**< 0.001**
Arthritis	**2.644**	**(1.098,6.369)**	**0.030**
Thrombocytopenia	**4.366**	**(1.165,16.366)**	**0.029**
Anti-nucleosome antibody	**2.927**	**(1.107,7.740)**	**0.030**
Anti-β2-glycoprotein I antibody (IgG)	**5.291**	**(1.224,22.875)**	**0.026**
Use immunosuppressant for initial treatment	**0.221**	**(0.091,0.540)**	**0.001**
Use Hydroxychloroquine for initial treatment	**0.267**	**(0.076,0.936)**	**< 0.001**
Patient's self-discontinuation of medicine maintenance therapy	**10.463**	**(3.786,28.912)**	**< 0.001**

OR odds ratio; *95%CI* 95% confidence interval

Table 3 Two subgroup analyses of patients with thrombocytopenia and arthritis at onset

	SLE patients with arthritis at onset			SLE patients with thrombocytopenia at onset		
	Flare group ($N = 67$)	Stable remission group($N = 42$)	P value	Flare group ($N = 19$)	Stable remission group($N = 7$)	P value
Age (Year), mean (SD)	43(13)	46(8)	0.008	41(14)	63(9)	0.067
Gender (female/male)	62/5	35/7	0.207	18/1	7/0	1.000
Disease duration (Month), mean (SD)	108.1(83.5)	72.8(41.6)	0.003	66.6(66.2)	88.6(71.1)	0.916
SLEDAI-2 K,mean (SD)	13.2(4.0)	13.7(4.2)	0.964	12.4(5.0)	17.4(3.4)	0.212
Initial organ damage						
Lupus nephritis	22(32.8)	21(50.0)	0.107	6(31.6)	5(71.4)	0.095
Neuropsychiatric lupus	4(6.0)	0	0.158	3(15.9)	0	0.540
Lupus pneumonia	2(3.0)	0	0.522	1(5.3)	0	1.000
Lupus related cardiac damage	0	1(2.4)	0.385	0	1(14.3)	0.269
Gastrointestinal damage	1(1.5)	0	1.000	1(5.3)	0	1.000
Initial treatment						
Glucocorticoid amount (mg/kg/d), mean (SD)	0.82(0.32)	1.05(0.47)	< *0.001*	1.0(0.36)	1.31(0.24)	0.050
Glucocorticoid cumulative at the time of achieving clinical remission (mg), mean (SD)	1653.7(942.4)	2384.7(1390.0)	< *0.001*	2215.7(1112.3)	3418.0(601.9)	0.005
Hydroxychloroquine, n (%)	54(80.6)	38(90.5)	0.188	15(78.9)	6(85.7)	1.000
Immunosuppressors, n (%)	30(44.8) [a]	28(66.7) [b]	0.031	**9(47.4)** [c]	**7(100.0)** [d]	0.023
Patient's self-discontinuation of medication maintenance therapy, n (%)	35(15.0)	0	< 0.001	8(42.1)	0	0.062

[a]: the immunosuppressors used by the patients included CTX (12 cases), MMF (6 cases), CsA (2 cases), AZA (4 cases), and MTX (6 cases); [b]: the immunosuppressors included CTX (14 cases), AZA (7 cases), and MTX (7 cases). [c]: the immunosuppressors included CTX (1 cases), MMF (1 case), CsA (1 case), AZA (3 cases), and MTX (3 cases); [d]: all patients were treated with CTX

was higher in the Stable remission group. The immunosuppressants used by the patient in the Flare group included CTX in 1, MMF in 1, CsA in 1, AZA in 3, and MTX in 3, while all patients with initial thrombocytopenia of the Stable remission group were treated with CTX.

Another subgroup analysis for patients with first-onset symptoms of arthritis, which were also divided into the Flare group and the Stable remission group. The SLE activity, organ damage, and treatment were compared in the patients with initial arthritis between the two groups, the result shows in (Table 3). Although the mean (SD) age of patients in the Flare group was lower than that of patients in the Stable remission group, the mean (SD) disease course of patients in the Flare group was longer than that of the Stable remission group. There was no statistical difference in clinical symptoms and organ damages between the two groups, however, the initial dose of glucocorticoids, glucocorticoid cumulative at the time of achieving clinical remission, and the proportion of using immunosuppressants in the Flare group were lower than those in the Stable remission group.

Figure 1 shows the Kaplan–Meier curves of the survival rate for patients with SLE who discontinued medicine maintenance therapy by themself and with regular medicine maintenance therapy, and the result showed they had a similar survival time [19.7 ± 0.9 years and 19.1 ± 0.7 years, respectively]. Five patients with SLE flare still die after received intensive treatment such as glucocorticoids or immunosuppressants again. The cause of death in the patients with SLE flare: central system involvement in 2, severe autoimmune pancreatitis in 1, severe pulmonary hypertension combine with infection in 1, diffuse alveolar hemorrhage with thrombocytopenia and infection in 1. The other patients with flare who had obtained stable condition after treatment and discharged from the hospital.

The occurrence of risk factors in different degrees of SLE flare

Among 121 patients with SLE flare, the proportion of patient's self-discontinuation of medicine maintenance therapy (55/93 vs 10/28, $P = 0.033$) and infection (47/93 vs 7/28, $P = 0.019$) in the severe flare group was higher than that in the mild to moderate flare group. There was no significant difference in the incidence of other risk factors between patients with mild to moderate flare and those with severe flare. (Table 4).

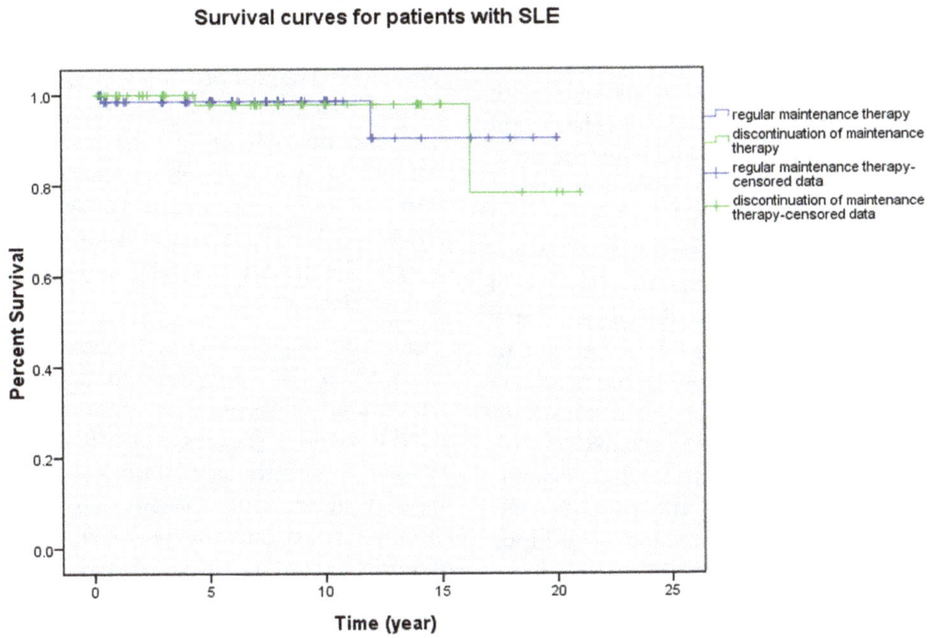

Fig. 1 Survival curves for patients with SLE who discontinued medicine maintenance therapy by themself and with regular medicine maintenance therapy (Log- Rank test $P = 0.949$)

Relationship between patient's self-discontinuation of medicine maintenance therapy and prognosis of SLE

Among the 121 patients with SLE flare, 65 patients discontinued of medicine maintenance therapy by themself, and the other 56 patients took the glucocorticoid regularly and maintained at the minimum dose (prednisolone ≤5 mg/d), with or without hydroxychloroquine or immunosuppressant. There was no significant difference between patients who discontinued medicine maintenance therapy by themself and received regular maintenance therapy in terms of age, sex, disease duration, SLEDAI-2 K score and therapeutic drugs at the time of onset. However, the proportion of patients with severe flare of SLE was 84.6% in patients who discontinued medicine maintenance therapy by themself, and the proportion of severe flare of SLE in patients with regular maintenance therapy was 67.9% ($P = 0.033$) (Table 4). There were still two patients discontinued medicine maintenance therapy by themselves, who had SLEDAI-2 K score of 0 and experienced SLE flare for pulmonary hypertension. The symptoms of these patients were relieved after the treatment with glucocorticoids and immunosuppressants. The mean (SD) of SDI values and the SDI increment (SDI_2-SDI_1) at the last hospitalization

Table 4 The occurrence of risk factors in different degrees of SLE flare

	Mild or moderate SLE flare (*n* = 28)	Severe SLE flare (*n* = 93)	*P*-value
Infection	**7(25.0)**	**47(50.5)**	**0.019**
Arthritis, n (%)	16(57.1)	51(54.8)	1.000
Thrombocytopenia, n (%)	6(21.4)	13(14.0)	0.378
Anti-nucleosome antibody, n (%)	9(32.1)	37(39.8)	0.513
anti-β2-glycoprotein I antibody (IgG), n (%)	5(17.9)	15(16.1)	0.779
Use immunosuppressant for initial treatment, n (%)	8(28.6)	41(44.1)	0.188
Use Hydroxychloroquine for initial treatment, n (%)	21(75.0)	77(82.8)	0.412
patient's self-discontinuation of medicine maintenance therapy, n (%)	***10(35.7)***	***55(59.1)***	***0.033***

of patients who discontinued medicine maintenance therapy by themself was 2.06 ± 1.45 (mean ± SD) points and 1.86 ± 1.26 (mean ± SD) points, respectively, which were significantly higher than those in patients with regular maintenance therapy ($P < 0.05$) (Table 5). In terms of clinical manifestations, the incidence of serositis, anemia associated with SLE, and pulmonary hypertension were higher in patients who discontinued medicine maintenance therapy by themself than in patients with regular maintenance therapy ($P < 0.01$) (Table 5), while the incidence of other clinical symptoms was not significantly different between the two groups of patients. In the patients who discontinued medicine maintenance therapy by themself, the main causes of anemia were autoimmune hemolytic anemia in 12, aplastic anemia in 2, anemia secondary to lupus nephritis in 16, chronic anemia in 6. In the patients with regular maintenance therapy, anemia secondary to lupus nephritis in 7, chronic anemia in 5, autoimmune hemolytic anemia in 2.

Effect of maintenance therapy time on the occurrence of pulmonary hypertension, anemia associated with SLE, and serositis at the flare of SLE

According to whether there is anemia, arthritis and pulmonary hypertension at the time of SLE flare, 121 patients were divided into a pulmonary hypertension group and a non-pulmonary hypertension group, a serositis group and a serositis-free group, or an anemia group and an anemia-free group, respectively. Age, disease duration, sex, SLEDAI-2 K score and initial treatment in each group are shown in (Table 6). The proportions of patients with regular maintenance therapy of less than 1 year, 2 years, 3 years, 4 years, and 5 years in each group are listed in (Table 6). Models for logistic multivariate regression analysis were established using pulmonary hypertension, anemia associated with SLE, and serositis as dependent variables and using age, sex, disease duration, SLEDAI-2 K score, initial treatment and regular maintenance therapy of less than 3 years as independent variables. The results showed that SLE patients with regular maintenance therapy of less than 3 years were more prone to pulmonary hypertension [odds ratio (OR) = 2.986, 95% confidence interval (CI) (1.087, 8.202)] ($P = 0.034$) (Table 7), SLE patients with regular maintenance therapy of less than 1 year were more prone to serositis [odds ratio (OR) = 5.764, 95% confidence interval (CI) (1.642, 20.241)] ($P = 0.006$). High SLE activity was a risk factor for the occurrence of anemia associated with SLE and serositis, with OR values of 1.134 (95% CI 1.059, 1.214) and 1.156 (95% CI 1.070, 1.248), respectively ($P < 0.001$) (Table 7).

Discussion

SLE often has a disease process of alternating flare and remission. The cohort study published by Conti et al. showed that the annual flare rate of SLE was 7 to 9.4% [18], and multiple studies have shown that Asian SLE patients have a more severe disease condition, higher flare rate and higher organ damage rate than Caucasian patients [19]. Therefore, it is worthwhile to search for the risk factors for SLE flare and clarify their impact on the prognosis of SLE.

Infection as an important cause of death in SLE patients [5, 6, 20], especially in developing countries. A subsequent meta-analysis published in 2016 [21] provided evidence regarding a significant increase of mortality due to infectious complications, showing 4.98-fold increase in mortality. Meanwhile, infectious agents, including viruses, bacteria, parasites, and fungus, are a pivotal factor for induction of autoimmunity [22], which could lead to SLE flare. Infection also could result in organ damage in SLE patients, and its risk and prevalence are much higher because of the combined with a defective immune system and use of immunosuppressive drugs [3, 22, 23]. Therefore, infection is always a vulnerable point in SLE patients. Early recognition is crucial when considering that this condition is preventable and treatable, especially in the use of appropriate immunosuppressive therapy.

In this study, the occurrence of thrombocytopenia at the onset of SLE was a risk factor for SLE flare, while a cohort study by Minowa et al. [24] show the same results. For SLE patients with organ damage, clinicians usually use a high glucocorticoid starting dose and often in combination with immunosuppressants to achieve the remission of SLE and reduce the possibility of flare [8, 25, 26]. However, if there is blood system involvement, such as thrombocytopenia, the application of immunosuppressants should be chosen more cautiously because of the adverse effects of bone marrow suppression. In this study, we conducted a subgroup analysis of SLE patients with thrombocytopenia, the results showed that the use of immunosuppressants in the Stable remission group was higher than that in the Flare group (7/7 vs 9/19, $P = 0.023$), and the use of cyclophosphamide was higher in the Stable remission group.

At the same time, our results suggest that that arthritis is also a risk factor for SLE flare, especially patients who are younger at the onset of SLE deserve more attention. In fact, in clinical practice, we have found that the severity of arthritis in SLE patients is relatively mild, and the rate of deformity is significantly lower than that of rheumatoid arthritis. In most cases, the symptoms are quickly relieved after glucocorticoid treatment, so these patients are often overlooked by clinicians, immunosuppressants would not be used for treatment. The

Table 5 The clinical characteristics in patients with SLE flare

	patient's self-discontinuation (*n* = 65 Case)	regular maintenance therapy (*n* = 56 Case)	*P*-value
Age (Year), mean (SD)	38.5(12.5)	41.6(13.7)	0.396
Gender (female/male)	61/4	52/4	1.000
Disease duration (Month), mean (SD)	91.6(82.3)	95.0(78.1)	0.926
SLEDAI-2 k of first onset (score), mean (SD)	10.9(3.8)	12.4(4.4)	0.072
Initial treatment			
glucocorticoid amount (mg/kg/d), mean (SD)	0.9(0.3)	1.0(1.3)	0.153
Hydroxychloroquine, n (%)	52(80.0)	46(82.1)	0.819
Immunosuppressive therapy, n (%)	27(41.5)	22(39.3)	0.854
Regular maintenance treatment	/	*56*	/
Prednisone(≤5 mg/d)	/	8	/
Prednisone(≤5 mg/d) + HCQ	/	20	/
Prednisone(≤5 mg/d) + HCQ + MMF	/	6	/
Prednisone(≤5 mg/d) + HCQ + AZA	/	9	/
Prednisone(≤5 mg/d) + HCQ + MTX	/	10	/
Prednisone(≤5 mg/d) + HCQ + CsA	/	2	/
Prednisone(≤5 mg/d)HCQ + FK-506	/	1	/
Characteristics of SLE flare			
Flare degree (mild moderate / severe, n/n)	*10/55*	*18/38*	*0.033*
SLEDAI-2 k (Score), mean (SD)	13.1(6.6)	10.5(5.6)	0.140
SDI_1, mean (SD)	0.20(0.44)	0.25(0.48)	0.270
SDI_2, mean (SD)	*2.06(1.45)*	*1.21(1.07)*	*0.042**
SDI increment [a], mean (SD)	*1.86(1.26)*	*0.96(0.89)*	*0.011**
Clinical symptoms of flare, n (%)			
Fever	16(24.6)	13(23.2)	1.000
Rash	17(26.2)	18(32.1)	0.548
Arthritis	12(18.5)	11(19.6)	1.000
oral ulcer	5(7.7)	5(9.0)	1.000
Serositis	*26(40.0)*	*9(16.1)*	*0.005**
Leukopenia [b]	15(23.1)	15(26.8)	0.677
Anemia associated with SLE [c]	*36(55.4)*	*14(25.0)*	*0.001**
Thrombocytopenia [d]	14(21.5)	12(21.4)	1.000
Vasculitis	10(15.4)	3(5.4)	0.086
Lupus nephritis	38(58.5)	23(41.1)	0.069
Neuropsychiatric lupus	11(16.9)	14(25.0)	0.368
Lupus pneumonia	12(18.5)	7(12.5)	0.456
Pulmonary hypertension	*17(26.2)*	*3(5.4)*	*0.003**
Lupus related cardiac damage	9(13.8)	4(7.1)	0.378
Lupus related gastrointestinal damage	8(12.3)	6(10.7)	1.000

N Number of cases; *SLEDAI-2 K* Systemic lupus erythematosus disease activity index-2000; *SDI* systemic lupus international collaborating clinics and the American College of Rheumatology diagnostic and therapeutic criteria committee damage index; *SDI_1* SDI at the time of complete or clinical response; *SDI_2* SDI at the last hospitalization; *HCQ* Hydroxychloroquine; *MMF* Mycophenolate mofetil; *AZA* Azathioprine; *MTX* Methotrexate; *CsA* Cyclosporine A; *FK-506* Tacrolimus. [a]: SDI_2-SDI_1, 'SDI at the last hospitalization' – 'SDI at the time of complete or clinical response'. [b]: white blood count < 4.0×10^9/L. [c]: hemoglobin < 110 g/L. [d]: platelet count < 100×10^9/L. *: $P < 0.05$

Table 6 Distribution of patients with SLE flare

	Pulmonary hypertension		Serositis		Anemia associated with SLE	
	Yes (*N* = 20)	No (*N* = 101)	Yes (*N* = 35)	No (*N* = 86)	Yes (*N* = 50)	No (*N* = 71)
Age (Year), mean (SD)	41.3(11.8)	39.7(13.4)	37.7(12.7)	40.9(12.3)	37.6(13.8)	41.6(12.5)
Gender (female/male)	20/0	93/8	34/1	79/7	47/3	66/5
Disease duration (Month), mean (SD)	109.6(79.5)	89.9(80.2)	93.1(85.3)	93.2(78.4)	86.3(71.1)	98.0(86.0)
SLEDAI-2 K,mean (SD)	12.1(8.0)	11.8(5.9)	15.2(5.5)	10.5(6.1)	14.4(5.8)	10.1(5.9)
Initial treatment						
Glucocorticoid amount (mg/kg/d), mean (SD)	0.80(0.22)	0.95(0.97)	0.89(0.34)	0.94(1.04)	0.88(0.37)	0.96(1.13)
Hydroxychloroquine, n (%)	18(90.0)	80(79.2)	30(85.7)	68(79.1)	43(86.0)	55(77.5)
Immunosuppressive therapy, n (%)	7(35.0)	42(41.6)	12(34.3)	37(43.0)	19(38.0)	30(42.3)
Regular maintenance treatment, n (%)	3(15.0)	53(52.5)	9(25.7)	47(54.7)	14(28.0)	42(59.2)
maintenance therapy < 1 year, n (%)	6(30.0)	14(13.9)	9(25.7)	11(12.8)	7(14.0)	13(18.3)
maintenance therapy < 2 years, n (%)	8(40.0)	20(19.8)	11(31.4)	17(19.8)	11(22.0)	17(23.9)
maintenance therapy < 3 years, n (%)	9(45.0)	25(24.8)	12(34.3)	22(25.6)	13(26)	21(29.6)
maintenance therapy < 4 years, n (%)	14(70.0)	84(83.2)	27(77.1)	71(82.6)	41(82.0)	57(80.3)
maintenance therapy < 5 years, n (%)	15(75.0)	86(85.1)	29(82.9)	72(83.7)	43(86.0)	58(81.7)

N Number of cases; *SLEDAI-2 K* Systemic lupus erythematosus disease activity index-2000

subgroup analysis of SLE patients with arthritis in our study also shows that the proportion of using immunosuppressants in the Stable remission group was much higher than that in the Flare group. SLE patients with arthritis but without organ damage might have received lower-dose glucocorticoid treatments or lack of immunosuppressants treatments, which leads to a higher possibility of flare. During follow-up, SLE patients with arthritis do not have the precise remission criteria similar as rheumatoid arthritis, which depends more on the subjective feelings of the patients, and then a considerable proportion of patients with arthritis may have prematurely down-dosed the immunotherapy strength of SLE before a true remission has been achieved, which eventually results in flare. A study also reveals that SLE patients with arthritis who discontinued or reduce MTX usage were more likely to flare [11].

Clinically, many SLE patients are SACQ. For these patients, it is believed that intensive treatment should not be administered for the purpose of turning serological indicators negative. Previous clinical studies have confirmed that AnuA as a diagnostic indicator of SLE have

Table 7 Risk factors of pulmonary hypertension, anemia and serositis in SLE flare

	Pulmonary hypertension		Anemia associated with SLE		Serositis	
	OR	95%CI	OR	95%CI	OR	95%CI
Age	1.007	(0.963,1.053)	0.978	(0.946,1.012)	0.979	(0.942,1.018)
Gender	0.000	/	0.480	(0.094,2.446)	0.177	(0.019,1.160)
Disease duration	1.000	(0.993,1.008)	1.002	(0.995,1.008)	1.003	(0.996,1.010)
SLEDAI-2 K	1.024	(0.942,1.113)	1.134	**(1.059,1.214)[e]**	1.156	**(1.070,1.248)[g]**
Glucocorticoid amount	0.577	(0.105,3.185)	0.784	(0.426,1.442)	0.889	(0.503,1.609)
Hydroxychloroquine	0.704	(0.217,2.290)	1.722	(0.602,4.963)	2.085	(0.637,6.821)
Immunosuppressive therapy	0.883	(0.299,2.606)	0.973	(0.423,2.236)	0.742	(0.294,1.874)
Regular maintenance treatment	**0.158**	**(0.043,0.577)[a]**	**0.319**	**(0.141,0.720)[f]**	**0.362**	**(0.145,0.908)[h]**
Maintenance therapy < 1 years	**4.000**	**(1.232,12.989)[b]**	0.687	(0.205,2.299)	**5.764**	**(1.642,20.241)[i]**
Maintenance therapy < 2 years	**3.208**	**(1.129,9.115)[c]**	0.799	(0.288,2.216)	2.283	(0.759,6.684)
Maintenance therapy < 3 years	**2.986**	**(1.087,8.202)[d]**	0.734	(0.266,2.022)	1.745	(0.584,5.215)
Maintenance therapy < 4 years	2.252	(0.627,8.089)	0.776	(0.254,2.374)	1.335	(0.403,4.420)

[a]: $P = 0.005$; [b]: $P = 0.021$; [c]: $P = 0.029$; [d]: $P = 0.034$; [e]: $P < 0.001$; [f]: $P = 0.006$; [g]: $P < 0.001$; [h]: $P = 0.030$; [i]: $P = 0.006$; *SLEDAI-2 K* Systemic lupus erythematosus disease activity index-2000

higher sensitivity compared with anti-SM antibodies and a specificity of higher than 90% [27]. It has a certain correlation with disease activity [27] and may be involved in the pathogenesis of organ damage in SLE patients. Our study suggests that AnuA may be a risk factor for SLE flare, so when AnuA in the serum of SLE patients are persistently positive, immunotherapy should not be terminated whether the patient has achieved clinical remission or not.

Anti-β2 glycoprotein-I (β2GPI) is one of the diagnostic antibodies of APS, which have also been detected in a large range of autoimmune diseases, such as SLE [28, 29] and so on. The mechanism of thrombosis induced via the action of anti-β2GPI has been described: this action is mediated by dimerization of β2GPI by platelet factor 4 (PF4) tetramers, dimerization takes place mainly in the presence of anti-β2GPI antibodies which in turn bind to the PF4/β2GPI complexes and activate platelets [29]. In our study, there were a total of 20 patients with IgG subtype of anti-β2GPI positive in the SLE flare group, among them, including 3 cases of hemolytic anemia, 3 cases of interstitial pneumonia, 3 cases of Raynaud's phenomenon, 2 cases of cerebral infarction, 3 cases of intestinal obstruction secondary to mesenteric vasculitis and thrombosis and 2 cases of pulmonary hypertension, which suggest that vascular disease or microvascular disease may be the main pathological basis of organ damage in these patients. Based on the pathogenic mechanism of anti-β2GPI in vitro, we speculate that it may induce thrombosis or micro thrombosis, which lead to chronic vascular disease and SLE flare. Taraborelli M' study reveal that a clinically significant antiphospholipid antibody profile is associated with an increased risk of organ damage accrual during a 15-year follow-up in SLE patients [30]. Although we also found that the positive rates of aCL and La in patients with SLE flare were higher than those in patients with SLE remission, multiple regression analysis showed that aCL and LA were not risk factors for SLE flare. It is possible that the binding ability of anti-β2GPI to the target antigen is different from that of other antiphospholipid antibodies, the specific mechanism remains to be studied.

In China, most SLE patients are treated with low-dose glucocorticoids or combined with hydroxychloroquine as maintenance therapy, when they reached clinical remission [2, 9]. Only a few patients are treated with hydroxychloroquine as maintenance therapy alone [9]. Most SLE patients will reduce or stop immunosuppressants when the disease is stabilized. Studies show that SLE patients with low-dose glucocorticoid as maintenance therapy have a significantly lower flare rate than patients with discontinuation of medicine maintenance therapy [31, 32]. In fact, most SLE patients require glucocorticoid maintenance therapy to achieve long-term clinical remission, and fewer than 15% of patients without glucocorticoid maintenance therapy have achieved 5-year clinical remission [33]. However, long-term glucocorticoid maintenance therapy greatly increases the incidence of complications, such as infection and osteoporosis, in SLE patients [34], which seriously affect the quality of life of patients. Therefore, the recommendations for the management of SLE suggest that glucocorticoids progressive tapering until withdrawal, when SLE patients reach to complete remission [8]. But little evidence on immunosuppressants withdrawal in remitted patients is available [11].

Patients reducing the dose or stopping a drug altogether is one of the most common causes of flare in Chinese patients with SLE [2]. Poor understanding of the disease and the glucocorticoids as well as the fear of adverse reactions of the drugs are the most common reasons for discontinuation of drug maintenance therapy [2]. Due to the restrictions of medical ethics, it is difficult for clinical research to prospectively observe the effect of termination of drug maintenance therapy on disease progression and long-term prognosis when SLE patients have reached clinical remission. Therefore, there are still many unanswered questions about maintenance therapies for SLE patients, such as whether the drugs can be terminated and what the indicators of drug termination are. This study found that for patients with flared SLE, patient's self-discontinuation of medicine maintenance therapy demonstrated higher severity of the disease and higher incidence of new organ damage, such as SLE related anemia, serositis and pulmonary hypertension.

It has been reported that the serositis usually related to SLE activity and severity [35–37], especially in nephropathy, interstitial lung disease, pulmonary hypertension and hematologic involvement [35]. Organ damage of SLE patients with serositis were generally more severe than patients without serositis [36]. In our study, we found that the probability of SLE patients complicated with serositis was significantly increased if the duration of medicine maintenance therapy less than 1 year. The systemic damage of SLE was induce by vasculitis and non-inflammatory vascular remodeling [38–40]. Vasculitis is significantly correlated with the activity of SLE [38], while the pathophysiological mechanisms of non-inflammatory vascular remodeling may play an important role when the course of the disease is longer [38, 40], which might act as a key factor in the choice of treatment strategy and the prognosis. Vascular remodeling erodes multiple organs throughout the body along the course of the disease, and they tend to become chronic, requiring long-term drug control or even life-long medication. Therefore, the maintenance therapy is important, and premature medicine withdrawal can cause irreversible organ damage and poor prognosis. In our study, if the duration of maintenance treatment less than 3 year, we found that the probability of SLE patients complicated with pulmonary hypertension was significantly increased. These results show that insufficient maintenance treatment may cause more severe SLE activity and organ damage. Meanwhile, more large-scale prospective researches are needed for further exploration.

Although there is no difference in the survival rate between SLE patients who discontinued medicine maintenance therapy by themself and received regular maintenance therapy. This may be related to the fact that the patients included in this study only experienced the first SLE flare. It is a limitation to evaluate the overall prognosis of SLE patients with drug withdrawal.

Conclusion

In conclusion, our study demonstrates that SLE patients with infection, thrombocytopenia, arthritic or positive AnuA/aβ2GPI(IgG) antibody have an increased risk of SLE flare. Therefore, special attention needs to be paid to these patients during remission. The use of immunosuppressors and hydroxychloroquine during the initial treatment of SLE can lower the risk of flare. Patients with discontinuation of medicine maintenance therapy are prone to more severe flares and organ damage, of which pulmonary hypertension being the most significant. According to the research results, we recommend that SLE patients have regular maintenance therapy for no less than 3 years during remission. Certainly, larger scale clinical studies will be conducive to point out the indication of drug withdrawal.

Abbreviations

SLE: Systemic lupus erythematosus; ACR: American College of Rheumatology; SLEDAI-2 K: Systemic lupus erythematosus disease activity index 2000; SDI: Systemic lupus erythematosus damage index; SACQD: Serological active clinical quiescent disease; ANA: Antinuclear antibodies; ds-DNA: Anti-double-stranded DNA antibodies; anti-RNP: Anti-ribonucleoprotein antibodies; anti-SM: Anti-Smith antibodies; anti-SSA: Anti-Sjogren's syndrome A antibodies; anti-SSB: Anti-Sjogren's syndrome B antibodies; AnuA: Anti-nucleosome antibodies; aCL: Anti-cardiolipin antibodies; anti-β2GPI: Anti-β2-glycoprotein I; LAs: Lupus anticoagulants; APS: Antiphospholipid syndrome; PF4: Platelet factor 4

Acknowledgments

The authors thank Dr. Fan Xu for his assistance with data analysis.

Authors' contributions

Contributors All authors as listed below, XZ, LZ, HR, RK, JC, HC, JL, were involved in all the following aspects of the research presented: Substantial contributions to the conception or design of the work, or the acquisition, analysis or interpretation of data. XZ was responsible for the intellectual content of the study. All authors read and approved the final manuscript.

References

1. Ugarte-Gil MF, Acevedo-Vásquez E, Alarcón GS, Pastor-Asurza CA, Alfaro-Lozano JL, Cucho-Venegas JM, et al. The number of flares patients experience impacts on damage accrual in systemic lupus erythematosus: data from a multiethnic Latin American cohort. Ann Rheum Dis. 2015;74(6): 1019–23. https://doi.org/10.1136/annrheumdis-2013-204620.
2. Zhang L, Luan W, Geng S, Ye S, Wang X, Qian L. Lack of patient education is risk factor of disease flare in patients with systemic lupus erythematosus in China. BMC Health Serv Res. 2019;19(1):378. https://doi.org/10.1186/s12913-019-4206-y.
3. Joo YB, Kim K-J, Park K-S, et al. Influenza infection as a trigger for systemic lupus erythematosus flares resulting in hospitalization. Sci Rep. 2021;11(1): 4630.
4. Liang H, Pan HF, Tao JH, Ye DQ. Causes and factors associated with frequent hospitalization in Chinese patients with systemic lupus erythematosus: an Ambispective cohort study. Med Sci Monit. 2019;25: 8061–8. https://doi.org/10.12659/MSM.919381.
5. Fei Y, Shi X, Gan F, Li X, Zhang W, Li M, et al. Death causes and pathogens analysis of systemic lupus erythematosus during the past 26 years. Clin Rheumatol. 2014;33(1):57–63. https://doi.org/10.1007/s10067-013-2383-3.
6. Ocampo-Piraquive V, Nieto-Aristizábal I, Cañas CA, Tobón GJ. Mortality in systemic lupus erythematosus: causes, predictors and interventions. Expert Rev Clin Immunol. 2018 Dec;14(12):1043–53. https://doi.org/10.1080/1744666X.2018.1538789.
7. Pons-Estel BA, Bonfa E, Soriano ER, Cardiel MH, Izcovich A, Popoff F, et al. First Latin American clinical practice guidelines for the treatment of systemic lupus erythematosus: Latin American Group for the Study of lupus (GLADEL, Grupo Latino Americano de Estudio del lupus)-Pan-American league of associations of rheumatology (PANLAR). Ann Rheum Dis. 2018; 77(11):1549–57. https://doi.org/10.1136/annrheumdis-2018-213512.
8. Gordon C, Amissah-Arthur MB, Gayed M, Brown S, Bruce IN, D'Cruz D, et al. The British Society for Rheumatology guideline for the management of systemic lupus erythematosus in adults. Rheumatology. 2018;57(1):e1–e45. https://doi.org/10.1093/rheumatology/kex286.
9. Gao D, Hao Y, Lin M, Xie W, Fan Y, Ji L, et al. Frequencies and predictors of the lupus low disease activity state and remission in treatment-naïve patients with systemic lupus erythematosus. Rheumatology (Oxford). 2020; 59(11):3400–7. https://doi.org/10.1093/rheumatology/keaa120.
10. Ruiz-Irastorza G, Ruiz-Estevez B, Lazaro E, Ruiz-Arruza I, Duffau P, Martin-Cascon M, et al. Prolonged remission in SLE is possible by using reduced doses of prednisone: an observational study from the lupus-cruces and lupus-Bordeaux inception cohorts. Autoimmun Rev. 2019;18(9):102359. https://doi.org/10.1016/j.autrev.2019.102359.
11. Zen M, Saccon F, Gatto M, Montesso G, Larosa M, Benvenuti F, et al. Prevalence and predictors of flare after immunosuppressant discontinuation in patients with systemic lupus erythematosus in remission. Rheumatology (Oxford). 2020;59(7):1591–8. https://doi.org/10.1093/rheumatology/kez422.
12. Hochberg MC. Updating the American College of Rheumatology revised criteria for the classification of systemic lupus erythematosus. Arthritis Rheum. 1997;40(9):1725. https://doi.org/10.1002/art.1780400928.
13. Bombardier C, Gladman DD, Urowitz MB, Caron D, Chang CH. Derivation of the SLEDAI:a disease activity index for lupus patients. Arthritis Rheum. 1992; 35(6):630–40. https://doi.org/10.1002/art.1780350606.
14. Gladman D, Ginzler E, Goldsmith C, Fortin P, Liang M, Sanchez-Guerrero J, et al. The development and initial validation of the systemic lupus international collaborating clinics and American College of Rheumatology damage index for systemic lupus erythematosus. Arthritis Rheum. 1996; 39(3):363–9. https://doi.org/10.1002/art.1780390303.
15. Zen M, Iaccarino L, Gatto M, Bettio S, Nalotto L, Ghirardello A, et al. Prolonged remission in Caucasian patients with SLE: prevalence and outcomes. Ann Rheum Dis. 2015;74(12):2117–22. https://doi.org/10.1136/annrheumdis-2015-207347.
16. Buyon P. Kim, et al. the effect of combined estrogen and progesterone hormone replacement therapy on disease activity in systemic lupus erythematosus: a randomized trial. Ann Intern Med. 2005;142(12 Pt 1):953–62. https://doi.org/10.7326/0003-4819-142-12_Part_1-200506210-00004.
17. Galiè N, Humbert M, Vachiery JL, et al. 2015 ESC/ERS guidelines for the diagnosis and treatment of pulmonary hypertension: the joint task force for the diagnosis and treatment of pulmonary hypertension of the European Society of Cardiology (ESC) and the European Respiratory Society (ERS): endorsed by: Association for European Paediatric and Congenital

Cardiology (AEPC), International Society for Heart and Lung Transplantation (ISHLT). Eur Respir J. 2015;46(4):903–75.

18. Conti F, Ceccarelli F, Perricone C, Miranda F, Truglia S, Massaro L, et al. Flare, persistently active disease, and serologically active clinically quiescent disease in systemic lupus erythematosus: a 2-year follow-up study. PLoS One. 2012;7(9):e45934. https://doi.org/10.1371/journal.pone.0045934.
19. Golder V, Connelly K, Staples M, Morand E, Hoi A. Association of Asian ethnicity with disease activity in SLE: an observational study from the Monash lupus clinic. Lupus. 2013;22(13):1425–30. https://doi.org/10.1177/0961203313500547.
20. Gladman DD, Hussain F, Ibañez D, Urowitz MB. The nature and outcome of infection in systemic lupus erythematosus. Lupus. 2002;11(4):234–9. https://doi.org/10.1191/0961203302lu170oa.
21. Lee YH, Choi SJ, Ji JD, Song GG. Overall and cause-specific mortality in systemic lupus erythematosus: an updated meta-analysis. Lupus. 2016;25(7):727–34. https://doi.org/10.1177/0961203315627202.
22. Esposito S, Bosis S, Semino M, Rigante D. Infections and systemic lupus erythematosus. Eur J Clin Microbiol Infect Dis. 2014;33(9):1467–75. https://doi.org/10.1007/s10096-014-2098-7.
23. Prabu V, Agrawal S. Systemic lupus erythematosus and tuberculosis: a review of complex interactions of complicated diseases. J Postgrad Med. 2010;56(3):244–50. https://doi.org/10.4103/0022-3859.68653.
24. Minowa K, Amano H, Ando S, Watanabe T, Ogasawara M, Kawano S, et al. Disease flare patterns and predictors of systemic lupus erythematosus in a monocentric cohort of 423 Japanese patients during a long-term follow-up: the JUDE study. Mod Rheumatol. 2017;27(1):72–6. https://doi.org/10.1080/14397595.2016.1192745.
25. Fanouriakis A, Kostopoulou M, Cheema K, Anders HJ, Aringer M, Bajema I, et al. 2019 update of the joint European league against rheumatism and European renal association-European Dialysis and transplant association (EULAR/ERA-EDTA) recommendations for the management of lupus nephritis. Ann Rheum Dis. 2020;79(6):713–23. https://doi.org/10.1136/annrheumdis-2020-216924.
26. Costedoat-Chalumeau N, Amoura Z, Hulot JS, et al. Low Blood Concentration of Hydroxychloroquine Is a Marker for and Predictor of Disease Exacerbations in Patients With Systemic Lupus Erythematosus. Arthritis &Rheumatism 2006;54(10):3284–3290, DOI: https://doi.org/10.1002/art.22156.
27. Ghiggeri GM, D'Alessandro M, Bartolomeo D, et al. An update on antibodies to Necleosome components as biomarkers of Sistemic lupus erythematosus and of lupus flares. Int J Mol Sci. 2019;20(22):5799. https://doi.org/10.3390/ijms20225799.
28. Willis R, Pierangeli SS. Anti-β2-glycoprotein I antibodies. Ann N Y Acad Sci. 2013 May;1285(1):44–58. https://doi.org/10.1111/nyas.12080.
29. Vlachoyiannopoulos PG, Routsias JG. A novel mechanism of thrombosis in antiphospholipid antibody syndrome. J Autoimmun. 2010;35(3):248–55. https://doi.org/10.1016/j.jaut.2010.06.015.
30. Taraborelli M, Leuenberger L, Lazzaroni MG, Martinazzi N, Zhang W, Franceschini F, et al. The contribution of antiphospholipid antibodies to organ damage in systemic lupus erythematosus. Lupus. 2016;25(12):1365–8. https://doi.org/10.1177/0961203316637431.
31. Galbraith L, Manns B, Hemmelgarn B, Walsh M. The steroids in the maintenance of remission of proliferative lupus nephritis (SIMPL) pilot trial. Can J Kidney Health Dis. 2014;1:30. https://doi.org/10.1186/s40697-014-0030-9.
32. Mathian A, Pha M, Haroche J, Cohen-Aubart F, Hié M, Pineton de Chambrun M, et al. Withdrawal of low-dose prednisone in SLE patients with a clinically quiescent disease for more than 1 year: a randomised clinical trial. Ann Rheum Dis. 2020 Mar;79(3):339–46. https://doi.org/10.1136/annrheumdis-2019-216303.
33. Steiman AJ, Urowitz MB, Ibañez D, Papneja A, Gladman DD. Prolonged clinical remission in patients with systemic lupus erythematosus. J Rheumatol. 2014;41(9):1808–16. https://doi.org/10.3899/jrheum.131137.
34. Mosca M, Tani C, Aringer M. Aringer. Withdrawal of therapy in non-renal systemic lupus erythematosus:is this an achievable goal? Clin Exp Rheumatol. 2013;31(4 Suppl 78):S71–4.
35. Zhao J, Bai W, Zhu P, Zhang X, Liu S, Wu L, et al. Chinese SLE treatment and research group (CSTAR) registry VII: prevalence and clinical significance of serositis in Chinese patients with systemic lupus erythematosus. Lupus. 2016;25(6):652–7. https://doi.org/10.1177/0961203315625460.
36. Man BL, Mok CC. Serositis related to systemic lupus erythematosus: prevalence and outcome. Lupus. 2005;14(10):822–6. https://doi.org/10.1191/0961203305lu2187oa.
37. Li LH, Pan HF, Li WX, Li XP, Xu JH, Ye DQ. Study on clinical features and complications with systemic lupus erythematosus (SLE) activity in Chinese Han population. Clin Rheumatol. 2009;28(11):1301–7. https://doi.org/10.1007/s10067-009-1240-x.
38. Tan Y, Yu F, Liu G. Diverse vascular lesions in systemic lupus erythematosus and clinical implications. Curr Opin Nephrol Hypertens. 2014 May;23(3):218–23. https://doi.org/10.1097/01.mnh.0000444812.65002.cb.
39. Sun F, Lei Y, Wu W, Guo L, Wang K, Chen Z, et al. Two distinct clinical phenotypes of pulmonary arterial hypertension secondary to systemic lupus erythematosus. Ann Rheum Dis. 2019;78(1):148–50. https://doi.org/10.1136/annrheumdis-2018-214197.
40. Prabu A, Gordon C. Pulmonary arterial hypertension in SLE: what do we know? Lupus. 2013;22(12):1274–85. https://doi.org/10.1177/0961203313505010.

Permissions

All chapters in this book were first published by BioMed Central; hereby published with permission under the Creative Commons Attribution License or equivalent. Every chapter published in this book has been scrutinized by our experts. Their significance has been extensively debated. The topics covered herein carry significant findings which will fuel the growth of the discipline. They may even be implemented as practical applications or may be referred to as a beginning point for another development.

The contributors of this book come from diverse backgrounds, making this book a truly international effort. This book will bring forth new frontiers with its revolutionizing research information and detailed analysis of the nascent developments around the world.

We would like to thank all the contributing authors for lending their expertise to make the book truly unique. They have played a crucial role in the development of this book. Without their invaluable contributions this book wouldn't have been possible. They have made vital efforts to compile up to date information on the varied aspects of this subject to make this book a valuable addition to the collection of many professionals and students.

This book was conceptualized with the vision of imparting up-to-date information and advanced data in this field. To ensure the same, a matchless editorial board was set up. Every individual on the board went through rigorous rounds of assessment to prove their worth. After which they invested a large part of their time researching and compiling the most relevant data for our readers.

The editorial board has been involved in producing this book since its inception. They have spent rigorous hours researching and exploring the diverse topics which have resulted in the successful publishing of this book. They have passed on their knowledge of decades through this book. To expedite this challenging task, the publisher supported the team at every step. A small team of assistant editors was also appointed to further simplify the editing procedure and attain best results for the readers.

Apart from the editorial board, the designing team has also invested a significant amount of their time in understanding the subject and creating the most relevant covers. They scrutinized every image to scout for the most suitable representation of the subject and create an appropriate cover for the book.

The publishing team has been an ardent support to the editorial, designing and production team. Their endless efforts to recruit the best for this project, has resulted in the accomplishment of this book. They are a veteran in the field of academics and their pool of knowledge is as vast as their experience in printing. Their expertise and guidance has proved useful at every step. Their uncompromising quality standards have made this book an exceptional effort. Their encouragement from time to time has been an inspiration for everyone.

The publisher and the editorial board hope that this book will prove to be a valuable piece of knowledge for researchers, students, practitioners and scholars across the globe.

List of Contributors

Philipp Klemm, Johanna Becker, Iris Aykara, Gabriel Dischereit, Elena Neumann, Ulf Müller-Ladner and Uwe Lange
Department of Rheumatology, Immunology, Osteology and Physical Medicine, Justus-Liebig-University Giessen, Campus Kerckhoff, Bad Nauheim, Germany

Thomas Asendorf
Department of Medical Statistics, University Medical Center Göttingen, Göttingen, Germany

Simon Parreau, Kim-Heang Ly and Anne-Laure Fauchais
Internal Medicine Department, Limoges University Hospital, 16 rue du Professeur Bernard Descottes, 87042 Limoges, France
EA 3842 - Cellular Homeostasis and Diseases, Faculty of Medicine, University of Limoges, 2 rue du Docteur Marcland, 87025 Limoges, France

Jérémie Jacques
Gastroenterology Department, Limoges University Hospital, 2 Avenue Martin Luther King, 87042 Limoges, France
BioEM, UMR 7252, CNRS, Limoges, France

Stéphanie Dumonteil, Sylvain Palat, Guillaume Gondran, Holy Bezanahary, Eric Liozon, Julie Azaïs and Stéphanie Colombie
Internal Medicine Department, Limoges University Hospital, 16 rue du Professeur Bernard Descottes, 87042 Limoges, France

Marie-Odile Jauberteau
EA 3842 - Cellular Homeostasis and Diseases, Faculty of Medicine, University of Limoges, 2 rue du Docteur Marcland, 87025 Limoges, France

Véronique Loustaud-Ratti and Sophie Geyl
Gastroenterology Department, Limoges University Hospital, 2 Avenue Martin Luther King, 87042 Limoges, France

Vikas Kumar Tiwari, Srishti Nanda, Suvercha Arya and Renu Bhatia
Pain Research and TMS Laboratory, Department of Physiology, All India Institute of Medical Sciences, New Delhi, India

Uma Kumar
Department of Rheumatology, All India Institute of Medical Sciences, New Delhi, India

Ratna Sharma
Stress and Cognition Electroimaging Laboratory, Department of Physiology, All India Institute of Medical Sciences, New Delhi, India

Senthil S. Kumaran
Department of Nuclear Magnetic Resonance and MRI Facility, All India Institute of Medical Sciences, New Delhi, India

Marina Maria Vieira de Figueiredo Caldas
Medicine Student, Federal University of Rio Grande do Norte, Natal, Rio Grande do Norte, Brazil

Kesley Pablo Morais de Azevedo, Ana Clara de França Nunes, Victor Hugo de Oliveira and Isac Davidson Santiago Fernandes Pimenta
Post-Graduation Program in Public Health (PPGS Col), Federal University of Rio Grande do Norte, Natal, Rio Grande do Norte, Brazil

Isabela Dantas Torres de Araújo
Post-Graduation Program in Dental Sciences, Federal University of Rio Grande do Norte, Natal, Rio Grande do Norte, Brazil

Francisco Alves Bezerra Neto
Department of Clinical Medicine, Federal University of Rio Grande do Norte, Natal, Rio Grande do Norte, Brazil

Ana Katherine da Silveira Gonçalves de Oliveira
Department of Tocoginecology, Post-Graduation Program in Health Sciences, Federal University of Rio Grande do Norte, Natal, Rio Grande do Norte, Brazil

Grasiela Piuvezam
Post-Graduation Program in Public Health (PPGS Col), Federal University of Rio Grande do Norte, Natal, Rio Grande do Norte, Brazil
Department of Public Health, Post-Graduation Program in Public Health (PPGSCol), Federal University of Rio Grande do Norte, Natal, Rio Grande do Norte, Brazil

Vanessa Posener de Andrade and Fernando Henrique Carlos De Souza
Division of Rheumatology, Faculdade de Medicina FMUSP, Universidade de Sao Paulo, Sao Paulo, SP, Brazil

Samuel Katsuyuki Shinjo
Division of Rheumatology, Faculdade de Medicina FMUSP, Universidade de Sao Paulo, Sao Paulo, SP, Brazil
Disciplina de Reumatologia, Faculdade de Medicina, Universidade de Sao Paulo, Av. Dr. Arnaldo, 455, 3° andar, sala 3184 - Cerqueira César, CEP: 01246-903, Sao Paulo, Brazil

Renata Casseb de Souza Carboni and Gustavo Luiz Behrens Pinto
Division of Rheumatology, Faculdade de Medicina FMUSP, Universidade de Sao Paulo, Av. Dr. Arnaldo, 455, 3° andar, sala 3184 - Cerqueira César. CEP: 01246-903, Sao Paulo, Brazil

Ming-Hui Hung and Ya-Chih Tien
Division of Allergy, Immunology and Rheumatology, Department of Internal Medicine, Changhua Christian Hospital, 135 Nanxiao St., Changhua City 500-06, Taiwan

Ying-Ming Chiu
Department of Allergy, Immunology, and Rheumatology, Tungs' Taichung MetroHarbor Hospital, 699, Sec. 8, Taiwan Blvd., Taichung City 43503, Taiwan

Laiana Schneider and Ricardo Xavier
Serviço de Reumatologia, Hospital de Clínicas de Porto Alegre, Universidade Federal do Rio Grande do Sul, 2350 Ramiro Barcelos St, Room 645, Porto Alegre, RS 90035-903, Brazil
Programa de Pós Graduação em Medicina: Ciências Médicas, Universidade Federal do Rio Grande do Sul, Porto Alegre, Brazil

Vanessa Hax
Serviço de Reumatologia, Hospital de Clínicas de Porto Alegre, Universidade Federal do Rio Grande do Sul, 2350 Ramiro Barcelos St, Room 645, Porto Alegre, RS 90035-903, Brazil

Natália Aydos Marcondes
Laboratório Zanol, Porto Alegre, Brazil

Isadora Flesch da Silva Moreira, Carolina Yuka Ueda and Rafaella Romeiro Piovesan
Faculdade de Medicina, Universidade Federal do Rio Grande do Sul, Porto Alegre, Brazil

María Alejandra Martínez-Ceballos, Juan Pablo Alzate-Granados and Natalia Aguilera
Research Division Fundación Universitaria de Ciencias de la Salud (FUCS), Bogotá, Colombia

Kenny Carolina Garzón-González
Internal Medicine Department, Fundación Universitaria de Ciencias de la Salud (FUCS). Hospital San José, Bogotá, Colombia

Jairo Cajamarca-Baron
Rheumatology Department, Fundación Universitaria de Ciencias de la Salud (FUCS), Bogotá, Colombia

Adriana Rojas-Villarraga
Research Institute, Fundación Universitaria de Ciencias de la Salud (FUCS), Bogotá, Colombia

Alexandre Moura dos Santos, Rafael Giovani Misse, Isabela Bruna Pires Borges, Bruno Gualano, Liliam Takayama and Rosa Maria R. Pereira
Division of Rheumatology, Faculdade de Medicina FMUSP, Universidade de Sao Paulo, Sao Paulo, Brazil

Alexandre Wagner Silva de Souza
Division of Rheumatology, Universidade Federal de São Paulo (UNIFESP), Sao Paulo, Brazil

Angela Shiratsu Yamada and Flavia Tasmim Techera Antunes
Molecular and Cellular Biology Applied to Health, Lutheran University of Brazil (ULBRA), Canoas, Brazil

Camila Ferraz
Human Molecular Genetics Laboratory, Lutheran University of Brazil (ULBRA), Canoas, Brazil

Daniel Simon
Molecular and Cellular Biology Applied to Health, Lutheran University of Brazil (ULBRA), Canoas, Brazil
Human Molecular Genetics Laboratory, Lutheran University of Brazil (ULBRA), Canoas, Brazil

Alessandra Hubner de Souza
Biochemical and Molecular Pharmacology from the Federal University of Minas Gerais, Belo Horizonte, Brazil

Sinem Can Oksay and Sami Hatipoglu
Dr. Sadi Konuk Training and Research Hospital Department of Pediatrics, Health Science University, Istanbul, Turkey

Hasan Dursun
Dr. Sadi Konuk Training and Research Hospital Department of Pediatric Nephrology, Health Science University, Istanbul, Turkey
Okmeydani Training and Research Hospital Department of Pediatric Nephrology, Health Science University, Kaptan Paşa Mahallesi, Darülaceze Cad. No: 25 Okmeydani, 34384 Şişli/Istanbul, Turkey

Sebnem Tekin Neijmann
Dr. Sadi Konuk Training and Research Hospital Department of Biochemistry, Health Science University, Istanbul, Turkey

Hülya Kaçmaz
Department of Pediatric Rheumatology, University of Health Sciences, Kanuni Sultan Süleyman Research and Training Hospital, Istanbul, Turkey

Esin Aldemir
Department of Pediatric Rheumatology, University of Health Sciences, Başakşehir Çam ve Sakura City Hospital, Istanbul, Turkey

Ayşe Tanatar and Nuray Aktay Ayaz
Department of Pediatric Rheumatology, Istanbul University Medical School, Istanbul, Turkey

Şerife Gül Karadağ
Department of Pediatric Rheumatology, Sadi Konuk Research and Training Hospital, Istanbul, Turkey

Hafize Emine Sönmez
Department of Pediatric Rheumatology, Kocaeli University, Istanbul, Turkey

Mustafa Çakan
Department of Pediatric Rheumatology, University of Health Sciences, Zeynep Kamil Research and Training Hospital, Istanbul, Turkey

Fatema T. Elgengehy, Sherif M. Gamal, Nesreen Sobhy and Tamer A. Gheita
Rheumatology and Rehabilitation Department, Cairo University, Cairo, Egypt

Ibrahem Siam
Internal Medicine Department, National Research Center, Cairo, Egypt

Ahmed M. Soliman
Dermatology and venereology Department, National Research Center, Cairo, Egypt

Ghada W. Elhady
Public Health Department, Cairo University, Cairo, Egypt

Leda Magalhaes Oliveira and Vera Lucia Szejnfeld
Rheumatology Division, Universidade Federal de Sao Paulo (UNIFESP), São Paulo, Brazil

Suely Roizenblatt
Department of Internal Medicine, Universidade Federal de Sao Paulo (UNIFESP), Rua Angelina Maffei Vita 670. CEP:01455070, Sao Paulo, SP, Brazil

Flavio Duarte Silva and Artur Rocha Correa Fernandes
Department of Diagnostic Imaging, Universidade Federal de Sao Paulo (UNIFESP), São Paulo, Brazil

Arnaldo Roizenblatt
Medical Student Universidade Federal de Sao Paulo (UNIFESP), São Paulo, Brazil

Edson Hernán Chiganer, Bruno Camargo Ochi and Carmen Flora Lessa
Department of Immunology and Histocompatibility Unity, Carlos G Durand Hospital, Díaz Vélez Avenue, 5044, C1405DCS Buenos Aires, Argentina

Odirlei Monticielo and Rafael Chakr
Serviço de Reumatologia, Hospital de Clínicas de Porto Alegre, Universidade Federal do Rio Grande do Sul, 2350 Ramiro Barcelos St, Room 645, Porto Alegre, RS 90035-903, Brazil
Faculdade de Medicina, Universidade Federal do Rio Grande do Sul, Porto Alegre, Brazil

Tamires Ferri Macedo and Roberta Kern Menna Barreto
Faculdade de Medicina, Universidade Federal do Rio Grande do Sul, Porto Alegre, Brazil

Natália Aydos Marcondes
Laboratório Zanol, Porto Alegre, Brazil

Isadora Carvalho Medeiros Francescantonio, Leandro Augusto Rodrigues dos Santos, Paulo Luiz Carvalho Francescantonio and Wilson de Melo Cruvinel
Pontifícia Universidade Católica de Goiás (PUC Goiás), Escola de Ciências Médicas, Farmacêuticas e Biomédicas, Avenida Universitária 1.440, Setor Universitário, Goiânia, GO, Brazil

Luiz Eduardo Coelho Andrade
Disciplina de Reumatologia, Escola Paulista de Medicina, Universidade Federal de São Paulo (UNIFESP), Divisão de Imunologia, Fleury Medicina e Saúde, São Paulo, SP, Brazil

Laiza Hombre Dias
Department of Clinical Medicine, Cassiano Antonio Moraes University Hospital / EBSERH, Federal University of Espírito Santo (Ufes), Av. Marechal Campos, 1468, Maruípe, Vitória, ES CEP: 29075-910, Brazil
Brazilian Society of Rheumatology, São Paulo, Brazil

Samira Tatiyama Miyamoto
Department of Integrated Health Education, Federal University of Espírito Santo (Ufes), Av. Marechal Campos, 1468, Maruípe, Vitória, ES CEP: 29075-910, Brazil

Raquel Altoé Giovelli
Brazilian Society of Rheumatology, São Paulo, Brazil
Department of Clinical Medicine, School of Sciences of Santa Casa de Misericórdia de Vitória (Emescam), Av. Nossa Senhora da Penha 2190, Vitória, ES 29045-925, Brazil

Caerê Iamonde Maciel de Magalhães
Federal University of Espírito Santo (Ufes), Av. Marechal Campos, 1468, Maruípe, Vitória, ES CEP: 29075-910, Brazil

Valeria Valim
Department of Clinical Medicine, Cassiano Antonio Moraes University Hospital / EBSERH, Federal University of Espírito Santo (Ufes), Av. Marechal Campos, 1468, Maruípe, Vitória, ES CEP: 29075-910, Brazil
Brazilian Society of Rheumatology, São Paulo, Brazil
Brazilian Sjögren Syndrome Commission, São Paulo, Brazil

Álvaro Henrique-Neto
Graduate Program in Internal Medicine, Ribeirão Preto Medical School, University of São Paulo, Ribeirão Preto, Brazil

Marianna Yumi Kawashima Vasconcelos and Giuliana Martinelli Dotoli
Graduate Program in Internal Medicine, Ribeirão Preto Medical School, University of São Paulo, Ribeirão Preto, Brazil
Center for Cell-Based Therapy, Ribeirão Preto Medical School, University of São Paulo, Ribeirão Preto, Brazil

Juliana Bernardes Elias Dias, Daniela Aparecida de Moraes and Luiz Fernando Weffort
Hospital das Clínicas da Faculdade de Medicina de Ribeirão Preto, Ribeirão Preto Medical School, University of São Paulo, Ribeirão Preto, Brazil

Maynara Santana Gonçalves
Center for Cell-Based Therapy, Ribeirão Preto Medical School, University of São Paulo, Ribeirão Preto, Brazil
Graduate Program in Oncology, Stem Cells and Cell Therapy, Ribeirão Preto Medical School, University of São Paulo, Ribeirão Preto, Brazil

Djúlio César Zanin-Silva
Center for Cell-Based Therapy, Ribeirão Preto Medical School, University of São Paulo, Ribeirão Preto, Brazil
Graduate Program in Basic and Applied Immunology, Ribeirão Preto Medical School, University of São Paulo, Ribeirão Preto, Brazil

Talita Graminha Zucoloto
Graduate Program in Internal Medicine, Ribeirão Preto Medical School, University of São Paulo, Ribeirão Preto, Brazil
Center for Cell-Based Therapy, Ribeirão Preto Medical School, University of São Paulo, Ribeirão Preto, Brazil
Hospital das Clínicas da Faculdade de Medicina de Ribeirão Preto, Ribeirão Preto Medical School, University of São Paulo, Ribeirão Preto, Brazil

Marília de Fátima Cirioli de Oliveira and Vanessa Cristina Leopoldo
Hospital das Clínicas da Faculdade de Medicina de Ribeirão Preto, Ribeirão Preto Medical School, University of São Paulo, Ribeirão Preto, Brazil
Ribeirão Preto School of Nursing, University of São Paulo, Ribeirão Preto, Brazil

Maria Carolina Oliveira
Center for Cell-Based Therapy, Ribeirão Preto Medical School, University of São Paulo, Ribeirão Preto, Brazil
Department of Internal Medicine, Ribeirão Preto Medical School, University of São Paulo, Avenida dos Bandeirantes 3900, Ribeirão Preto, SP 14048-900, Brazil

Jamil Natour
Rheumatology Division, Universidade Federal de São Paulo - Escola Paulista de Medicina (Unifesp-EPM), Sao Paulo, SP 04023900, Brazil

Luiz Claudio Lacerda Rodrigues
Rheumatology Division, Universidade Federal de São Paulo - Escola Paulista de Medicina (Unifesp-EPM), Sao Paulo, SP 04023900, Brazil
Faculdade de Medicina Santa Marcelina, Sao Paulo, Brazil

Damla Cankurtaran, Nihal Tezel, Buse Ercan, Sadik Yigit Yildiz and Ece Unlu Akyuz
Department of Physical Medicine and Rehabilitation, University of Health Sciences Diskapi Yildirim Beyazit Training and Research Hospital, Altındag, 06080 Ankara, Turkey

Juliana Rosa Pires Vieira and Andréa Toledo de Oliveira Rezende
Postgraduate Program in Health Sciences, School of Medicine of the Universidade Federal de Goiás (UFG), Goiânia, Brazil

Marcos Rassi Fernandes
Postgraduate Program in Health Sciences, School of Medicine of the Universidade Federal de Goiás (UFG), Goiânia, Brazil
Department of Orthopedics/Traumatology, School of Medicine of the Universidade Federal de Goiás (UFG), Goiânia, Brazil

Nilzio Antonio da Silva
Postgraduate Program in Health Sciences, School of Medicine of the Universidade Federal de Goiás (UFG), Goiânia, Brazil
Rheumatology Service of Hospital das Clínicas, School of Medicine of the Universidade Federal de Goiás (UFG), Goiânia, Brazil

Deise Marcela Piovesan, Vanessa Barrili Busato, Romulo Gomes da Silveira, Aline Defaveri do Prado, Sheila Hickmann, Guilherme Kopik Bongiorno, Camila de David Cruz, Sheron Zamboni, Julio César Simon and Markus Bredemeier
Rheumatology Service at Hospital Nossa Senhora da Conceição (HNSC), Grupo Hospitalar Nossa Senhora da Conceição (GHC), Avenida Francisco Trein, 596, 3 Andar, Porto Alegre, Rio Grande do Sul, Brazil

Cynthia Goulart Molina-Bastos and Marcelo Rodrigues Gonçalves
Federal University of Rio Grande do Sul (UFRGS), Porto Alegre, Rio Grande do Sul, Brazil
TelessaúdeRS, Federal University of Rio Grande do Sul (UFRGS), Porto Alegre, Rio Grande do Sul, Brazil

Xiaohong Zeng, Ling Zheng, Hongbing Rui, Rihui Kang, Junmin Chen, Huaning Chen and Jizan Liu
Department of Rheumatology, the First Affiliated Hospital of Fujian Medical University, 20 Chazhong Road, Fuzhou 350005, Fujian, China

Index

www.ingramcontent.com/pod-product-compliance
Lightning Source LLC
La Vergne TN
LVHW082218200926
848484LV00008B/2275